Pathologies of Speech Systems

Edward D. Mysak, Ph.D.

Professor of Speech Pathology
Chairman, Department of Speech
  Pathology and Audiology
Teachers College, Columbia University
Fellow of the American Speech and
  Hearing Association
New York, New York

D1613540

The Williams & Wilkins Company
Baltimore, Md.

Library of Congress Cataloging in Publication Data

Mysak, Edward Damien, 1930–
    Pathologies of speech systems.

    Includes index.
    1.   Speech, Disorders of. I. Title. [DNLM: 1. Speech disorders. WM475 M998p]
RC423.M85   616.8′55   75-9771
ISBN 0-683-06162-3

Composed and printed at the
Waverly Press, Inc.
Mt. Royal and Guilford Aves.
Baltimore, Md. 21202, U.S.A.

In memory of my parents,
Charles and Mary Mysak, who
placed love of God and
their seven children above
all else.

Preface

The growth and development of the field of speech pathology and audiology in the United States may be estimated in many ways. Some of the more important of these include: (a) the great increase in the number of training programs offering master's and doctorate degrees in the field; (b) the establishment of the American Boards of Examiners in Speech Pathology and Audiology; (c) the rapid growth in membership in the American Speech and Hearing Association; and (d) the great increase in the establishment and expansion of speech pathology and audiology services in school and in rehabilitation and medical center settings.

Concomitant with the growth and development of the field has been the rapid increase in the amount and type of responsibility of the speech and hearing clinician. He may be required to diagnose difficult and relatively unfamiliar speech-hearing complexes and to report his findings in multidisciplinary conferences composed of various medical and health-related specialists. He also finds it important to understand more fully the contributions of these various health-related specialists to any one client with multiple problems. Because of these increased responsibilities, speech pathologists require a deeper understanding and knowledge of those structures and functions that comprise the speech systems and of those bodily anomalies and diseases that may affect any part of those systems.

The purpose of this book therefore is to assist the speech and hearing clinician assume his broadened clinical responsibilities by: (a) discussing in detail the major speech systems; (b) identifying the wide range of human disorders and diseases that may affect the speech systems; and (c) presenting principles of examining and treating those systems. Hopefully, the information presented in this book will also motivate the clinician to ask important theoretical and practical research questions.

The book should be of value both as a text for students of speech pathology and audiology and as a manual for practicing clinicians. It should also serve as a good source of information on speech disorders for physicians, dentists, psychologists, social workers, and other health-related professionals.

For originally stimulating a deep interest in studying the organs of speech and thereby contributing much to the material in this book, the author remains indebted to his late teacher, colleague, and friend, Dr. Robert W. West.

Gratitude is also expressed to Theresa M. Mysak for her support, patience, and understanding and to Damien and Blaise Mysak for their forbearance during the period of the project; and to Mrs. Mary Katanik and Mr. Robert M. Tucker for their excellent typing of many drafts of the original manuscript.

E. D. M.

1975

Contents

Introduction

General texts of speech pathology written in the United States are organized customarily according to various types of recognized speech disorders, that is, according to manifest speech symptoms or dysfunctions. Hence, one usually finds chapters on disorders of articulation, of voice, or of language, or on stuttering. Occasionally, rather than such descriptive terms, one encounters etiologic or partially etiologic terms such as dysarthria, dyslalia, or dysphasia as chapter headings. This focus on the disordered output of the speech system, with slight regard for the structure and function of the various systems responsible for the disordered output, has contributed little to the speech and hearing clinician's knowledge of how various systems serve speech functioning. In addition, such a focus has encouraged some clinicians to limit their diagnostic procedures to merely identifying or confirming speech symptoms. As a result, "type-therapy programs," which aim at the disordered output as such rather than at a disorder of a particular speech system within a particular individual, predominate.

This book, which is organized differently, provides information not usually found in any planned or consistent fashion in the general literature of American speech pathology. Individual chapters are devoted to the six major systems believed to make up the total speech system, that is, the receptor, transmitter, higher-order integrator, lower-order integrator, effector, and sensor systems. Information in the chapters relates to important topics in the field, for example, speech disorder simplexes vs. complexes, classification of disorders, individual vs. group diagnosis, individualized vs. type therapy, preventive speech pathology and audiology, and future efforts at training clinicians.

SPEECH DISORDER SIMPLEXES VS. COMPLEXES

Continued expansion and development of the field of speech pathology and audiology means that an increasing number of clinicians will practice in medical and rehabilitation centers. Speech and hearing clinicians will thus be confronted more frequently with speech disorder complexes rather than with simplexes. By simplexes we mean those speech disorders that appear in relative isolation, for example, articulation or voice cases, and are also relatively specific to the speech system involved. Such cases are frequently encountered in college speech and hearing centers as well as in school settings. Complexes, on the other hand, refer to speech disorders that reflect combinations of symptoms, for example, respiratory and phonatory disorders or respiratory, phonatory, and articulatory disorders, and to disorders that may be part of greater conditions reflecting perceptual, intellectual, and socioemotional symptomatology. Such cases are more frequently found in special classes and schools, as well as in medical and rehabilitation centers.

In order to deal with such complexes, the speech clinician needs to know more about the various speech systems of which the total system is composed. Further knowledge of and competencies in diagnostic procedures are also required. Each chapter in this book includes, therefore, information both on the types of disorders within any particular system and on the diseases and disorders affecting it.

CLASSIFICATION OF DISORDERS

Nomenclature and classification of disorders of speech are important because they (a) facilitate inter- and intraprofessional communication, (b) facilitate the study of disorders by allowing an ordering and grouping of them, and (c) contribute to and customarily precede the discovery of causes of disorders. An ideal system of classifying disorders is one in which the terms would carry information on clinical manifestations, underlying tissue pathology, and etiology. Terms currently used to describe speech disorders are used in different ways by specialists and also lack uniformity of linguistic etymology.

Hopefully, a classification system based on speech systems, as used in this book, should contribute to the better understanding of speech systems and their disorders and to the further development of diagnostic and therapy procedures.

INDIVIDUAL VS. GROUP DIAGNOSIS

An increasing number of workups of complicated speech cases are being done by teams of specialists. Within a hospital or rehabilitation center, it is becoming more frequent that individuals with speech and hearing symptoms are evaluated by a speech pathologist and audiologist in addition to a pediatrician or internist, an otolaryngologist, and a social worker. In some cases, further examinations and evaluations are provided by a neurologist, a physiatrist, a psychiatrist, a psychologist, and a vocational counselor. Such workups are usually discussed at team conferences where group diagnoses and therapy plans may be formulated.

Material in this book should help the speech and hearing clinician to function more effectively in cooperative diagnostics and in multidisciplinary staff conferences. With the help of information presented here, clinicians may collect more often the kind of speech, hearing, and language data that will support more directly diagnoses of speech symptoms that are, in fact, secondary to, for example, minimal brain dysfunction, mental retardation, or childhood psychosis. Various diagnostic approaches such as differential, treatment, or provocative diagnoses, or diagnosis by exclusion are also discussed.

INDIVIDUALIZED VS. TYPE THERAPY

Information provided herein should also encourage the development of regimens of individualized therapy rather than what may be termed programs of type therapy. Individualized therapy derives from an in-depth study of the speech disorder of a particular individual, at a particular age, of a particular sex, in a particular home situation, in a particular school or job setting, and so on. Type therapy stems from the simple identification of the client as a stutterer or a voice case. For example, after the clinician identifies the client as a voice case, he reviews material in reference works on therapy techniques for voice disorders. This tendency for many clinicians, especially new ones, to apply type therapies may be a by-product of the manner in which many courses and training programs in speech pathology and audiology are organized and conducted.

In the pages that follow, the clinician is encouraged to orient his view of each case toward the individual rather than the group. That is, however important the results of studies that utilize groups of stutterers to establish measures of central tendency and dispersion relative to any particular piece of stuttering behavior, the clinician is encouraged to see his particular case as unique, one that requires careful study and analysis. A benign consequence of such an orientation should be an increased tendency for clinicians to develop programs of individualized speech therapy. Such programs may include a particular kind of parental counseling and home activity as well as a particular kind of speech therapy. At times speech therapy may be provided alone; at others it may precede, follow, or supplement some other form of therapy. Interim speech therapy may be considered while an individual awaits, for example, placement in a special school or surgery. Indicators of the time and type of speech therapy, whether preventive, causal, symptom, compensatory, or supportive, should also be considered.

PREVENTIVE SPEECH PATHOLOGY AND AUDIOLOGY

Increased knowledge of the speech systems, of speech disorder complexes, and of individualized therapy programs should contribute to increased knowledge and awareness of preventive speech pathology and audiology. Surprisingly, little in the way of organized material exists in our literature in the important area of prevention.

Efforts are made in this book to provide as much information as possible on preventive measures relative to each of the speech systems. Primary and secondary prevention considerations are discussed. Primary preventive measures are directed at: (a) facilitating the development of speech and hearing, and (b) preventing the onset of various speech and hearing disorders. Secondary preventive measures are directed at: (a) providing optimal speech conditions for infants who present a high risk of suffering from future speech and hearing problems, such as infants with congenital cleft palate and cerebral palsy; (b) recommending speech and hearing checks for all children between 30 and 36 months for purposes of early detection of, and attention for, speech problems; and (c) reducing the social, emotional, and educational repercussions as well as secondary speech symptoms arising from already existing speech and hearing problems. Also, in the interests of furthering the effectiveness of both primary and secondary preventive measures, an important need exists to educate lay as well as professional individuals concerning speech and hearing processes, their disorders, and their treatment.

TRAINING

The book also provides pertinent information for supervisors of speech and hearing services in hospital and rehabilitation centers who have responsibility over speech and hearing interns. Ideas herein should not only assist such supervisors in assuming their clinical responsibilities more fully but should also assist them in instructing their interns in those responsibilities.

Finally, because many new practical and theoretical concepts are discussed, those readers who seek areas to explore and hypotheses to test should not be disappointed.

1

Speech Systems

As preparation for the chapters that follow, Chapter One is devoted to a detailed description of the speech systems. The structure and function of each component of the entire system are described first and then intra- and intersystem relationships and influences are discussed.

COMPONENTS OF THE SYSTEMS

At least six systems are identifiable within the speech organism. They are the receptor, transmitter, higher-order integrator, lower-order integrator, effector, and sensor systems (Fig. 1.1). Each of these systems is interrelated and interdependent and contains its own complex subsystems. Altogether they are responsible in man for the functions of speech reception, perception, comprehension, formulation, production, control, and monitoring.

Speech Receptor System

Under normal circumstances speech reception is a bisensory function; the ear receives sound pressure energy associated with speech events, and the eye receives radiant energy in connection with speech-associated articulatory movements, facial expressions, and body postures and movements. These two receptors, as do other sense organs, have two essential mechanisms: " . . . One is responsible for its specific sensitivity to a particular kind of stimulation and involves some physical or chemical change, and the other, responsible for converting this change into the code of nerve impulses . . . " (Wyburn, 1960, p. 34). Speech information, in a face-to-face situation, is generated via the synthesis of verboacoustical and verbovisual (articulatory, facial, hand, and body movements) code.

Spoken symbols that describe an emergency situation of some kind more clearly and quickly represent that situation for a listener if the listener also views the excited articulatory movements, the tense facial expressions, and the hand and body movements of the speaker. Similarly, spoken words of endearment are usually more effective when the speaker's facial expressions and hand and body movements are also viewed. Hence, the communicative index of television, motion film, or

1

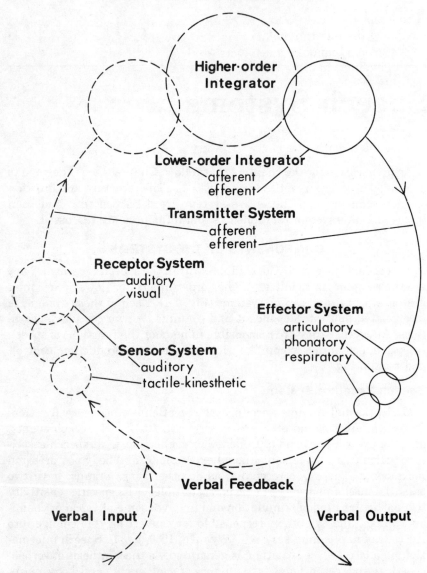

Higher-order Integrator

Lower-order Integrator
afferent
efferent

Transmitter System
afferent
efferent

Receptor System
auditory
visual

Effector System
articulatory
phonatory
respiratory

Sensor System
auditory
tactile-kinesthetic

Verbal Feedback

Verbal Input

Verbal Output

Figure 1.1. Interrelated and interdependent speech systems.

live theater is greater than that of radio, oral reading, or silent film. Audition remains, however, the dominant sensory modality for the reception and perception of speech signals.

In certain situations compensatory functioning of the speech receptor is required. For example, congenitally blind individuals may receive and process speech signals in a unisensory, auditory fashion rather efficiently, or deaf individuals may learn to receive and process speech signals via the eye. Because of the basic acoustical nature of spoken language, the blind individual, since he utilizes the auditory receptor, learns spoken language much more easily and efficiently than does the deaf individual. In other situations secondary speech receptors, such as the cutaneous sense organs of touch and pressure, may be utilized. These mechanoreceptors of compensatory speech signals can mediate what may be called skin or tactile communication. In this regard, man's fingertips, palms of the hand, lips, and tongue are claimed to be regions of maximum tactile sensitivity (Wyburn *et al.*, 1964, p. 18).

Vibration, a form of discontinuous pressure, has been considered for use in developing some form of vibratized skin language because it is a good attention-demanding stimulus. Wyburn *et al.* (1964, pp. 19–20) believe that, because vibration may be represented by at least four dimensions, intensity, duration, frequency, and locus, it may be the most suitable of all the cutaneous sense modalities for codification and some kind of interpretation. The authors report that such a vibratized alphabetical code was developed and that an individual was trained to interpret vibratized language at a rate of 35 lettered words per minute with 90% accuracy.

Anatomical boundaries and further comments on normal and compensatory functions of the speech receptor system will be outlined next. In brief, the primary system is composed of a mechanoreceptor and a photoreceptor to receive and convert auditory and visual stimuli (Fig. 1.2). The secondary system is composed of mechanoreceptors of touch, pressure, and kinesthesis. All parts of the speech receptor system are peripheral to the central nervous system.

Auditory Speech Receptor. The auditory speech receptor is made up of the outer, middle, and inner ear. Components of the receptor include: the auricle, external and internal auditory meatuses, eustachian tube, tympanic membrane, ossicular chain, tensor tympani and stapedius muscles (and associated peripheral branches of the trigeminal and facial nerves), and the cochlea, including the organ of Corti.

Visual Speech Receptor. The visual speech receptor normally works in conjunction with the auditory speech receptor. Parts of the receptor include: eyelids, eyeballs (cornea, sclera, iris, lens, aqueous and vitreous humors, choroid and ciliary bodies), medial, external, inferior, and superior rectus muscles, inferior and superior oblique muscles, peripheral oculomotor, trochlear, and abducens nerves, and the retinae.

As indicated, functioning of the audiovisual speech receptor involves the simultaneous reception and nerve impulse coding of auditory and visual events associated with the speech act. The visual speech receptor processes not only articulatory movements and face, hand, and body language but may also process compensatory finger spelling and manual sign language.

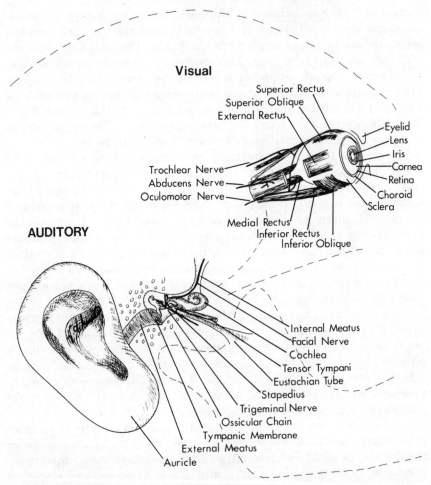

Figure 1.2. Speech receptor: auditory and visual components.

Tactile and Kinesthetic Communication Receptors. The tactile receptor includes skin and mucous membrane, hair roots, corpuscles of Meissner, Pacinian corpuscles in regions of the mandible, lips, tongue, soft palate, fingertips, palms of the hand, and areas of the thorax. The kinesthetic receptor may receive muscle-joint sensations from movements of the speech articulators that have been imposed by another individual, for example, a speech clinician.

Tactile-kinesthetic communication receptors may be used singularly or in combination as compensatory sensory channels for interpersonal communication. Subsumed under the category of tactile or skin communication are braille reading, palm writing, and the decoding of vibratized skin language. Touch-pressure-movement stimulation is used as supplementary stimulation to audiovisual stimuli during the use of Young's (1965) familiar motokinesthetic approach to speech therapy. Skin and movement language could also serve supplementary as well as major functions in communicating with, for example, the deaf or the congenitally deaf-blind. "Probably the greatest development of the tactile sense ever attained was by Helen Keller, blind and deaf from infancy, whose very comprehensive knowledge of the world was gained entirely from her sense of touch and her sense of smell" (Wyburn, 1960, p. 38).

Speech Transmitter System

The speech transmitter system has at least two roles. It has an afferent role in transmitting the code of nerve impulses generated by the speech receptors to central parts of the speech system. Such inflow is conveyed over lower and upper sensory neurons connected by various synapses and relay stations along the neural pathways. The amount and type of transmutation of particular inflows that accompany their transmission is open to question. Afferent inflow may be selectively filtered and routed at different levels of its ascent into the central nervous system, depending on the situation. The system also has an efferent role in transmitting patterns of motor impulses from the central speech system to the peripheral speech effector system. Such neural outflow is conveyed over upper and lower motor neurons connected by various synapses and relay stations, and such outflow may also be transmuted at different levels of its descent. More will be said about the effects of transmutations of afferent inflow or efferent outflow in this chapter in the section on lower-order speech integration.

With respect to the relationship between the receptor and transmitter systems, if the speech receptors are not receiving and converting stimulation into codes of nerve impulses, there is little value or need for the afferent transmission system. On the other hand, if the transmitter system is dysfunctioning or nonfunctioning, the pattern of nerve impulses generated at the receptors will carry reduced significance or none at all for various central speech regions. Similar relationships exist between the efferent transmission system and the speech effector system. Afferent speech transmission is below the level of speech perception, that is, the nerve impulses are being processed prior to their recognition as meaningful patterns of speech stimuli. Analogously, efferent speech-signal transmission is below the level of outflow patterning, that is, it is concerned with conveying the patterns of motor impulses that have already been organized in higher centers.

A description of the anatomical boundaries and further comments on the function of the afferent and efferent speech transmitter systems follows. Simply, the transmission system is composed of sensory and motor projection fibers and their relay centers. Portions of the system are within the central nervous system, in the form of upper sensory and motor neurons, and portions are outside of the central nervous system, in the form of lower sensory and motor neurons and the associated autonomic nervous system. The latter portion makes up the peripheral nervous system of the speech transmitter.

Afferent Speech Transmitter. The afferent speech transmitter includes the primary auditory and visual transmission pathways and the secondary tactile and kinesthetic transmission pathways.

The auditory speech transmitter (Fig. 1.3) is composed of those structures that Goodhill and Guggenheim (1971, p. 279) identified as comprising the transmissive neural pathway, including the neural auditory

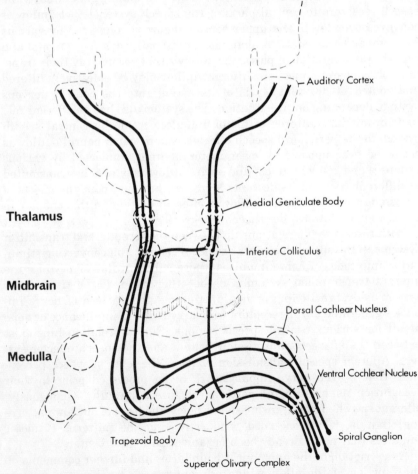

Figure 1.3. Speech transmitter: auditory tracts.

pathway, which is central to the organ of Corti. Relay centers in the pathway to the auditory cortices, in addition to the ganglion cells within the cochlea, include the ventral and dorsal cochlear nuclei and the superior olive and trapezoid body at the level of the medulla, the inferior colliculi at the midbrain level, and the medial geniculate body at the thalamic level. Wyburn *et al.* (1964, p. 57) report that a characteristic of the auditory pathway is its complexity, with up to six or more relaying stations as compared to the usual up to four well-defined neuron relays of other somatic sensory systems. Some fibers cross at the level of the pons, and from this level on transmission is binaural and brain centers receive speech information from both ears (Hardy, 1956). Auditory impulses also reach the brain by the reticular activating system and hence can produce arousal reactions; auditory impulse patterns in the brain also initiate localization movements (Wyburn *et al.*, 1964, pp. 56–57). Conjugate movements of the eyes in response to sound are reflexes mediated by branches of the auditory pathway being connected to nuclei of the abducent, oculomotor, and trochlear nerves via the superior olive (Gatz, 1966, p. 67). The central auditory system also includes cerebrifugal control mechanisms that can regulate the sensory responses of the receptors and lower neurons, that is, activity at any level of the auditory system can be modified by response to events in both higher and lower centers and by preceding auditory or other sensory stimuli.

The visual speech transmitter (Fig. 1.4) is composed of the two optic tracts, including the crossed fibers from the nasal half of each contralateral retina and the uncrossed fibers from the temporal half of each ipsilateral retina up to the lateral geniculate bodies of the thalamus, and the final visual pathways to the visual cortices in the occipital lobes. Other fibers of the optic tract form connections with neurons in the midbrain region concerned with reflex control of pupillary size and eyeball movements (Wyburn *et al.*, 1964, p. 107). Also important is the visual fixation reflex (Gatz, 1966, p. 8) involved with making the adjustments responsible for bringing a desired image into identical positions on each retina after the head and eyes have moved in its direction and also allows for reflexly holding a moving object of interest in view by causing appropriate turning movements of both eyes. The afferent path of the reflex is from the retina to the visual cortex; the efferent path is from the occipital lobe to the superior colliculi and eventually to the nuclei of cranial nerves III, IV, and VI.

The primary role of the afferent transmission system is to conduct verboacoustic and verbovisual information to appropriate higher centers for purposes of speech perception. However, many of the auditory and visual relay centers mediate certain kinds of behaviors that are also important to speech perception. These behaviors may be viewed as reflecting lower-order integration of speech information and are dis-

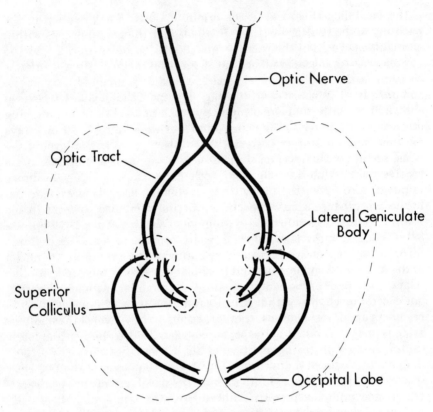

Figure 1.4. Speech transmitter: visual tracts.

cussed in the next section of the chapter devoted to the speech integrator system.

The tactile-kinesthetic communication transmitters serve the compensatory speech receptors concerned with touch, pressure, and movement stimuli. As with the audiovisual transmitter system, the major role of the compensatory transmission system is to convey impulses to higher levels of the nervous system so that the perceptualizing process may take place. The system is comprised of the peripheral and central sensory neurons that serve parts of the thorax, fingertips, palms of the hands; and the mandible, lips, teeth (trigeminal nerve), palate (palatine nerve), and tongue (trigeminal and glossopharyngeal nerves). Two relay systems, the medial lemniscal and spinothalamic systems, convey impulses from touch, pressure, and movement receptors primarily to the contralateral somatic sensory center of the cerebral cortex (Wyburn *et al.*, 1964, pp. 27–35). Touch and kinesthesis are served by the medial lemniscal system. The thalamus is an important relay center for this afferent inflow. Sensory impulses reach the cortex via the direct routes of the medial lemniscal and spinothalamic systems and also via the reticular activating system, or secondary ascending systems. These secondary sensory pathways are considered to be " . . . activating mechanisms alerting the cortex to a state of awareness" (Wyburn *et al.*, 1964, p. 35).

In addition to its possible function in compensatory communication and as a system to supplement audiovisual speech stimuli, the tactile-kinesthetic transmitter system is utilized in speech control and monitoring functions. Control and monitoring functions are discussed in detail in the section of this chapter devoted to the speech sensor system.

Efferent Speech Transmitter. The efferent speech transmitter is composed of all the peripheral and central motor neurons supplying respiratory, phonatory, resonatory, and articulatory mechanisms. This efferent system includes the pyramidal and striatal extrapyramidal systems and their descending relay stations.

The pyramidal system appears in animals with well-developed cerebral cortices and may be considered a part of the "new motor system." It consists of the descending fibers of the motor area of the brain. The motor cortices of the brain are in the right and left frontal lobes and include certain areas anterior to the Rolandic fissure. The two motor strips primarily control contralateral body parts; the larynx and tongue are represented in the lowest part of the strip, followed in a superior sequence by the face, thumb, hand, forearm, arm, thorax, abdomen, etc. Because of the complex development of motor control of the hand, tongue, and larynx, especially for linguistic purposes, the areas serving these functions are disproportionately large.

The extrapyramidal system, or "old motor system," is composed of the corpus striatum and subthalamus (Gatz, 1966, p. 118). It becomes subordinate to the more recently evolved pyramidal system. Most mammals are able to use the striatal system for habitual or semiautomatic activities even after the motor cortex has been removed, for example, in the case of the cat. Humans, however, are much more dependent on the pyramidal system and suffer severe loss of motor function when it is damaged. Gatz (1966, p. 118) indicates that, in order for the pyramidal system to function appropriately, it requires the cooperation of the vestibular system together with proprioception, the cerebellar system, and the corpus striatum (all are extrapyramidal systems). The striatal extrapyramidal system includes the caudate nucleus, the lenticular nucleus (including the putamen and globus pallidus), and the subthalamus. Efferent outflow from the corpus striatum or basal ganglia is believed to emanate from the globus pallidus. Pallidal fibers enter the region of the subthalamus and some reach the thalamus; some pallidal fibers also descend from the subthalamus and enter into the area of the red nucleus. Connections exist between caudate nucleus and the putamen, between the putamen and the globus pallidus, between the substantia nigra and both the putamen and the globus pallidus, and between the thalamus and the caudate nucleus. Connections are also supposed to exist between the premotor cortex and the basal ganglia.

Comparatively little is known about the operation of the corpus striatum during normal motor activity. The caudate nucleus and putamen are presumed to inhibit the globus pallidus, which is considered to act as a facilitator of motor activity. Facilitation of the premotor and motor cortex by the globus pallidus is via thalamic projection fibers, and facilitation of motor activity of lower neurons of the spinal cord is via the subthalamus, the prerubral field, the reticular formation of the midbrain, and reticulospinal tracts (Gatz, 1966, p. 120). Zemlin (1968, p. 526) states, "The extrapyramidal tract is indirectly associated with voluntary movements." In coordination with the pyramidal system, it " . . . makes possible . . . fine, smooth, voluntary motor activities . . . ." Zemlin states further, "Inasmuch as the pyramidal and extrapyramidal tracts are combined functionally into a complex servomechanism, we ought not to attempt to dichotimize them into strictly separate systems."

The primary role of the efferent transmission system is to conduct patterns of nerve impulses, organized by higher speech centers, over upper and lower motor neurons to respiratory, phonatory, resonatory, and articulatory mechanisms for the specific purpose of producing speech events. However, as in the case of afferent transmission, various relay centers are involved with this transmission, and in the case of efferent transmission, there are "old" as well as "new" motor systems involved. For example, lesions of the new motor system may result in hypo- or hypertonicity of the articulatory mechanism, while lesions in the old system may cause "freezing," tremors, athetotic or choreiform movements, or festinating movements of the articulatory mechanism. The specific role of the pyramidal system in the nervous supply of respiratory, phonatory, resonatory, and articulatory mechanisms is discussed next.

The respiratory speech transmitter (Fig. 1.5) is part of the corticospinal tract. It represents those pyramidal fibers and their lower motor neurons that supply the muscles of vegetative and speech breathing. The tract descends from the cerebral cortex to the spinal cord via the internal capsule, cerebral peduncle, pons, pyramid, pyramidal decussation (some fibers do not decussate), and lateral corticospinal tract. Zemlin's (1968, p. 527) motor nerve supply for muscles of breathing, including muscles possibly used in compensatory breathing, includes cervical nerves I through VIII and thoracic nerves I through XII.

The phonatory, resonatory, and articulatory speech transmitter (Fig. 1.6) is part of the corticobulbar tract. It represents those pyramidal fibers and their lower motor neurons that supply the muscles of phonation, resonation, and articulation. The fibers of the tract begin their

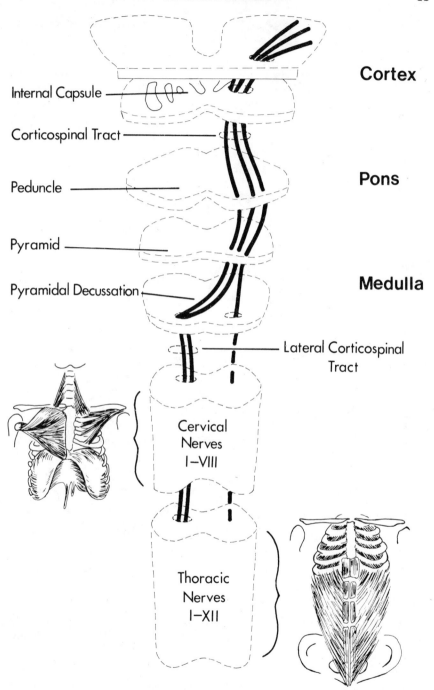

Cortex

Internal Capsule

Corticospinal Tract

Peduncle

Pons

Pyramid

Pyramidal Decussation

Medulla

Lateral Corticospinal Tract

Cervical Nerves I–VIII

Thoracic Nerves I–XII

Figure 1.5. Speech transmitter: respiratory tracts and nerves.

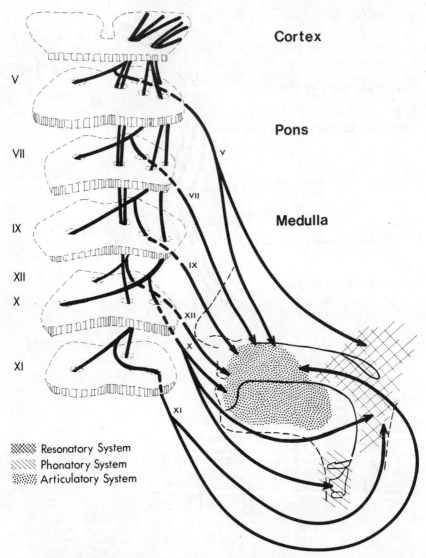

Figure 1.6. Speech transmitter: phonatory, resonatory, and articulatory tracts and nerves.

descent with the fibers of the corticospinal tract but take a different path at the level of the midbrain and terminate on the nuclei of the various cranial nerves. The cranial nerve supplying the phonatory mechanism is cranial nerve X or the vagus; those supplying the resonatory mechanism (including nasal vs. non-nasal sound distinctions) are branches of cranial nerves X, V (trigeminal), and XI (accessory), and those supplying the articulatory mechanism are cranial nerves V, VII (facial), IX (glossopharyngeal), X, XI, and XII (hypoglossal). Most of the corticobulbar fibers cross, but uncrossed fibers also exist. For example, articulatory and phonatory muscles appear to benefit from bilateral representation, and hence a unilateral lesion of the corticobulbar tract (upper motor neuron) is not expected to cause permanent dysarthria (Brain and Walton, 1969, p. 98) or dysphonia (Greene, 1957, p. 153).

In summary, the primary role of the respiratory, phonatory, resonatory, and articulatory transmitters is to convey nervous impulses, organized by higher speech centers, to the speech effectors for the purpose of creating speech events. However, as in the case of afferent transmission, various kinds of influences are brought to bear on the efferent outflow as it descends to the effectors, and these influences are important to final speech production. These influences may be viewed as reflecting lower-order integration of speech output, analogous to the previously discussed lower-order integration of speech input. They are discussed further in the following section.

Speech Integrator System

The speech integrator system can be divided into two parts. The lower-order integrator is used in an automatic, subconscious manner and has both speech input and output roles. The higher-order integrator is used in a less automatic, less organized, and more conscious manner and is involved with complicated comprehension and formulation speech functions; it represents the "thinking" level of speech integration, while the lower-order integrator represents the "doing" level of speech integration.

Structure and Function of the Lower-Order Speech Integrator. The function of lower-order, afferent integration is to adjust and facilitate speech input signals and includes system arousal and selective attention processes; the function of lower-order, efferent integration is to adjust and facilitate speech output signals and includes coordinating and refining processes.

The ascending reticular activating system may be identified with lower-order afferent integration of speech input. In West's (1968, pp. 27–30) discussion of various centers of speech control or integration, he compares the reticular system to the cerebellum. The cerebellum, according to West, "sorts out the neuromuscular components of motor acts," while the reticular system "sorts the various sensory inputs." By the process of inhibition and selection, " . . . the listener selects from the sounds that strike his ear those that make intrinsic meaning and those which are compatible with the visible patterns on the lips, face, and hands of the person who is making the noises."

Further, in the section on afferent transmission of speech signals it may be recalled that auditory inflow also initiated arousal and localization behavior, conjugate movements of the eyes, and cerebrifugal impulses that could regulate sensory responses of the receptor and lower neurons, while visual inflow also initiated visual fixation and optokinetic reflexes.

Hence, as speech information is being conveyed, mechanisms involved with lower-order afferent integration are activated and these mechanisms are responsible for, so to speak, turning on, tuning in, and fine tuning of the speech system. These adjustments make important contributions to speech reception, transmission, and eventual perception. More specifically, speech signals impinging upon the auditory and visual systems initiate transmission processes that, in turn, contribute to the process by activating lower-order afferent integration mechanisms. Auditory mechanisms contribute to transmission and perception of speech signals by: (a) orienting the head, ears, and eyes toward the source of speech signals, (b) stimulating auditory arousal mechanisms, and (c) generating efferent impulses to regulate responsiveness of the auditory system at any level of the ascent pathway. Visual mechanisms contribute to transmission and perception of speech signals by: (a) allowing for retinal localization of the speaker's face, his expressions, and his hand and body movements; and (b) eliciting optokinetic reflexive activity that allows the listener optically to follow speech articulatory movements.

In short, lower-order afferent integration involves audiovisual localization of the speech signals, arousal and sensitizing of the audiovisual system, and audiovisual tracking of the speech information.

The basal ganglia, cerebellum, midbrain, and minor speech hemisphere may be identified as brain regions that have a function in lower-order efferent integration of speech output.

West and Ansberry (1968, pp. 28–29) identify the basal ganglia (the authors include the thalamus and striate bodies) as the seats of control for emotional reactions such as crying, laughing, sobbing, frowning, smiling, and sneering, " . . . as well as of impulses that condition the vocal organs and give emotional color to the voice." The cerebellum, whose important function in speech control and monitoring is discussed in the section devoted to the speech sensor system, also has an important role in lower-order efferent integration of speech output. West and Ansberry (1968, pp. 29–30) identify the important role of the cerebellum in mediating compensatory movements. Such compensatory movements allow the speech output to remain relatively intact while concomitant movements, which might affect the speech mechanism, are taking place, for example, head turning or nodding, arm movements, and so on. West and Ansberry also identify the important role of the cerebellum in maintaining appropriate muscle tonus throughout the body. Hypotonia is associated with cerebellar involvement, for example, and may influence the speech mechanism in a negative manner.

In the discussion section of a chapter by Lilly (1967, p. 18), Dr. H. W. Magoun speaks of a central neural mechanism for vocal expression in man that serves "nonverbal affective communication." He believes that there is a subcortical mechanism for faciovocal expression in the middle brain stem that manages " . . . vocal and related mimetic responses involved in the expression of affective states . . . ." According to Magoun, "Midbrain lesions in man may impair such behavior without impairment of his speech. Conversely, widespread bilateral cortical injury in man may be followed by a pathologic exaggeration of laughter and crying, interpreted as release of lower functions from higher inhibition." This subcortical mechanism for nonverbal communication is functional at birth, and this fact can certainly be attested to by young parents.

The speech function of the minor or right hemisphere was described by Jackson (1931). He identified the aphasic utterances of emotional speech, recurrent utterances, and jargon as manifestations of release of lower functions from higher inhibition in aphasia.

Information on minor hemisphere speech function was offered by Falconer (1967, pp. 185–203) through his study of seizure-related speech phenomena. He describes two types of ictal (epileptic) speech manifestations: ictal dysphasia, which is discussed in the next portion of the chapter concerned with higher-order speech integration, and ictal speech automatisms. Speech automatisms may be observed at the beginning of or during a seizure and are characterized by the use " . . . of identifiable words or phrases which are linguistically correct but for which the patient is subsequently amnesic." Falconer's study of ictal speech manifestations in 100 consecutive patients with temporal-lobe epilepsy revealed and suggested the following: (a) ictal speech automatisms are common, may be evoked by seizures originating in either hemisphere, but occur slightly more frequently with seizures originating in the minor hemisphere; and (b) since ictal speech automatisms occur slightly more often with involvement in the minor hemisphere, the responsible discharges apparently leave the traditional speech hemisphere undisturbed, and hence homologous areas in the minor hemisphere may be responsible for these speech automatisms.

Falconer believes that his findings support the view held by Jackson that the right half of the brain is for the automatic use of words, while the left half of the brain is for both automatic and voluntary use. In Jacksonian terms, ictal speech automatisms may be considered as release of automatic verbal phenomena, or a positive symptom, while ictal dysphasia, or the disturbance or loss of voluntary verbal function, may be considered a negative symptom.

Hence, lower-order efferent speech integration appears to be responsible for various types of verbal stereotypy as well as for the coordination of pyramidal and extrapyramidal systems at various levels in the descent pathway. Such integration is responsible for: (a) producing fine, smooth, and accurate movements; (b) coordinating respiratory, phonatory, resonatory, and articulatory movements; (c) permitting the motor speech system to function concomitantly with movements of the head, hand, foot, and so on; and (d) providing for appropriate paralanguage (tonal and kinetic).

Structure and Function of the Higher-Order Speech Integrator. The higher-order speech integrator is the "brain" of the central neural mechanisms devoted to speech function. Higher-order speech integration embraces speech perception and speech comprehension and formulation, including elaboration, interpretation, memory, retrieval, and response functions. Some of these functions are utilized in inner speaking or verbal thinking, and all may be involved in actual speaking.

The neuropsychology of the central speech system has been discussed for a long time. Various means have been utilized to help determine the location, composition, and functioning of components of the central neural speech mechanisms. Among these means are: (a) the evaluation of disordered speech of neurological patients and attempts to correlate the speech deficits with lesions found in postmortem studies; (b) the use of intracarotid amytal speech testing on certain neurological patients; (c) the evaluation of speech disturbances during focal epilepsy involving various parts of the brain; (d) the stimulation of vocalization and interference with speech as a function of electrostimulation of various cortical regions in patients undergoing special neurosurgery; (e) the evaluation of the type and permanence of language disturbance in children who suffered brain trauma; (f) the correlation of motor development, brain maturation, and language development; and (g) split-brain and dichotomous listening experiments. Since most of the methods mentioned involve the study of individuals suffering from various types of brain disease, the findings relative to central brain mechanisms underlying speech function must be qualified accordingly.

Studies correlating language symptoms with postmortem findings were reviewed by Roberts (see Penfield and Roberts, 1959, Ch. 4). Results of this extensive review of the literature are summarized by the following comments. (a) Motor components of speech are more involved the closer the lesion is to the posterior part of the third frontal convolution (Broca's area). (b) Speech comprehension is more affected the more the posterior superior temporal region is involved (Wernicke's area). (c) Reading and writing are more affected the nearer the lesion is to the area of junction of the parietal, temporal, and occipital lobes.

Intracarotid amytal speech testing and effects of electroconvulsive shock treatment (EST) on language function have been utilized to help determine which cerebral hemisphere subserves speech function.

The use of the sodium amytal test introduced by Wada (1949) has generally shown speech function to be unilaterally represented and almost always in the left hemisphere. Rossi and Rosadini (1967, pp. 167–184) reported on their use, over a 5-year period, of intracarotid injection in determining lateralization of speech mechanisms and its relation to handedness. The investigators point out that one limitation to carotid-amytal speech testing is that a global impairment of sensory as well as motor speech usually follows the functional inactivation of a large part of the dominant hemisphere. Of a total of 126 patients studied, 115 were right-handed, 8 were left-handed, and 3 could not be clearly classified. Bilateral intracarotid injections were administered to 49 cases and unilateral injections were administered to 77 cases for a total of 175 examinations. In the great majority of cases, the investigators believed that motor rather than sensory speech mechanisms were affected by the amytal test. Because of various complications, only 84 patients were finally used for the analysis of speech dominance.

Left carotid injection produced "aphasia" in 91.6% of the cases, and right carotid injection produced it in 5.9% of the cases. In one case, both left and right carotid injections failed to produce speech disturbances, while in another case, speech disturbance followed injection into either the left or right side. In summary, the investigators believe their findings suggest the following: (a) the possible independence of speech and hand dominance, (b) that left-handed persons may show right-sided speech representation, (c) the rare occurrence of ipsilateral speech representation in right-handers, and (d) the possibility of bilateral representation of speech in adults.

Milner (see Rossi and Rosadini, 1967, pp. 178–179) also reported on 18 of 212 cases who apparently reflected bilateral speech representation under amytal speech testing; however, because of differences in speech disturbance depending on the hemisphere blocked, it is suggested that in such cases the hemispheres may participate in the verbal function in somewhat different ways.

Cohen *et al*. (1968) reported a study using EST applied either to the left, right, or both cerebral hemispheres of neurologically normal patients being treated for affective depression. They evaluated the differential effects on certain verbal and nonverbal associative tasks during a postictal (postconvulsive) period. Consistent with the expected functional asymmetry linking the left hemisphere with verbal skills, subjects did more poorly on the verbal task following bilateral EST or EST to the left hemisphere; findings on the nonverbal task were consistent with the expected functional asymmetry linking the right hemisphere to nonverbal skills.

Speech manifestations during seizures involving certain brain areas were divided into at least two types by Penfield and Roberts (1959, pp. 87–88). Vocalization, a positive effect, occurs with epileptic discharge in the Rolandic or supplementary motor area of either hemisphere or in subcortical areas. Loss of ability to understand speech, one of the negative effects, occurs with epileptic discharge in the dominant hemisphere. Interference with primary auditory mechanisms, another negative effect, may occur with epileptic discharge in either hemisphere or in subcortical areas. According to Roberts, it is not always possible to determine whether primary audition or auditory comprehension is involved. "The disturbance in language may occur as an aura, during the seizure, or postictally. Disturbance in comprehension, reading, motor speech, or writing may occur with seizures originating in the temporo-parietal or Broca's or supplementary motor area of the dominant hemisphere. The focus of the seizure discharge may be adjacent to a speech area in so-called silent areas of cortex . . .."

Ictal dysphasia was also discussed by Falconer (1967, pp. 185–203). It is characterized by " . . . an inability on the part of the patient to express himself by the correct words while he is still conscious and without impairment of articulation or hearing." It occurs while the patient is aware of his surroundings, and the language disturbance can be recalled by the person. Such speech disturbances can be observed at the start of a seizure, during a minor seizure without loss of consciousness, or following a seizure when consciousness is regained.

Ictal dysphasia is usually associated with seizures in the dominant hemisphere, and hence the ictal discharges are apparently disturbing the traditionally accepted speech centers.

Many neurologically intact individuals who suffer from migraine headaches may also report aphasic-like interference with motor language function, or migrainous dysphasia, usually of a paraphasic variety. Such minor speech "fluffing" may precede, be concomitant with, or follow the actual headache. Migraine headache phenomena have no doubt contributed to the origin of phrases such as, "I have such a headache I can't see straight" (visual aura) or, "I can't talk straight" (transient paraphasia).

Speech manifestations during electrostimulation of the brain prior to surgery for relief of "focal cerebral seizures" were studied by Penfield and Roberts (1959). Before entering the discussion proper, it would be well to comment on some of Penfield and Robert's (1959, Ch. 2) concepts of brain physiology. Penfield and Roberts believe that there is a level of integration within the central nervous system that is higher than that found in the cerebral cortex, and it probably resides in the diencephalon or higher brain stem (which includes the thalamus, midbrain, and part of the pons). They define this central coordinating and integrating mechanism as a centrencephalic system, which consists of " . . . all those areas of subcortical gray matter (together with their connecting tracts) which serve the purposes of inter-hemispheral integration and intra-hemispheral integration" (p. 21).

Further, each functional subdivision of the cerebral cortex may be considered as an outward projection of some area of gray matter in the brain stem. Thus, the anterior frontal cortex could be viewed as an elaboration from the dorsal-medial nucleus of the thalamus, and much of the temporal cortex could be viewed as an elaboration from the pulvinar and the posterior part of the lateral nucleus of the thalamus. Penfield and Roberts (pp. 25–27) consider the motor function of the cortex is " . . an arrival platform and a departure platform . . . . Its function is to transmit and possibly transmute, with the aid of second-ary motor areas, the patterned stream of impulses which arises in the centrencephalic system and passes on out to the target in voluntary muscles." The somatic sensory area on the postcentral gyrus is also considered to function as a transmitting strip. "The somatic sensory stream which comes in from the skin, muscles, and joints of the body goes to the postcentral gyrus . . . after ganglionic interruption in the lateral nucleus of the thalamus. But it must, therefore, return inward to join the centrencephalic system along a post-cortical limb . . . ."

With that much information on Penfield and Roberts' concepts of brain physiology, let us return to the discussion of speech manifesta-tions resulting from electrostimulation of the brain during special neuro-surgery. Since the patients were fully conscious during the surgery for relief of focal cerebral seizures, it was possible to discover what parts of the cortex were devoted to speech function (Penfield and Roberts, 1959, p. 5). Only local anesthesia was used during the osteoplastic craniotomy which " . . . does away with the pain of the procedure and yet leaves the brain normally active . . . ." Electrical stimulation of the brain was found to produce at least two speech phenomena: it either arrested or interfered with the speech of the patient (negative effect), or, during silence, it elicited vocalization in the form of a sustained "vowel cry" that at times included a consonant (positive effect). Intelligible words were not evoked in silent patients.

Positive speech effects were produced by the investigators during stimulation of the Rolandic area (precentral and postcentral gyri for lips, jaw, and tongue) and the supplementary area (superior and medial aspects of the intermediate precentral region of Campbell). Such posi-tive effects occurred during stimulation of either dominant or nondomi-nant motor areas.

Negative speech effects included such phenomena as complete arrest, hesitation, slurring, distortion of speech, and repetition of words. In addition, " . . . inability to name with retained ability to speak, confusion of numbers while counting, and misnaming with or without perseveration have occurred during electrical interference of the left Broca's, inferior parietal-posterior temporal, and supplementary motor areas" (Penfield and Roberts, 1959, p. 133). On rare occasions such effects were elicited during stimulation of the right hemisphere. Since the effects of the current applied in the dominant hemisphere to any of the three areas were similar, it was suggested "that these three areas are connected by transcortical and subcortical pathways in a single system."

Hence, the left hemisphere may continue to subserve speech function even after one part of the speech area is damaged. However, the investigators (Penfield and Roberts, 1959) state, "The three speech areas . . . are of different values. The posterior, or parieto-temporal, area is the most important. The anterior, or Broca's, area is the next most important but is dispensable in some patients, at least. The superior, or supplementary motor, area is dispensable but probably is very important after damage to one of the other speech areas" (p. 189). They hypothesize that the functions of all three cortical speech areas in man are coordinated by projections of each to parts of the thalamus. Further, the investigators believe that total destruction of the posterior cortical speech area or of the underlying posterior portion of the thalamus would produce global aphasia.

In summary, Penfield and Roberts, who have apparently come closest in recent times to what might be called the "speech brain," or, in terms of this section of the chapter, the higher-order speech integrator, offer the following information on its structure and function. (a) The speech hemisphere is almost always the left. (b) The speech brain is represented by a corticothalamic unit composed of left cortical areas, related thalamic regions, and interconnecting tracts. The cortical areas include a *posterior cortical speech area* (posterior parts of first, second, and third temporal convolutions behind the vein of Labbé, the supramarginal gyrus, and the angular gyrus), the most important; the *anterior cortical speech area* (Broca's area including the three gyri anterior to the precentral face area), the next in importance; and the *superior cortical speech area* (supplementary motor area on the medial and a little on the superior aspect of the hemisphere in front of the precentral foot area), the least important. The posterior speech area probably has projection connections with the pulvinar and the nucleus lateralis-posterior of the thalamus, and the anterior speech area with the centrum medianum and medial-dorsal nucleus of the thalamus. Connections between the pulvinar and centrum medianum make possible a functional interrelationship between the posterior and the anterior speech areas. Figure 1.7 shows Penfield's corticothalamic speech unit.

The neurodynamics of speech comprehension and formulation may be explained in the following manner. Speech comprehension is the result

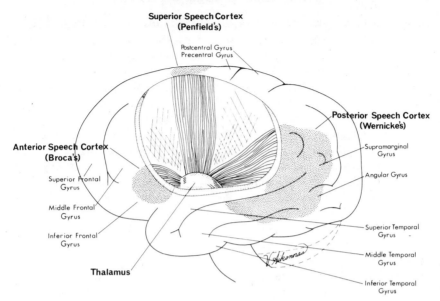

Figure 1.7. Speech integrator (higher-order): Penfield's cortico-thalamic speech unit.

of receiving auditory impulses in both hemispheres and in the higher brain stem and during interaction between thalamic areas and the posterior speech area. Motor speech is the result of interaction between the anterior speech area (or, if that area is damaged, some other speech area of the left hemisphere) and the higher brain stem and the transference of the impulses produced by this interaction to the motor cortex of either hemisphere, and finally to the lower motor neurons of the speech musculature.

Recovery of language following childhood brain trauma sheds light on the plasticity of the speech cortex of children. Remarkable recovery of language in children following disease or injury to the left speech cortex was reported by Penfield and Roberts (1959, p. 240). Examples of complete transfer of speech function from left to right hemispheres in children under three or four years are numerous. Penfield (1966, p. 222) reported that damage to the major or posterior speech area will result in aphasia; however, if it occurs before the age of ten or twelve, the homologous area in the minor hemisphere will assume the speech function within a year or more. Such a transfer does not occur in adult life.

Lenneberg (1969) reports that lesions of the left hemisphere in children under two years are of no more consequence to future language development than are lesions of the right hemisphere. Transient aphasias may be expected in children who experience brain trauma following the onset of language but before the age of four; if the right hemisphere remains intact, however, language is usually quickly regained. Lenneberg also states that language-disturbing lesions acquired " . . . before the very early teens also carry an excellent prognosis . . . ."

Following are two other concepts of Lenneberg's that have pertinence to speech theory. (a) If the lesion in the left hemisphere is incurred early enough, " . . . the right hemisphere remains competent for language throughout life." This may explain why certain adults who undergo left cerebral hemispherectomies may recover various degrees of language function (i.e., the hemispherectomy may have been performed to remedy a condition that began during the preteen years). (b) Recovery from childhood aphasia is best explained not as a "taking over" by the right hemisphere but rather as a reflection that language functions are not as yet limited to the left hemisphere during the early years of speech activity, that is, there is bilateral cerebral functioning for speech until the brain reaches full maturity. This latter point may explain why in some cases language may be disturbed by interference with the function of either hemisphere in certain individuals who, for example, undergo sodium amytal speech testing.

Findings on the possible speech role of specific cortical and subcortical regions also contribute to our knowledge of the speech brain. Certain kinds of verbal behavior have been ascribed to various regions of the brain such as the arcuate fasciculus, the angular gyrus, the parietal lobes, the left frontal dominant cortex, the temporal lobes, and the thalamus.

The speech function of the arcuate fasciculus was discussed by Konorski (1967) and by Geschwind (see Lilly, 1967, p. 17). The arcuate fasciculus connects the posterosuperior temporal region and the lower frontal region via a tract that apparently runs backward around the posterior end of the Sylvian fissure and then forward in the lower parietal lobe, finally reaching the frontal lobe. According to Konorski, "Lesions sustained in the posterior part of the first temporal gyrus and/or in the white substance beneath the supramarginal gyrus give rise to a special type of aphasia . . . of which the chief symptom is the strong impairment of repetition of words heard, although comprehension of these words . . . is preserved" (p. 244). He calls this type of aphasia auditory-verbal aphasia.

The role of the angular gyrus and the limbic system in language learning was reported by Geschwind (see Roberts, 1966, pp. 26–31). He stated that " . . . in order to learn language we must be able to form nonlimbic cross-modal associations." (The limbic system is that portion of the brain that is supposed to represent survival of individual or species behavior.) For example, man can form visual-auditory or tactile-auditory associations, that is, man can associate the sight or feel of an object with its spoken name. On the other hand, monkeys can form rather easily visual-limbic, tactile-limbic, and auditory-limbic associations but not associations between two nonlimbic stimuli. Geschwind believes that the anatomical substrate for this capacity in man is the angular gyrus or "the association area of association areas."

The role of the parietal lobes in the neurology of language has also received specific attention. Hécaen (1967, pp. 146–166) reported on his studies of the posterior region of the parietal lobe, together with the parieto-temporo-occipital junction centered mainly around the supramarginal gyrus and the angular gyrus. Hécaen also summarized what is known of the symptoms associated with damage to this zone, in either major or minor hemispheres, and discussed the relationships of parietal pathophysiology and speech and language function.

He cites the following kinds of possible relationships that have been reported: (a) parietoangular gyrus softening (due to Sylvian artery pathology) and aphasia of Wernicke (alexia predominating); (b) temporoangular gyrus softening and aphasia of Wernicke; (c) damage to the angular gyrus and amnesic aphasia; (d) parietal injury and verbal perseveration, stutter-like symptoms, and word and sentence distortion; (e) upper parietal and temporal lobe damage and sensory aphasia; and (f) injury to the angular and supramarginal gyri and central aphasia (i.e., that aphasia in which all language mechanisms are defective). Considering reported findings as well as his own, Hécaen believes " . . . that parietal aphasia is especially characterized in verbal amnesia, alexic disorders, and agraphia predominate in the setting of moderate sensory aphasia. There are likewise often expressive difficulties called parietal stuttering." (p. 152).

The possible role of the left anterior frontal region in language function is also interesting. Milner (1967, p. 131), in describing effects of left frontal lobectomy, indicates that " . . . one of the first things one notices about such patients is their lack of spontaneous speech." Impairment of spontaneous narrative speech has also been reported in patients with tumors in the dominant frontal lobe. Such patients reflect reduced spontaneous verbal expression but are not considered aphasic in the usual sense of the term. The symptom of reduced or lack of spontaneous speech appears to represent a pathological form of what the present writer (Mysak, 1966, p. 32) referred to as alloplastic verbal behavior. An individual who exhibits such behavior is one who customarily depends on his interactant to initiate and sustain a conversation, while an individual who reflects autoplastic verbal behavior is one who customarily initiates and sustains a conversation. Exaggerations of both modes of speech behavior may accompany various kinds of neuro- or psychopathologies.

Milner (1967, pp. 122–145) reported on a 15-year study of temporal lobe function in man. All patients studied underwent unilateral brain surgery for relief of focal cerebral seizures originating in early life. In both left and right temporal lobectomies, some excisions extended laterally to include the transverse gyri of Heschl; on the mesial surface, removals always included the amygdala but varied in the degree to which they involved the hippocampus. Since care is taken not to invade primary speech areas in the left hemisphere procedures, lasting aphasias are not produced by the surgery.

Some of the effects of right temporal lobectomy include impairment of auditory discrimination of tonal patterns and of tone quality and impairment of tonal memory. Impairment of verbal memory, whether it is tested by recognition, free recall, or associative learning tasks, results from left temporal lobectomy. Since individual variation existed in verbal memory capacity among the left temporal group, Milner subdivided the group into those where the hippocampus was destroyed or not and those where Heschl's gyrus was spared or not, that is, by extent of removal. This further analysis revealed that larger lesions on the left are associated with greater degrees of impairment of verbal memory. The suggestion that left hippocampectomy may increase the verbal learning deficit was also appreciated.

With respect to areas involved in verbal memory, Falconer (1967, p. 200) cites " . . . the hippocampal structures, the mammillary bodies, the connecting systems in the fornix tracts, and the mammillothalamic bundles" as structures thought to be responsible for the laying down of memory. Also, in the discussion section of Falconer's chapter, Magoun commented, "There are a number of indications that while the hippocampus and the temporal lobe may be instrumental in the initial induction of memory, the long-time storage of memory and its availability for retrieval subsequently becomes much more widely distributed in the cortex."

Finally, information on thalamic influence on speech has been acquired from electrostimulation studies and from the effects of thalamic lesions. In this regard, it may be recalled that Penfield and Roberts view the primary speech areas as a corticothalamic unit. Purpura (see Darley and Millikan, 1967, p. 49) also believes that specific and nonspecific thalamic nuclear organizations have regulating or influencing effects on the behavior of motor cortex units. As for subcortical participation in speech mechanisms, Purpura stated that " . . .stimulation of . . . ventrolateral nuclear groups of the thalamus as well as some related basal ganglia structures may severely disturb the ordering and motivational factors of speech." Arrest of speech during thalamic stimulation, language disturbance with lesions of the thalamus, and transient aphasias following thalamic surgery for parkinsonism have also been reported. The question of the precise thalamic role in language is far from settled as reflected by the differing views presented by various authorities in an issue of *Brain and Language* (Vol. 2, No. 1, 1975) devoted entirely to the thalamus and language. A summary table of the possible speech roles of various cortical and subcortical areas within the major speech brain is presented in Figure 1.8.

Components of Major Speech Brain (Usually the Left Hemisphere)	Speech Role
Cortical areas:	
Posterior parts of first, second and third temporal convolutions behind the vein of Labbé, the supramarginal gyrus, and the angular gyrus (Penfield's posterior speech cortex)	Speech comprehension and formulation
Broca's area, including the three gyri anterior to the precentral face area (Penfield's anterior speech cortex)	Speech formulation
Supplementary motor area on the medial, and a little on the superior aspect of the hemisphere in front of the precentral foot area (Penfield's superior speech cortex)	Speech formulation
Junction of parietal, temporal, and occipital lobes	Reading and writing
Arcuate fasciculus, which connects the posterosuperior temporal region and the lower frontal region via a tract that apparently runs backward around the posterior end of the Sylvian fissure and then forward in the lower parietal lobe, finally reaching the frontal lobe (from Konorski)	Repetition of words heard
Angular gyrus, or the association area of association areas (from Geschwind)	Allows man to associate, for example, the sight or feel of an object with its spoken name, or, in short, allows language learning
Anterior frontal region (from Milner)	Spontaneous narrative speech
Temporal lobe (from Milner, Falconer)	Verbal memory
Subcortical areas:	
Centrum medianum and medial dorsal nucleus of the thalamus (in association with anterior speech cortex; from Penfield)	Contributes to speech formulation
Pulvinar and posterior part of the lateral nucleus of the thalamus (in association with posterior speech cortex; from Penfield)	Contributes to speech comprehension and formulation
Amygdala and hippocampus (in association with temporal lobe; from Milner)	Contributes to verbal memory
Ventrolateral nucleus of thalamus (from Purpura)	Contributes to ordering and motivational factors of speech

Figure 1.8. Speech integrator (higher-order). A summary table showing speech roles of various cortical and subcortical regions.

Studies correlating physical and brain maturation with language development have contributed information on the physical requirements needed before one may expect speech to emerge. Lenneberg (1969) reported " . . . that language development correlates better with motor development than it does with chronological age." Lenneberg relates simple comprehension and the use of first words with the capacity to stand and to walk with assistance. Similarly, the present writer (Mysak, 1961), in discussing the concept of the organismic development of spoken language, emphasized the interrelatedness and interdependence of the developments of the general motorium (e.g., capacities to sit, stand, walk), the perceptorium (auditory, visual, tactual perceptual processes), and speech mechanisms.

Lenneberg also believes that it is possible to relate language development to certain physical measures of brain maturation, just as it is possible to relate it to chronological age or motor development. He believes, for example, that language emerges when the gross weight of the brain, neurodensity in the cerebral cortex, or the changing weight proportions in either gray or white matter have reached at least 65% of their mature values.

Investigations of monaural and dichotic listening and results of interhemispheric disconnection have provided important data to our understanding of central auditory processing of speech information. Carhart (see Hirsh, 1967, p. 34) pointed out that unilateral lesions within the central auditory system (beyond the cochlear nuclei but at brain stem or temporal lobe levels) could interfere with speech comprehension in the contralateral ear. Such findings lead Carhart to the opinion that " . . . we do not have balanced bilateral representation of the neural code for unilaterally heard speech."

Studies of interhemispheric disconnection syndromes in individuals who underwent commissurotomies have shown that, to a large extent, the disconnected hemispheres continue to function normally. Miller *et al.* (1968) indicated that only the left hemisphere, in the typically right-handed person, " . . . appears capable of propositional speech and writing. The . . . right hemisphere does show some rudimentary verbal comprehension but emits few if any words." Because visual and tactile stimuli have contralateral representation, patients cannot name or describe objects in the left visual field or those handled by the left hand, that is, " . . . the commissurectomized patient is able to tell us in any detail only about sensory information that has reached his verbally dominant left hemisphere."

Sperry and Gazzaniga (1967, pp. 108–121) reported on further studies of the cerebral disconnection syndrome in man that have caused them to modify somewhat their initial views of the syndrome. (a) They confirm that visual stimuli such as words, letters, phrases, and numbers, flashed to the right half visual field, that is, the right half visual field-speaking hemisphere (left hemisphere) combination, can be read by the subjects; whereas in a left half visual field-nonspeaking hemisphere (right hemisphere) combination, the subject appears to be alexic and word blind. (b) When visual stimuli such as objects and colors are presented to the right half visual field-speaking hemisphere combination, the subject can describe in speech and writing what he saw; he cannot do so when the stimuli are presented to the left half visual field-nonspeaking hemisphere combination. (c) With respect to stereognostic perception, subjects also name and describe objects well that are presented to the right hand-speaking hemisphere combination but not to the left hand-nonspeaking hemisphere combination. The investigators concluded that, in all their patients (all right-handed), speech and writing appear firmly confined to the left hemisphere. However, since the patients apparently lack the capacity for verbal expression in the minor hemisphere, the results do not necessarily prove that the non-speaking hemisphere does not comprehend verbal material.

Therefore, the investigators sought to determine whether the minor hemisphere is capable of any language comprehension by modifying their testing procedures. Instead of requesting the subject to report by speaking or writing what he sees flashed into his left half visual field-nonspeaking hemisphere combination, he is asked to find a matching object (without the aid of vision), and under these conditions he gives a correct response. Such correct matching object responses are obtained for both half visual fields; however, only the left hand can be used to identify objects flashed to the left visual field, and only the right hand can be used to identify objects flashed to the right field. Cross combinations do not work. From such tests and others, the investigators conclude that the minor hemisphere senses, perceives, learns, and remembers stimuli in the visual, tactual, and auditory spheres, even though it is unable to talk or write about such experiences.

According to the investigators, the nonspeaking hemisphere has at least a moderate vocabulary, since it apparently understood many nouns, complex phrases, and not so simple definitions. Further, subjects were able to read and comprehend printed words with the minor as well as the major hemisphere. The minor hemisphere spelled on a very low level (unscrambling cut-out letters three to four inches high with the left hand); however, calculations appear restricted almost entirely to the major hemisphere.

The implication of these findings to speech theory is that the speech formulation function is basically lateralized, while the speech comprehension function is bilaterally represented. The researchers pointed out that such findings may help explain why some aphasics are not able to evoke the name of an object but can comprehend its name and why severe comprehension disorders are more rare then severe expression disorders.

Audition, unlike vision or somesthesis, is represented bilaterally at every stage of the afferent pathway, that is, either hemisphere is able to hear through either ear. Miller *et al.* (1968) undertook an experiment with commissurotomized patients and found " . . . near-complete suppression by the left or speaking hemisphere of input from the left ear." Four groups of subjects were studied: commissurotomized patients (for control of severe convulsive disorders), normal control subjects, a group of patients with right temporal lobectomies, and a group of patients with left temporal lobectomies. Complete excision of the transverse gyri of Heschl was reported in the two lobectomy groups.

All groups performed a dichotic-listening experimental task and a monaural listening control task. In the dichotic-listening task different digits are presented simultaneously (in groups of three pairs) to the two ears via a dual channel tape recorder with stereophonic earphones. Following each group of six digits, the subject is asked to report all numbers heard, irrespective of order. In the monaural condition, all six digits are presented to one ear.

Results under the experimental conditions were as follows. Normal subjects showed a slight but significant superiority in the right ear. Patients with left temporal lobectomy showed a slight impairment in the test as a whole, and patients with right temporal lobectomy showed an accentuation of the right-ear superiority found in the normals. The ear difference in the commissurotomized patients was much more marked than in the lobectomized patients; these patients reported very few digits from the left ear. In contrast to the suppression of the input from the left ear under dichotic stimulation, none of the commissurotomized patients showed abnormal differences in performance of the two ears under monaural conditions. The authors conclude, "The suppression of ipsilateral input in the presence of a competing stimulus from the contralateral ear provides clear behavioral evidence of the dominance of the contralateral auditory projection system in man. . . ."

Kimura and Folb (1968) reported that previous dichotic-listening studies have indicated right ear superiority for speech sounds (digits, words, nonsense syllables) and left ear superiority for musical and other nonspeech sounds. These auditory asymmetries appear only with dichotic presentation of stimuli and appear to be due to ". . . advantageous neural connections of each ear with the opposite cerebral hemisphere." These findings point to a division of labor between hemispheres in processing verbal and nonverbal stimuli.

Kimura and Folb wanted to explore whether highly unfamiliar and meaningless sounds would be processed as other speech sounds. They recorded trisyllabic nonsense words and presented them backwards and dichotically to a group of undergraduate students. Results again reflected right ear superiority; hence, backwards speech sounds are apparently processed by neuropsychological systems overlapping those for normal speech sounds.

The final portion of this section of the chapter devoted to the structure and function of the higher-order speech integrator describes the critical blood supply to the central neural speech mechanisms.

Cerebral arteries and veins are important to the neurology and pathophysiology of language since they convey the blood that brings food and oxygen to the nervous cells of which the central speech system is composed. The three cerebral arteries are the anterior, middle, and posterior cerebral arteries. The anterior and middle cerebral arteries are branches of the internal carotid artery; the posterior cerebral artery forms from the basilar artery (Gatz, 1966, pp. 113–114).

The middle cerebral artery and its cortical branches supply the insula and the lateral surface of the frontal, parietal, occipital, and temporal lobes. The lenticulostriate arteries are small branches of the middle cerebral artery that supply the internal capsule. Hemorrhage of one of the branches of the lenticulostriate arteries into the internal capsule could cause complete hemiplegia. An occlusion of the main trunk of the middle cerebral artery in the speech hemisphere produces paralysis of the opposite side of the body, hypesthesia, partial hemianopia, and general aphasia. Occlusion of individual cortical branches of the middle cerebral artery will cause more limited symptoms; for example, involvement of the left inferior frontal branch might produce weakness of the lower part of the right face and tongue and motor aphasia. The middle cerebral artery of the speech hemisphere, then, can be viewed as the "speech artery."

In a study of angiographic patterns of cerebral veins, Di Chiro (1962) reported on the vein of Labbé. He found that the vein of Labbé in the speech hemisphere was larger than the vein of Trolard; he found the reverse in the nonspeech hemisphere.

The next system to be discussed is directly responsible for the production of the verboacoustic code organized by the higher-order speech integrator and conveyed by the efferent speech transmitter.

Speech Effector System

The speech effector system is composed of respiratory, phonatory-resonatory, and articulatory mechanisms. These mechanisms, in order, produce the speech airstream, create and modify laryngeal tone, and create additional speech sounds. The patterned neural impulses from the efferent transmitter system drive the various speech effectors. The quality of the end-product of speech formulation and efferent transmission processes is, to a major extent, in proportion to the integrity of the various speech effectors.

Respiratory Speech Effector (Fig. 1.9). Zemlin (1968, Ch. 2) de-

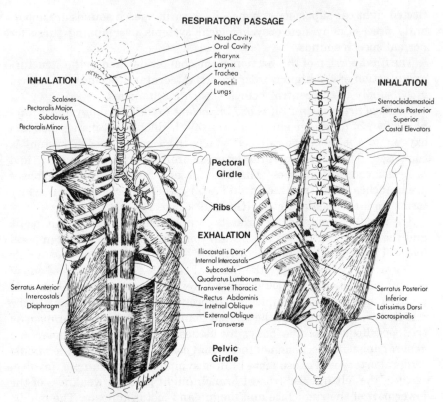

Figure 1.9. Speech effector: respiratory components.

scribed respiratory mechanisms in terms of: (a) the respiratory passage, which includes the nasal and oral cavities, pharynx, larynx, trachea, bronchi, and lungs; (b) the skeletal framework for the breathing mechanism, which includes the spinal column, the rib cage, the pectoral girdle, and the pelvic girdle; (c) the muscles of inhalation, including the diaphragm, the pectoralis major and minor, the subclavius, the serratus anterior, the intercostal muscles, the costal elevators, the serratus posterior of the thorax, the sternocleidomastoid and scalenes of the neck, and the latissmus dorsi and sacrospinalis of the back; and (d) the muscles of exhalation, including the internal and external obliques, the transversus and rectus of the abdomen, the transversus, subcostals, and internal intercostals of the thorax, the iliocostalis dorsi, and the quadratus lumborum of the back.

The function of the respiratory speech effector is to produce the speech airsteam. However, the respiratory system produces at least two types of airsteams, vegetative and speech. A discussion and differentiation of these two breathing functions is appropriate here.

Mysak (1971, pp. 674–675) reported that infantile (under six months) vegetative respiration is characterized by nasal intake, a diaphragmatic-abdominal breathing pattern, and cycles that are comparatively shallow and of a high frequency. After six months, the pattern evolves into a mixed one in which the diaphragm and thorax participate and cycles become deeper and slower. Thoracic breathing is predominant at about seven years. Frequency of respiration, breaths per minute (bpm), for the first through the sixth month ranges from 21 to 58 bpm; from the first half to the second year of life, from 19 to 45 bpm; for the fifth through the tenth years, 15 to 31 bpm; and for the tenth through fifteenth years, 14 to 31 bpm. Vegetative breathing rates for mature individuals average about 12 bpm.

Cerebral control of breathing mechanisms is required to modify vegetative into speech breathing patterns. Speech breathing is characterized by a shift from a nasal inflow-outflow pattern to an oral inflow-outflow pattern and a shift from rather equal inspiratory-expiratory phases to a comparatively short and rapid inspiratory phase followed by a long and slow expiratory phase (i.e., from a 1:1 type inflow-outflow ratio to a 3:1 to 10:1 inflow-outflow ratio). In short, medullary vegetative breathing may be described as a nasal-symmetrical pattern, and cerebral speech breathing may be described as an oral-asymmetrical pattern.

Generally, if an individual possesses an adequate respiratory mechanism for vegetative breathing, his respiratory speech effector should also be adequate. Also, it apparently makes little difference to speech function whether the individual utilizes a predominantly diaphragmatic-abdominal pattern (inhalation marked by protrusion of anterior abdominal wall) or a thoracic pattern (inhalation marked by a lateral expansion of the thorax). In most individuals inspiratory activity is accompanied by expansion in the abdominal area as well as in the upper and lower thoracic areas. Occasionally, the region of predominant expansion appears to be in the extreme upper chest area, and hence the pattern has been termed clavicular breathing. Clavicular breathing in voice cases may be discouraged, since many believe it may contribute to throat tension and an inadequate speech airstream.

The vocal tract, or that part of the speech mechanism above the level of the focal folds, includes pharyngeal, mouth, and nasal cavities and is capable of modifying and adding to the speech sounds generated by the vocal folds. Both the modifying and adding functions may be viewed as speech sound articulation. For purposes of this discussion of the speech effector system, however, speech tone generation and modification will be viewed as a function of phonatory and resonatory mechanisms, and the addition of speech sounds to the modified or unmodified speech airstream will be viewed as a function of the articulatory mechanism. Such a division of labor in speech sound production results in some overlap in the discussions of resonatory and articulatory structures.

Phonatory-Resonatory Speech Effector (Fig. 1.10). The phonatory-resonatory speech effector is composed of the sound generator, or larynx, and the sound resonating and modifying system or the pharyngeal, nasal, and mouth cavities. Major components of the larynx include: (a) nine cartilages, which are the thyroid (1), cricoid (1), epiglottis (1), arytenoid (2), corniculate (2), and cuneiform (2); (b) extrinsic laryngeal musculature (at least one attachment to structures outside the larynx), including digastric, stylohyoid, mylohyoid, geniohyoid, sternohyoid, omohyoid, thyrohyoid, and sternothyroid muscles; and (c) intrinsic laryngeal musculature, including thyroarytenoid, posterior cricoarytenoid, lateral cricoarytenoid, interarytenoid, and cricothyroid muscles.

Both extrinsic and intrinsic muscles may influence laryngeal function; however, the control of sound production is primarily a function of the intrinsic muscles. Extrinsic muscles support, fix, elevate, or depress the larynx. Intrinsic laryngeal muscles may be indentified as abductors (posterior cricoarytenoid muscle), adductors (lateral cricoarytenoid and

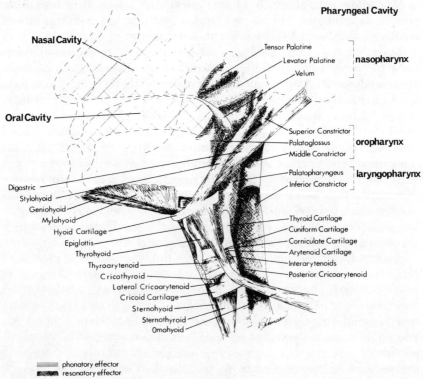

Figure 1.10. Speech effector: phonatory-resonatory components.

interarytenoid muscles), or relaxer-tensors (thyroarytenoid and cricothy-roid muscles).

Resonation and modification of the laryngeal tone is a function of the resonators of the vocal tract. Major components of the resonator mecha-nism include: (a) the velopharyngeal closure mechanism, composed of the velum, the laryngopharynx, oropharynx, and nasopharynx and its related musculature (that is, the levator palatine, tensor palatine, palatoglossus, and palatopharyngeus of the soft palate), and the infe-rior, middle, and superior constrictor muscles of the pharynx; (b) the fauces; and (c) the oral, buccal, and nasal cavities.

In terms of function, the phonatory mechanism can produce varying pitch levels primarily by modifying glottic tension and mass and can vary loudness by altering the factors of subglottal pressure, airflow rate, and glottal resistance. The resonatory mechanism, which amplifies and varies the laryngeal tone, functions by modifying the size, shape, and tension of the pharynx and by coupling the pharynx with the nose or mouth. The coupling of the oro- and the nasopharynx is essential to the production of the nasal sounds [m, n, ŋ].

Articulatory Speech Effector (Fig. 1.11). The articulatory speech effector is composed of those structures of the vocal tract capable of modifying further the laryngeal tone and of creating speech sounds in addition to those generated at the level of the vocal cords. Major struc-tures of the articulatory mechanism include: the lips, face, and associ-ated musculature, the mandible and associated musculature, the teeth, palate, and associated musculature, and the tongue and associated musculature.

The lips and face are discussed in terms of the muscles of which they are composed. Muscles of the lips (Zemlin, 1968, pp. 258–260) include: the orbicularis oris, which closes and puckers the lips; transverse muscles, which pull the lips against the teeth; angular muscles, used in produc-ing smile and frown movements; and vertical muscles, used in produc-ing facial expression and in compressing corners of the mouth. Facial muscles (Zemlin, 1968, pp. 260–262) include: the buccinator, which presses the lips and cheeks against the teeth and pulls the corners of the mouth laterally; the risorius, which helps pull the corners of the mouth laterally; the quadratus labii superior, which is the principal elevator of the upper lip; the zygomatic, which pulls the angle of the mouth upward and laterally; the quadratus labii inferior, which draws the lower lip downward and laterally; the mentalis, which everts the lower lip; the triangularis, which either depresses the angle of the lip or assists in compressing the lips; the canine, which draws the corner of the mouth upward and assists in closing the mouth; the incisivis labii superior, which pulls the corner of the mouth medially and upward; and the incisivis labii inferior, which draws the corner of the mouth medially and downward.

Facial and lip muscles contribute to the production of vowels, bilabial, and labiodental speech sounds and to speech communication in general by providing the visual components of speech sound production and appropriate accompanying facial expressions.

The mandible contains the lower teeth and points of attachment for lingual and other musculature. Elevation and depression are primary mandibular movements; however, the jaw may also be protruded, retruded, or moved laterally. Muscles involved in mandibular depression are the digastricus, the mylohyoid, the geniohyoid, and the external pterygoid muscle. Muscles involved in mandibular elevation are the masseter, temporalis, and internal pterygoid muscles.

The mandible, and its component lower teeth, contributes to speech production by modifying the shape of the oral cavity and by contributing to the production of vowels and consonants requiring either wide or narrow mouth openings. It may also play an important role as a compensator for restricted lingual movements.

The teeth in the upper and lower dental arches and the occlusion of

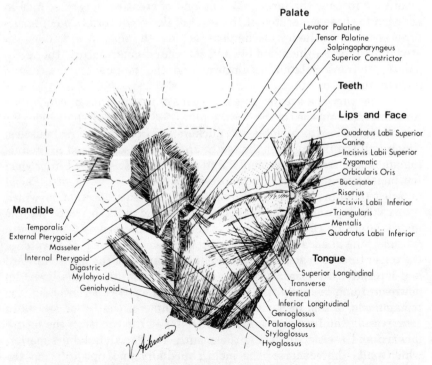

Figure 1.11 Speech effector: articulatory components.

these arches are important in normal speech articulation. Deciduous dental arches contain 10 teeth in the mandibular arch and 10 teeth in the maxillary arch, for a total of 20 teeth. Each dental quadrant contains a central and lateral incisor, a cuspid or canine, and two molars. Deciduous teeth erupt between approximately the first 6 to 24 months of life. Permanent dental arches contain 16 teeth in the mandibular arch and 16 teeth in the maxillary arch, for a total of 32 teeth. Each dental quadrant contains a central and lateral incisor, a cuspid or canine, two bicuspids or premolars, and three molars. Permanent teeth erupt between approximately 6 and 21 years of age. Normal occlusion of the dental arches is marked by three relationships: (a) the normal relationship of the first permanent molars, that is, when the mesiobuccal cusp of the maxillary first molar occludes in the buccal groove of the mandibular first molar; (b) the normal overjet by the maxillary teeth, that is, when the teeth in the maxillary arch overhang the teeth in the mandibular arch labially and buccally; and (c) the normal overbite of the maxillary anterior teeth, that is, when the maxillary incisors overlap the mandibular incisors by one-third of the mandibular incisor crowns (Bloomer, 1971, pp. 727–728).

The function of teeth and dental arches in speech sound articulation is related to the manner in which they contribute to the opening or constricting of the oral exit for the speech airstream or as articulatory bases or cues for the tongue and lips; in short, teeth and their occlusion may have direct or indirect effects on speech production. For example, in the formation of bilabial sounds the dental arches form a base for the compressing lips; in the formation of labiodental and linguadental sounds the anterior teeth function as fellows with the upper lip and tongue, respectively, in constricting the oral exit for the purpose of creating labiodental and linguadental fricative sounds; and in the formation of sibilants the approximating arches may serve as cues for the tongue and also as obstructions to assist in creating the desired linguaalveolar or linguapalatal fricative sounds.

The palate and associated musculature, in terms of articulatory function, include the alveolar process that houses the teeth, the palatine processes that form the bony roof of the mouth, and the velopharyngeal closure mechanism. Velopharyngeal closure is effected by movements of various muscles in at least two and in some cases three directions, that is, by superior, mesial, and anterior movements. Upward, backward, and spreading movements of the velum are effected by action of the levator and tensor palatine muscles. Mesial movement of the lateral pharyngeal walls of the nasopharynx is effected by action of the salpingopharyngeal muscle, and anterior movement of the posterior pharyngeal wall is effected by action of the superior constrictor muscles. The anterior movement is not usually active under normal circumstances but may become active in a compensatory role in cases of velar insufficiency.

The palate and associated musculature contribute to the articulatory function by: (a) separating oral and nasal chambers and allowing the build-up of intraoral breath pressure for the production of pressure sounds; (b) coupling oral and nasal chambers for the production of nasal sounds; and (c) providing articulatory contact points for the production of lingua-alveolar, linguapalatal, and linguavelar sounds.

The tongue and associated musculature, the last articulator to be discussed, are considered to be the most important. The tongue may be divided into four sections: the tip, or that part nearest the front teeth; the blade, or that part just below the alveolar ridge; the front, or that part below the hard palate; and the back, or that part below the soft palate. The extrinsic muscles of the tongue include the genioglossus, styloglossus, palatoglossus, and hyoglossus muscles; they, in turn, contribute to lingual protrusion, retrusion, and depression, lingual elevation and retrusion, elevation of the back of the tongue, and retrusion and depression of the tongue. The intrinsic muscles of the tongue include the superior longitudinal, inferior longitudinal, transverse, and vertical muscles; they, in turn, contribute to shortening or turning the tip and lateral margins upward, shortening or drawing the tip downward, narrowing and elongating, and flattening the tongue.

The tongue contributes to vowel production by altering the resonance characteristics of the oral cavity. By acting as a valve to impede the outgoing speech airstream, it contributes to the production of linguadental, lingua-alveolar, and linguapalatal fricatives and affricates. By redirecting the speech airstream the tongue contributes to the production of the lateral and retroflex sounds, and by temporarily stopping the speech airstream it contributes to the production of lingua-alveolar and linguavelar plosives.

More detailed discussions of respiratory, phonatory, and articulatory mechanisms may be found by referring to appropriate sections in books by Zemlin (1968), Judson and Weaver (1965), and Kaplan (1960).

Speech Sensor System

The speech sensor system is the last of the six major systems of which the speech organism is composed; it is involved with the function of intrapersonal speech perception. The system is responsible for automatically controlling and monitoring not only what has been said, the spoken symbol, but also how the symbol has been said, or the phonatory, articulatory, rate, and rhythm aspects. Control and monitoring of the content of spoken symbols depend on auditory feedback, while control and monitoring of the manner of symbol production depend not only on auditory but also on tactile and kinesthetic feedbacks.

Speech control is manifested by the control that is simultaneous to the speech act, whereas speech monitoring implies the control that follows the act. Also, speech control functions can only be engaged when actual speech is being produced, whereas speech monitoring functions may also be engaged during inner speech.

Auditory Speech Sensor. The auditory sensor is composed of: the outer, middle, and inner ear components, described in the section on the auditory speech receptor; the neural auditory pathway, including relay centers within the cochlea, medulla, and at the midbrain and thalamic levels described in the section on the auditory speech transmitter; and the auditory reticular system and thalamic and posterior cortical speech areas, described in sections on lower-order and higher-order auditory speech integration.

As previously indicated, the auditory sensor monitors self-produced verboacoustic code as well as at least certain aspects of how this code is actually produced by phonatory and articulatory mechanisms. In terms of content of spoken code, the system monitors and triggers the correction of mistaken utterances, for example, giving someone the wrong name, address, or telephone number. In terms of how the code is produced, the system controls and monitors pitch, loudness, quality, and durational aspects of voicing, and speech rate, rhythm, and articulation.

The importance of the auditory system as a control mechanism is supported by numerous studies based on the investigation of effects on speech output of experimentally manipulating auditory speech feedback. For example, it was found that voice level varies inversely as a function of changing the level of an individual's personal voice feedback (Black, 1954) and that a rise in speaking fundamental frequency and speech loudness, a decrease in speech rate, and the elicitation of speech sound repetitions may result from an electronically-induced retardation in intrapersonal, auditory speech feedback (Black, 1950; Lee, 1951; Fairbanks and Guttman, 1958).

Tactile-Kinesthetic Speech Sensor. The tactile-kinesthetic sensor utilizes touch, movement, and position sensations in contributing to the control and monitoring of speech articulation. It is composed of the sensory end-organs and the peripheral and central sensory neurons associated with important articulatory structures such as the lips, face, mandible, and teeth (trigeminal nerve), the palate (palatine nerve), and the tongue (trigeminal and glossopharyngeal nerves). Touch and movement sensations are conveyed primarily to the contralateral somatic sensory center of the cerebral cortex via the medial lemniscus and thalamocortical fibers to the postcentral gyrus of the parietal lobe. The ventroposterior medial nucleus of the thalamus is an important relay center.

Not all proprioceptive impulses that reach the central nervous system (CNS) are routed to the sensory perception centers of the brain. Some are distributed to areas that do not function at a conscious level, and these impulses contribute to mechanisms of automatic motor control (Gatz, 1966, p. 16). Thus proprioception may be divided into cortical and cerebellar systems. Proprioceptive impulses ascend via spinocerebellar tracts to the cortex of the cerebellum. The cerebellum receives immediate reports of the progress of movements and of the activity of muscle groups over the spinocerebellar tracts, and as a function of these reports, the cerebellum is capable of ensuring smoother and more accurate movements by altering the action of muscle groups. Since, under ordinary circumstances, tactile-kinesthetic-controlling influences over speech are basically "subconscious," the cerebellum is considered a most important part of the speech sensor system and is discussed further.

The cerebellum may be viewed as being composed of three lobes: the anterior, middle, and posterior. "The evolution of the cerebellum advanced with the link up with the muscle and joint proprioceptors by way of the spinocerebellar tracts which terminate largely in the cortex of the anterior and posterior lobes, grouped together as the old or paleocerebellum" (Wyburn, 1960, p. 61–62). The neocerebellum, the middle lobe and the most recently evolved portion, is the lobe involved in the interconnection between the cerebellum and the cerebrum. Cutaneous sense organs send impulses to the cerebellum via arcuate fibers of the gracile and cuneate nuclei; connections with the auditory and visual systems also exist. Cerebellar efferent tracts originate from the dentate nucleus of the neocerebellum, partly terminating in the red nucleus of the midbrain but mainly in the thalamus, and from there projecting to the premotor and motor cortex of the cerebrum. Efferent fibers also emanate from the fastigial nucleus of the paleocerebellum and pass to the reticular formations of the brain stem and to the vestibular nucleus. Thus, the cerebellum receives inflow from the general proprioceptors, the vestibular system, cutaneous and special senses, and the cerebral cortex and sends outflow to motor units of the spinal cord, to the brain stem, and to the cerebral cortex (pp. 62–63).

As indicated, cerebellar activity is at a subconscious level and is involved with equilibrium, posture, and movement; consequently, cerebellar disorders are marked by problems in balance, muscle tonus, and movement. "The cerebral cortex is responsible for the executive planning of any movement, but its successful accomplishment requires the co-operation of the cerebellum" (Wyburn, 1960, p. 66). In terms of the control and monitoring functions of the cerebellum, the present author, reporting on Ruch's concepts of cerebellar activity, wrote that the cerebellum ". . . may receive signals from the cortex which represent the prescribed movement, and proprioceptive feedback signals from the muscles which represent the actual movement. Upon comparison . . . , if a discrepancy is found between prescribed and actual movements, appropriate error signals are then sent to the motor cortex which, in turn, alters its signals to the muscles . . ." (Mysak, 1966, p. 26). Related to the above is a statement made by Teuber (1967), when he conjectured about the significance of potential shifts in the brain, which precede a voluntary movement, to the physiologic understanding of active movements, including the production of speech. He said, ". . . I like to think that some of these curious electrophysiologic antecedents of overt action reflect not just the neural 'command' to the musculature but the concomitant presetting of cerebral systems for the expected consequence of the impending action, so that the result can be compared, centrally, with the intent" (p. 215).

The importance of tactile-kinesthetic feedback to speech control and monitoring is demonstrated in various ways: (a) personal dental experiences where Novocain may temporarily reduce articulatory accuracy, (b) articulatory disturbances associated with cerebellar involvement, and (c) studies that have reported that experimentally induced disturbances in tactile-kinesthetic feedback affected articulatory functioning (McCroskey, 1958; Ringel and Steer, 1963).

Visual Speech Sensor. Under special circumstances, for example, in a speech therapy situation, the visual system may be utilized as a supplementary or compensatory channel for the control and monitoring of articulatory activity. The visual speech sensor is made up of the components already described in the sections on the visual speech receptor and transmitter.

In the therapy situation, a client may be asked to observe in a mirror how the clinician produces a certain sound and then to watch his own articulators as he attempts to reproduce the articulatory postures and movements, or he may be asked to observe the visual aspects of his error-sound production as demonstrated by the clinician's imitation of it.

Appendix A, which summarizes the composition of the speech receptor, transmitter, higher- and lower-order integrator, effector, and sensor systems, certainly reflects the concept that speech behavior is one of the highest and most complicated forms of human behavior. Even a cursory glance at the table reveals that individuals who are interested in preparing for work in basic or applied research or in clinical work in the speech and hearing field must acquire knowledge and mastery of a most complex system if they are to be most effective in their pursuits.

INTRA- AND INTERSYSTEM FUNCTIONS AND RELATIONSHIPS

As a consequence of describing the speech functions of the receptor, transmitter, higher- and lower-order integrator, effector, and sensor systems, certain speech concepts emerge that are worthy of further elaboration. These are: (a) redundancy in speech system functioning, (b) adjustment and facilitation of speech input and output signals, (c) interdependence in functioning of speech systems, and (d) presence of major and minor speech brains.

Redundancy in Speech System Functioning

The concept of speech "back-up" systems has important implications for speech diagnostic and therapy procedures.

Speech Input Processing. In the sections on speech receptor and transmitter systems, it was pointed out that speech reception and afferent transmission is basically an audiovisual phenomenon, and, therefore, that auditory and visual receptor-transmitter mechanisms are complementary. That is, speech information is most efficiently received as a function of synthesizing verboacoustical and verbovisual codes. However, it is also possible to process adequately verboacoustic code alone, and from that standpoint the visual speech system becomes supplementary. Further, when only the auditory system is used because of blindness, or only the visual system because of deafness, or only the tactile-kinesthetic system because of deafness and blindness, the speech system is operating in a back-up or compensatory fashion.

Speech Output Patterning. In terms of speech output at least two forms may be recognized, the spontaneous and nonspontaneous forms. Spontaneous speech describes the normal process where the speaker transmutes thoughts into words automatically, that is, without apparently thinking of the words. For example, someone requests directions to some place and the communicant briefly considers certain spatial concepts and immediately begins verbalizing them. Nonspontaneous speech describes output that is preformed. For example, it is the type of speech produced when someone has asked you to pronounce a word differently, or when saying just the right words is important and hence inner speech rehearsal takes place, or when one echoes another speaker. It is hypothesized that different neurodynamics underlie spontaneous and nonspontaneous speech outputs.

In this regard, certain clinical cases may improve when producing certain forms of nonspontaneous speech; for example, stutterers may become more fluent when asked to echo another's speech or when reciting from memory, clutterers may become more intelligible when asked to "slow down," parkinsonian patients may become more intelligible when asked to "overarticulate," or misarticulators may pronounce their error sounds in standard fashion when asked to reproduce the sound immediately after the clinician.

The redundancy concept is also reflected by the fact that phonatory and articulatory mechanisms benefit from bilateral cerebral representation, and therefore unilateral central lesions are not expected to produce permanent dysphonia or dysarthria.

Speech Integration. The back-up principle is seen is central processing and elaboration mechanisms by (a) the existence of at least three cortical speech areas, and (b) the potential for bilateral cerebral functioning for speech, possibly during the first 10 or 12 years but much more likely during the first four or five years.

Speech Control and Monitoring. Speech articulation and speech-time factors may be controlled and monitored by either the auditory and(or) tactile-kinesthetic sensors. Depending upon the individual, the elimination or disturbance of one or the other of the sensors may or may not seriously affect the accuracy of speech articulation and time. Also, the visual speech sensor may be utilized as a supplementary or compensatory sensor in the control and monitoring of articulatory behavior. The content of spoken symbols is primarily monitored by the auditory sensor; however, compensatory monitoring appears possible here too, as in the case of deaf individuals who have learned to use speech communication.

Also of interest with respect to the control and monitoring of articulation is the concept of conscious and subconscious speech sensor activity. Under ordinary circumstances, tactile-kinesthetic control and monitoring of articulation is subconscious, that is, the speaker is not aware of the touch and movement sensations that are being processed to maintain accurate articulation. Subconscious sensor activity is considered to be a function of the cerebellar division of the system, while conscious sensor activity is considered to be a function of the cortical division. The concept of subconscious and conscious speech sensor activity has clinical implications. For example, under bilateral white noise, which reduces the efficiency of the auditory and more conscious sensor for control of speech-time factors, many stutterers will experience fluency; or, when certain dysarthrics are asked to voluntarily produce harder articulatory contacts for the purpose of "amplifying" sensory feedback, they may become more intelligible. In these examples, improvement in speech may be a function of utilizing more efficient sensor systems. This discussion of subconscious and conscious speech sensor activity also has implications for the previous discussion on spontaneous and nonspontaneous speech.

Adjustment and Facilitation of Speech Input and Output Signals

The concept of adjustment and facilitation of audiovisual speech input and of speech output is important for the better understanding of normal speech and hearing development and for the diagnosis of unusual speech and hearing disorders.

Speech Input Adjustment and Facilitation. Processing of audiovisual speech input is accompanied by various activities within the auditory and visual systems that make important contributions to speech signal reception, afferent transmission, and perception. This lower-order integrator functioning includes: (a) orienting the head, ears, and eyes to the source of the speech signals; (b) stimulating arousal and selective attention mechanisms; (c) generating auditory efferent impulses to regulate responsiveness at any level of the auditory system; (d) allowing for retinal fixation of articulatory movements and facial expressions; and (e) eliciting optokinetic activity that enables the listener to visually follow speech-associated movements.

Speech Output Adjustment and Facilitation. Patterning of speech output requires the coordination of pyramidal and extrapyramidal systems. Cooperation of the extrapyramidal systems at various levels of the cerebrifugal pathway allows for (a) the production of fine, smooth, and accurate movements, and (b) the coordination of the various speech effectors, that is, the respiratory, phonatory, resonatory, and articulatory effectors.

Problems in input adjustment and facilitation may include difficulty in achieving and maintaining auditory attention, while problems in output adjustment and facilitation may include difficulty in coordinating articulatory and phonatory mechanisms or articulatory and resonatory mechanisms or may result in tremors or athetotic or choreiform movements of the articulators.

Interdependence in Functioning of Speech Systems

The concept of interdependence in functioning of speech systems represents one aspect of the complexity of the systems in normal or disordered states. Clinicians need to remind themselves of this complexity and of the possible pitfalls of reducing highly-involved problems of speech communication into simple terms, or, in other words, the tendency to indulge in "clinical reductionism." Some of these speech-system complexities are touched upon below.

Receptor and Afferent Transmitter Systems. The efficiency of audiovisual speech transmission is dependent on the efficiency with which auditory and visual speech receptors receive and convert speech signals into appropriate codes of nerve impulses. Therefore, when any one individual is experiencing difficulty in receiving verboacoustic code, for example, one of the questions that must be answered is whether the difficulty is reflective of receptor or transmitter involvements or combinations of these involvements.

Afferent Transmitter and Lower-Order Afferent Integrator Systems. The efficiency of audiovisual speech transmission is also dependent, to an important extent, on the efficiency of lower-order afferent integration. Afferent integration involves functions such as auditory and visual localization of the source of speech information, arousal and sensitization of audiovisual speech systems, and audiovisual tracking of speech information. Hence, if any one individual appears to be experiencing difficulty in processing speech information, one question that must be answered is whether the problem is reflective of transmitter or lower-order afferent integrator involvements or combinations of these involvements.

Lower-Order Afferent and Higher-Order Integrator Systems. The efficiency of higher-order integration of speech information, that is, speech perception and comprehension functioning, is dependent to an important extent on the efficiency of lower-order afferent integrator activity. That is, how much of a particular problem in speech perception or comprehension is a function of difficulty in making expected associations to, or interpretations and elaborations of, well-received speech signals, and how much is a function of problems in lower-order integration processes?

Higher-Order Integrator and Lower-Order Efferent Integrator Systems. Efficiency in transmitting speech signals formed in the higher-order integrator is dependent on the integrity of the lower-order efferent integrator. That is, how much of a particular problem in speech production is a function of difficulty in generating and organizing appropriate patterns of output (higher-order memory and retrieval functions), and how much is a function in adjusting and facilitating the development of these patterns (lower-order integration)?

Efferent Transmitter and Effector Systems. The manifestation of efficient efferent transmission processes is dependent on the intactness of the speech effector system. Hence, if an individual is encountering difficulty in speech production, one question that must be answered is whether the problem is relective of a transmitter or an effector problem or some combination of these.

Effector and Sensor Systems. Finally, the efficiency of the verboacoustic code being utilized and the quality of its production is also dependent on the sensor systems. Accordingly, when one is confronted with a problem in production, one complicated question that needs to be answered is, how much of the difficulty may be due to the effectors, transmitters, or formulation processes and how much is due to control and monitoring functions?

Major and Minor Speech Brains

The final concept to be discussed concerns the functioning of a major speech brain and a minor speech brain, as well as bilateral cerebral functioning for speech. Information reviewed here has important implications for the normal development of speech and for its disorders and therapy.

Major Speech Brain. The major speech brain is almost always the left, irrespective of handedness; however, occasionally right brainedness for speech is found. The major speech brain is represented by three cortical areas, related thalamic regions, and interconnecting tracts. The major speech brain may continue to subserve language function even after one part of it is damaged. Potential for transferability of the major speech brain from the left to the right hemisphere is present during the early years of life. The major speech brain is responsible for speech comprehension and formulation.

Regions within the major speech brain that appear to have special functions are: (a) the *arcuate fasciculus,* which allows for simple repetition of syllables, words, or phrases heard; (b) the *angular gyrus,* or the "association area of association areas," which allows for the formation of nonlimbic cross-modal associations and verbal memory; (c) the *posterior parietal zone,* which has a role in speech comprehension and verbal memory; (d) the *anterior frontal region,* which allows for spontaneous narrative speech; (e) the *temporal lobe,* which serves the function of verbal memory; (f) *Broca's area,* which subserves speech expression; and (g) *Wernicke's area,* which subserves speech comprehension.

Minor Speech Brain. The minor speech brain is almost always the right. It appears capable of a certain amount of speech comprehension and of mediating speech automatisms and also appears dominant for musical and other nonspeech sounds.

Bilateral Speech Function. During early childhood both hemispheres are equipotential for speech function; specialization of function takes place gradually as the individual matures up to puberty. Occasionally, however, bilateral representation for speech may be found in the adult. Early damage to the major speech brain may result in establishing permanently the potential for either hemisphere to serve as the major speech brain. Both hemispheres appear capable of speech comprehension.

In conclusion, this chapter reveals the complexity of the speech system. Only the boundaries of the system appear rather well defined at this time. Providing well-established details for the structure and function of the system and its parts will require a great deal of further study of it during normal function, during dysfunction, and under imaginative experimental conditions.

REFERENCES

Black, J. W., The effect of delayed sidetone upon vocal rate and intensity. J. Speech Hear. Disord., 16, 56–60 (1950).

Black, J. W., The loudness of sidetone. Speech Monogr., 21, 301–305 (1954).

Bloomer, H. H., Speech defects associated with dental malocclusions and related abnormalities. In L. E. Travis (Ed.), Handbook of Speech Pathology and Audiology. New York: Appleton-Century-Crofts (1971).

Brain, W. R., and Walton, J. N., Diseases of the Nervous System. London: Oxford University Press (1969).

Cohen, B. D., Noblin, C. D., and Silverman, A. J., Functional asymmetry of the human brain. Science, 162, 475–477 (1968).

Darley, F. L., and Millikan, D. H. (Eds.), Brain Mechanisms Underlying Speech and

Language. New York: Grune and Stratton (1967).

Di Chiro, G., Angiographic patterns of cerebral convexity veins and superficial dural sinuses. Amer. J. Roentgenol. Radium Ther. Nucl. Med., 87, 308–321 (1962).

Fairbanks, G., and Guttman, N., Effects of delayed auditory feedback upon articulation. J. Speech Hear. Disord., 1, 12–22 (1958).

Falconer, M. A., Brain mechanisms suggested by neurophysiologic studies. In F. L. Darley and C. H. Millikan (Eds.), Brain Mechanisms Underlying Speech and Language. New York: Grune and Stratton (1967).

Gatz, A. J., Manter's Essentials of Clinical Neuroanatomy and Neurophysiology. Philadelphia: F. A. Davis Company (1966).

Geschwind, N., and Levitsky, W., Human brain: left-right asymmetries in temporal speech region. Science, 161, 186–187 (1968).

Goodhill, V., and Guggenheim, P., Pathology, diagnosis, and therapy of deafness. In L. E. Travis (Ed.), Handbook of Speech Pathology and Audiology. New York: Appleton-Century-Crofts (1971).

Greene, Margaret, C. L., The Voice and its Disorders. London: Pitman Medical Publishing Co., Ltd. (1957).

Hardy, W. G., Problems of Audition Perception and Understanding. A Keynote Address at the 1956 Summer Meeting of the Alexander Graham Bell Association for the Deaf, Los Angeles, Reprint No. 680. Washington, D. C.: The Volta Bureau (1956).

Hécaen, H., Brain mechanisms suggested by studies of parietal lobes. In F. L. Darley and C. H. Millikan (Eds.), Brain Mechanisms Underlying Speech and Language. New York: Grune and Stratton (1967).

Hirsh, I. J., Information processing in input channels for speech and language: The significance of serial order of stimuli. In F. L. Darley and C. H. Millikan (Eds.), Brain Mechanisms Underlying Speech and Language. New York: Grune and Stratton (1967).

Jackson, J. H., Selected Writings of John Hughlings Jackson, Vol. 2, In J. Taylor (Ed.). London: Hodder and Stoughton (1931).

Judson, L. S. V., and Weaver, A. T., Voice Science. New York: Appleton-Century-Crofts (1965).

Kaplan, H. M., Anatomy and Physiology of Speech. New York: McGraw-Hill (1960).

Kimura, D., and Folb, S., Neural processing of backwards speech sounds. Science, 161, 395–396 (1968).

Konorski, J., Integrative Activity of the Brain. Chicago: The University of Chicago Press (1967).

Lee, B. S., Artificial Stutter. J. Speech Hear. Disord., 16, 53–55 (1951).

Lenneberg, E. H., On explaining language. Science, 164, 635–643 (1969).

Lilly, J. C., Dolphin vocalization. In F. L. Darley and C. H. Millikan (Eds.), Brain Mechanisms Underlying Speech and Language. New York: Grune and Stratton (1967).

McCroskey, R., The relative contribution of auditory and tactile clues to certain aspects of speech. South. Speech J., 24, 84–90 (1958).

Miller, B., Taylor, L., and Sperry, R. W., Lateralized suppression of dichotically presented digits after commissural section in man. Science, 161, 184–186 (1968).

Milner, B., Brain mechanisms suggested by studies of temporal lobes. In F. L. Darley and C. H. Millikan (Eds.), Brain Mechanisms Underlying Speech and Language. New York: Grune and Stratton (1967).

Mysak, E. D., Organismic development of oral language. J. Speech Hear. Disord., 26, 377–384 (1961).

Mysak, E. D., Speech Pathology and Feedback Theory. Springfield, Ill.: Charles C Thomas (1966).

Mysak, E. D., Cerebral palsy speech syndromes. In L. E. Travis (Ed.), Handbook of Speech Pathology and Audiology. New York: Appleton-Century-Crofts (1971).

Penfield, W., Speech, perception and the uncommitted cortex. In J. C. Eccles (Ed.), Brain and Conscious Experience. New York: Springer-Verlag (1966).

Penfield, W., and Roberts, L., Speech and Brain Mechanisms. Princeton, N. J.: Princeton University Press (1959).

Ringel, R. L., and Steer, M. D., Some effects of tactile and auditory alterations on speech output. J. Speech Hear. Res., 6, 369–378 (1963).

Roberts, L., Central brain mechanisms in speech. In E. C. Carterette (Ed.), Brain Function: Speech Language and Communication. Los Angeles: University of California Press (1966).

Rossi, G. F., and Rosadini, G., Experimental analysis of cerebral dominance in man. In F. L. Darley and C. H. Millikan (Eds.), Brain Mechanisms Underlying Speech and Language. New York: Grune and Stratton (1967).

Sperry, R. W., and Gazzaniga, M. S., Language following surgical disconnection of the hemispheres. In F. L. Darley and C. H. Millikan (Eds.), Brain Mechanisms Underlying Speech and Language. New York: Grune and Stratton (1967).

Teuber, H., Lacunae and research approaches to them. 1. In F. L. Darley and C. H. Millikan (Eds.), Brain Mechanisms Underlying Speech and Language. New York: Grune and Stratton (1967).

Wada, J., A new method for the determination of the side of cerebral speech dominance: A preliminary report on the intracarotid injection of sodium amytal in man. Med. Biol., 14, 221–222 (1949).

West, R. W., and Ansberry, M., The Rehabilitation of Speech. New York: Harper and Row (1968).

Wyburn, G. M., The Nervous System. New York: Academic Press (1960).

Wyburn, G. M., Pickford, R. W., and Hirst, R. J., Human Senses and Perception. Toronto: University of Toronto Press (1964).

Young, E. H. Moto-kinesthetic approach to the prevention of speech defects, including stuttering. J. Speech Hear. Disord., 30, 269–273 (1965).

Zemlin, W. R., Speech and Hearing Science: Anatomy and Physiology. Englewood Cliffs, N. J.: Prentice-Hall (1968).

2

Evaluation and Diagnosis of Disorders of Speech Systems

An important purpose of this book is to assist the speech and hearing clinician to develop further his diagnostic and rehabilitative competencies through a better understanding of the speech systems. The purpose of this chapter is to discuss general principles and approaches to the evaluation of these systems.

EVALUATION OF SPEECH SYSTEMS

The suggested sequence in evaluating speech systems is based on the principle of parsimony. That is, while the adequacy of spoken language is being evaluated, an assessment of its production may also be made; hence, if the higher-order integrator is being examined for processing, storing, retrieving, and utilization functions and appears adequate, and if the manner of speech production also appears adequate, then little need exists to examine formally the other systems. However, if speech production deficiencies are detected, then the clinician should proceed to examine the lower-order integrator, receptor, effector, transmitter, and sensor systems.

The suggested examination techniques that follow are functionally- or conversationally-oriented. Verbal testing tasks described should be age-appropriate and adjusted to the individual's eductional and socioeconomic status. Interpretation of the results from a number of the examinations recommended requires clinical judgment and some experience, because either the examinations are not easily amenable to standardization or hard data on norms are still not available. A form for recording a general examination of the systems is found in Appendix B.

HIGHER-ORDER SPEECH INTEGRATOR

Higher-order speech integration is involved with verbal comprehension, formulation, and thinking. Verbal thinking embraces such functions as verbal sequencing, association, elaboration, interpretation, retention, and recall, or all those functions that may be associated with inner speech behavior.

Historical and Normative Data

In collecting pertinent history about the development of speech one should keep a quotation from West and Ansberry (1968) in mind. "That child will develop speech earliest and best whose environment is one that provides . . . (a) rich experience with good speakers, both children and adults, (b) real need for, and pleasure to be derived from, oral communication on the part of the child, and (c) rewards for, and encouragement of, day-by-day improvement in his speech" (p. 50).

In cases of adult language dysfunction, information should be sought on the individual's educational level, the number of languages used, whether the individual was primarily "a talker" or "a listener," his inclination for narrative speech, and his ability to engage in perceptual (easily imagined) and conceptual (abstract) verbalization.

Pertinent normative data with respect to the development of verbal behavior include: (a) indications of cerebral lateralization, (b) correlation of preverbal and early verbal behaviors with general motor development, and (c) indication of increasing functions and complexity of verboacoustic and verbomotor behaviors.

Cerebral lateralization and the development of a major speech hemisphere may be inferred from the child's use of spoken language and his showing preference for a lead hand and foot at about 2 or 3 years of age.

At about 6 to 9 months, auditory behavior marked by localization of the maternal voice and vocalization characterized by repetition of self-produced sounds (lalling) are correlated with the development of crawling and sitting. At about 9 to 12 months, verboacoustic development, manifested by the child's ability to respond to the calling of his name, "no," and simple "give me" requests, and vocalization characterized by the ability of the child to imitate sounds made by others (echolalia) are correlated with the development of standing. At about 12 to 18 months, verboacoustic development, manifested by the child's ability to follow simple requests and directions, and verbomotor development, marked by the intentful use of a few single words, are correlated with the development of walking.

Continued development of verbomotor behavior is characterized fundamentally by intraverbalizing, or the out loud verbalization of perceptual processes, and the expression of wants and needs up to about 3 years; by emerging interverbalizing behavior, or the verbal sharing of percepts with others, and by the expression of criticism, commands, requests, threats, and questions at 3 to 5 years; and, finally, by the emergence of conceptual intercommunication by 7 or 8 years (Mysak, 1961).

Examination Procedures

Examination of the higher-order integrator should include an attempt to determine whether cerebral lateralization for speech function has taken place. Functions of the higher-order integrator that should be evaluated are (a) perception-comprehension with its automaticity and complexity aspects; (b) verbal thinking with its sequencing, association, elaboration, interpretation, retention, recall, and motor programing aspects; and (c) formulation-production with its automaticity and complexity aspects. The individual's "verbotype" should also be evaluated. (Verbotype is an invented term used to denote the predominant verbal style of an individual.)

Major Speech Brain. Establishment of a major speech brain may be inferred when spoken language abilities appear normal. A direct test for the presence of a major hemisphere may be accomplished through the use of the carotid-amytal speech test, a test that must be conducted by a physician and for which there must be good reason.

Supplementary data to support the establishment of cerebral lateralization may be drawn from tests of eyedness, tonguedness (Froeschels, 1959), and earedness. Ear dominance may be evaluated through dichotic listening tests. Eyedness may be determined by the predominant use of one eye over the other in repeated eye-sighting tasks. Right or left tongue dominance may be inferred from differential performances on tongue clicking (as in calling a horse) and (or) during the rapid, serial production of [t ʌ] or [d ʌ] when the tongue is pointed in the direction of the right or left canine and premolars.

Speech Perception Comprehension. Automaticity and the complexity level of verbal comprehension may be evaluated through informal conversation and simple contextual testing. Simple comprehension and its automaticity can be estimated by observing the client during informal verbal exchanges about family members, school, job, hobby, and so on. Does he appear to understand easily and well or does he need to listen to each word and to have the words spoken slowly? Is the individual capable of simple speech comprehension (perceptual level) but shows difficulty when the topics are shifted to more complex ones such as politics, philosophy, or religion (conceptual level)?

Contextual testing supplements the information gathered via the conversational mode; this technique utilizes persons and things in the immediate environment of the individual being tested. Simple comprehension and its automaticity may be sampled by requesting the individual to point, as quickly as possible, to body parts, articles of clothing, parts of the room, room furniture, or objects and persons in the room. Asking the individual to point quickly to all things in the room that may be worn, sat upon, used to write with, used to hold water, and so on, is a more complex comprehension task.

Speech Formulation-Production. Automaticity and the complexity level of verbal formulation may also be evaluated through conversational and contextual testing modes. Simple formulation and its level of automaticity may be observed during informal conversation about familiar topics such as those suggested previously. Again, does he appear to formulate responses easily and well, or does he appear to speak in a nonspontaneous fashion similar to one learning to speak a foreign language? With respect to complexity of utterances, is he capable of only single word, phrasal, or simple sentence responses, or is he capable of narrative speech responses? Also, can he talk about easily imagined things (perceptual verbalization) as well as about ideas such as honesty and patriotism (conceptual verbalization)?

In contextual testing, formulation-production and its automaticity and complexity may be judged by requesting the individual to name body parts and objects that the examiner points to as quickly as possible (relatively simple) and by requesting the individual to tell you how various objects in the room are used (more complex). Ability for narrative speech may be estimated by presenting the individual with speech continuation tasks, for example, "The phone just rang and a strange voice on the other end began. . ."

Verbal Thinking. Retention and recall aspects of verbal thinking may be judged by having the client repeat progressively longer verbal units (retention), and by responding to sentence completion tasks (recall). They can also be tested by having the client withhold his response to a question by the examiner until the examiner provides a signal (retention and recall). Presenting a client with a progressively longer series of instructions (for example, "get up, go to the door, open it . . .") is another way of judging verbal retention. Having the client paraphrase short stories that are read or spoken by the examiner, or having him answer questions about them, is still another way of assessing verbal retention and recall capacities.

Verbal sequencing behavior may be judged by having the individual unscramble nonsequential syllables of a word or words of short sentences. Association, elaboration, and interpretation functions may be judged by having the individual respond to restricted word association tasks such as requests for synonym or antonym responses (association); by requesting word or proverb definitions (interpretation); by having the individual carry out requested acts that require verbal thinking, for example, "each time I tap the table once, you will . . . , each time I tap the table twice you will . . ."; by having the individual reformulate his responses to questions in specific ways, for example, "provide more detail"; and by requesting short impromptu talks on various topics that are presented (elaboration).

Many of these verbal tasks overlap, and information being collected in one area also provides information in other areas of verbal function.

Verbotype. Judging whether the individual exhibits a balance between initiating and maintaining conversational leads (autoplastic verbal behavior) and following conversational leads (alloplastic verbal behavior) may be of clinical value. Also, does he manifest speaking and listening behaviors that tend to maintain verbal interaction (regenerative verbal behavior) or to limit verbal interaction (degenerative verbal behavior)?

In addition to alloplastic and autoplastic and regenerative and degenerative verbotypes, other verbal styles, suggested in Spiegel's (1959, pp. 924–926) discussion of faulty interpersonal communication, should be identified.

Destructive communication is characterized by hostile communication with or without intent such as verbal ridicule, shouting down the communicant, hostile silence, and hostile paralanguage (as exhibited by voice tone, facial expressions, gestures). Such verbal behavior by the speaker may, in turn, disrupt the listener's speech patterns.

Authoritarian communication may take the form of implying to the listener that he must listen and may talk only when requested; or may be characterized by speech designed to exhibit the speaker's intellectual authority; or may be characterized by the speaker's reacting in a belittling fashion to the responses of the listener.

Disjunctive communication is that type in which the predominant purpose appears to be to confuse, disrupt, or divide. Techniques are used that tend to interfere with the flow of language such as introduction of semantic confusion and the use of the irrelevant and impertinent questions.

Pseudocommunication is characterized by guarded and restricted communication and by pretended communication; it may be used when the speaker wishes to keep from communicating his personal feelings, for example, when indulging in social chit-chat.

Noncommunication is characterized by a sense of the nonrelatedness of the communicant in spite of a continuing verbal exchange. A feeling that the listener is absent is frequent in interactions with such individuals. Such a verbal style is to be distinguished from resistant communication where there is a sense of an active rejection or denial of free verbal exchange.

Typing someone as a destructive-communication verbotype or a disjunctive-communication verbotype, for example, is justified only when one form of oral communication or another predominates or is present in exaggerated form in the speech style of the individual. Increasing one's sensitivity to verbotypes may help the clinician to identify speech problems associated with emotional disorders or to explain why a particular client is not progressing in his individual or group therapy.

Formal Tests. Numerous formal tests are available to the clinician that may provide useful information in some areas of verbal functioning. Most have been described and commented upon in at least two places (Johnson *et al.*, 1963, Ch. 7; Darley, 1964, Ch. 2). In the childhood area, there are receptive vocabulary tests such as the Peabody Picture Vocabulary Test (Dunn, 1959), the Ammons Full-Range Picture Vocabulary Test (Ammons and Ammons, 1948), the Illinois Test of Psycholinguistic Abilities (McCarthy and Kirk, 1961), the Verbal Language Development Scale (Mecham, 1959), and tests of grammatical functioning (Lee and Canter, 1971; Carrow, 1974). Tests for language impairment in adults include: the Language Modalities Test for Aphasia (Wepman and Jones, 1961), the Minnesota Test for Differential Diagnosis of Aphasia (Schuell and Jenkins, 1959), and Examining for Aphasia (Eisenson, 1954). Another test for aphasia that is being used more frequently is the Porch Index of Communicative Ability (Porch, 1967).

When using formal tests, the clinician should remind himself that only a sample of some language functions is being collected, and in an artificial situation. Also, the clinician needs to remind himself of the value of collecting language samples that are representative of what the individual's spoken language is like in everyday speaking situations.

LOWER-ORDER SPEECH INTEGRATOR

Broadly interpreted, lower-order speech integration is concerned with automatic tuning and fine tuning of verbal input and output. Lower-order integration is also responsible for mediating the tonal and kinetic paralinguistic features of verbal input or output. Those features include: appropriate body postures and facial expressions in response to certain input; and appropriate body postures, hand gestures, facial expressions and pitch, loudness, quality, and speech-time patterns associated with certain output.

Historical and Normative Data

Whether the child is aroused easily by, and attends selectively to, audiovisual speech input represents behavioral information of pertinence to the normal development of speech input adjustment and facilitation processing.

For example, did a nearby soft voice succeed in quieting the infant during the first weeks of life? Did the maternal voice elicit stare or smile behavior in the infant at about 3 months; did the maternal voice elicit immediate localizing behavior in the infant at about 6 months; and was there a tendency for the infant to localize the face visually and to track speech-associated movements of the face and articulators? Also, did the child respond to the calling of his name at about 9 to 12 months? Further, in line with the discussion of Fisch (1964) on functions of listening, did the child, in response to speech signals, orient his head and body toward its source, and did he keep still to eliminate body movement noises? Was he able to inhibit reactions to competing stimuli while listening?

Relative to the development of speech output patterning, historical information should be sought with respect to the smoothness and ease of the child's babbling, lalling, echolalia, jargon, and early verbal behavior; any tendency toward speech deterioration under emotional situations and during periods of concomitant motor behavior; the appropriateness of affect and muscle tonus during various speaking situations; and the use of automatic speech such as social gesture speech (I'm sorry," "Im fine," "Good morning,"etc.), memorized speech (counting, reciting days of the week, etc.), and emotional utterances.

Similar information should be sought with reference to older children and adults who suffer disorders of speech communication and where input processing or output patterning functions are suspected.

Examination Procedures

Input Processing. Adjustment and facilitation aspects of speech input processing that should be evaluated are: (a) arousal, localizing, fixing, and tracking capacities of the audiovisual system; and (b) capacity to sustain selective attention to audiovisual events under competing signal conditions.

Arousal to and localizing and fixing of the source of speech signals and the tracking of them may be judged by unexpectedly addressing a client who has been waiting in the examining room for a period of time and has been encouraged to keep busy in some way (e.g., with play objects or magazines). The quickness with which the client localizes and fixes the examiner's face and the accuracy with which he follows the examiner's question or request are the criteria by which to judge arousal, fixing, and tracking phenomena. The client's capacity to track visually the examiner's speech-associated articulatory movements, facial expressions, hand gestures, and body movements should be assessed.

The capacity for selective attention to speech signals may be estimated by observing listening efficiency of the client as he listens to speech (a) presented simultaneously with background music, and (b) presented simultaneously with background voices.

Output Patterning. Adjustment and facilitation aspects of speech output patterning that should be evaluated are: (a) the appropriateness of tonal and kinetic paralanguage, and (b) the capacity of the speech system to compensate during concomitant motor behavior. The development or status of certain reflexes, articulatory differentiation, articulopraxis, articulatory diadochocinesis, and automatic speech behavior should also be assessed.

The presence or absence of certain respiratory, laryngeal, or oropharyngeal activities; the degree of differentiation of the articulators; the adequacy of articulopraxis and laryngopraxis; and the adequacy of articulolaryngeal diadochocinesis may be judged in the following way.

In the case of the young client, the examiner should investigate for persisting infantile breathing activities and for infantile feeding reflexes such as the rooting, lip, mouth-opening, biting, suckling and chewing reflexes. The author has described these activities in some detail elsewhere (Mysak, 1968, pp. 69–71). In the case of the older client, the examiner should determine whether there has been a release of these activities as a result of the disorder presented by the client. Respiratory immaturity is characterized by high rates of breaths per minute (bpm) (e.g., averaging 30 to 35 bpm or more); shallow breathing cycles; predominant use of diaphragmatic-abdominal patterns; and vegetative breathing (nasal-symmetrical pattern) rather than speech breathing (oral-asymmetrical pattern) during speech attempts. Persistence or release of infantile breathing or feeding reflexes during speech attempts interferes with speech function.

Articulatory differentiation is assessed by judging the client's ability to move (a) the lips (pucker, spread movements) in isolation from the tongue and mandible, (b) the mandible (flexion, extension) in isolation from the lips and tongue, and (c) the tongue (elevation and depression) in isolation from the lips and mandible. The test for lips and tongue differentiation is done with the mandible held in a midopen position so that the examiner may view the appropriate articulators. Differentiation of the articulators should be complete by the time children complete speech sound development. Problems with differentiation in children aged seven or eight or dedifferentiation symptoms in adults may be of clinical significance.

Laryngopraxis, or the ability of the individual to initiate and cease phonation quickly and easily, is basic to speech function. Laryngopraxis may be tested by having the client produce on-off phonations of various vowels at a rate of at least one per second. The ability to coordinate movements of the articulators is also basic to speech function. Articulopraxis is tested by having the client produce various combinations of two, three, and four syllables. Syllable combinations to be coordinated are developed in a front to back sequence including bilabial, labiodental, linguadental, lingua-alveolar, lateral, linguapalatal, retroflex, and linguavelar articulatory positions. The first task involves coordinating laryngeal and articulatory mechanisms by producing voiced-voiceless syllable combinations as in [bʌ - pʌ, vʌ - fʌ, ðʌ - θʌ, dʌ - tʌ, ʒʌ - ʃʌ, gʌ - kʌ]. Ease and accuracy of voicing and unvoicing are evaluated, not speed of production. Each combination of two syllables is produced about five times each. Testing of intra-articulatory coordination begins with uttering combinations of two syllables with base [bʌ] as in [bʌ - vʌ, bʌ, - ðʌ, bʌ - dʌ, bʌ - lʌ, bʌ - dʒ, bʌ - rʌ, bʌ - gʌ]. The two-syllable combinations are varied so that each type of syllable serves as a base syllable. Various combinations of three and four syllables are then tested. Children that are 8 years old should be able to produce well combinations of four syllables.

Articulolaryngeal diadochocinesia or the ability of the individual to produce syllabic sequences at certain minimum rates is also basic to good speech function. Stoudt (1967) reviewed research and norms related to speech-sound diadochocinesia and as a result drew three conclusions: (a) rate of diadochocinesia increases as a function of age up to about 18 years; (b) norms for rate of movement can be established at various age levels for males and females; and (c) no significant difference in diadochocinesia is apparent between normal speakers and speakers described as having functional articulatory defects.

In clinical evaluations of speech-sound diadochocinesia, the examiner should consider the rate of syllable repetition, the evenness of rhythm of production, and the duration of the rhythmic production (at least 10 seconds). Positive findings are reflected by significant deficits in any one of these aspects. With respect to mean rate of syllable repetitions for [pʌ, tʌ, or kʌ], 7- to 11-year-olds may average about 40 repetitions for 10 seconds, whereas adults may average about 55 repetitions for 10 seconds. Children may reach the fifties and adults may reach the sixties or seventies.

In evaluating tonal and kinetic paralanguage, the following questions may be asked: How appropriate is kinetic paralanguage (facial expressions, hand movements, and body postures) with respect to what is being said? Are exciting, happy, sad, or dull topics accompained by appropriate tonal paralanguage (speech pitch, loudness, quality, and time patterns)?

Compensations within the speech system during concomitant motor behavior may be judged by asking the following questions: Can the client speak while walking? Is he able to continue speaking while engaged in some motor task such as sharpening a pencil, tying a shoelace, setting a watch, threading a needle? Are articulation, voicing, or time factors noticeably affected when the client lateralizes, ventroflexes, or dorsiflexes his head?

Automatic speech behavior may be judged by observing the ease and automaticity with which the client responds to questions and comments such as "How are you," "Good morning" (social gesture speech) and to requests to count, give the days of the week, months of the year and sing happy birthday (memorized speech). The amount and appropriateness of the use of curse words and sterotyped phrases of dejection or elation (emotional utterances) are also observed.

SPEECH RECEPTOR

Reception of speech-associated auditory and visual stimuli and their conversion into appropriate codes of neural impulses are the functions of the primary receptor system.

Historical Data

In addition to the historical data to be sought regarding audition when exploring the lower-order integrator, the following information should be gathered when investigating the auditory and visual receptors:

Any family incidence of hearing loss due to otosclerosis or due to congenital malformations of the auricle, external auditory canal, tympanic cavity, and cochlear aplasia. The presence of maternal rubella during the first trimester and the presence of Rh incompatibility are also pertinent. Additional noteworthy medical history includes: (a) otitis externa, (b) otitis media with spontaneous or operative perforations (paracentesis, myringotomy) of the tympanic membrane, (c) mastoidectomy, (d) Ménière's disease, (e) viral infections, (f) bacterial diseases, (g) infantile hypoxia or anoxia, (h) head trauma, and (i) noise trauma. Treatment history including the use of ototoxic drugs, such as dihydrostreptomycin, neomycin, and kanamycin, should also be noted.

Both ocular and cortical vision are necessary in order for the visual receptor to make its contribution to the reception of audiovisual speech signals. Information on eye movements as well as vision should be sought (Paine and Oppé, 1966, pp. 99–124).

History of pertinence relative to the visual receptor includes: presence of congenital cataracts (opacity of lens or its capsule) due to maternal rubella, early development of cataracts associated with galactosemia or Lowe's oculorenal dystrophy, later development of cataracts associated with Down's syndrome and myotonic dystrophy; presence of retinal diseases such as retrolental fibroplasia, choreoretinitis, congenital retinal colobomata, retinal angiomatosis, retinitis pigmentosa; congenital conditions associated with paralysis of eye movements such as the syndromes of Moebius, Gerhardt, Duane; acquired conditions associated with paralysis of eye movements such as the syndromes of Benedikt, Weber, Millard and Gubler, Foville, Raymond-Cestan; congenital or early presence of strabismus (nonparallelism of the ocular axes); and the presence of pathologic nystagmus (involuntary movements of the eyes) such as ocular nystagmus due to blindness or serious cases of visual impairment acquired early in childhood, congenital nystagmus, vestibular nystagmus due to disease of the semicircular canals or vestibular nerves, and cerebellar nystagmus due to cerebellar disease.

More specifically concerned with the function of the eye as a speech receptor is history concerning the use of vision and eye movements in speech reception. For example: did the child stare at or smile at mother's face while she engaged in speech play with the infant at about 3 months? From about 6 to 9 months, could the child immediately localize mother's voice and study her face and could the child visually discriminate different faces? From about 9 to 12 months, did the child echo or imitate sounds made by others and was this imitation accompanied by visual tracking of the oral movements of the speakers? During the 1- to 3-year-old period, did the child often enter the "communispheres" (Mysak, 1968, p. 81) of speakers (distance of an arm's length or so up to 12 feet from speakers) and speak and listen and visually scan speaker's faces?

Much more data need to be gathered with regard to the role of the visual receptor in speech sound maturation, in speech comprehension, and in the comprehension of kinetic paralanguage.

Examination Procedures

The auditory speech receptor is examined by observation of the pinna, the external auditory meatus, the tympanic membrane and by standard audiometry. The visual speech receptor is examined by observing the position of the eyes at rest and movements of the eyes, and by visual acuity in response to speech-associated articulatory movements and facial expressions.

Auditory Receptor. The integrity of the auricle, the patency of the external auditory meatus, and the normalcy of the tympanic membrane of each ear should be evaluated prior to the actual measurement of the individual's hearing. An examination of these structures plus the tympanic cavity, ossicular chain, and Eustachian tube should be done by the otologist prior to audiometric evaluation.

Audiometric procedures, which are designed to determine type and degree of impairment, should be performed including pure tone audiometry via air and bone conduction and speech audiometry including speech reception and speech discrimination testing. In addition, impedance testing, tests of recruitment such as the alternate binaural loudness balance test (ABLB), hypersensitivity to intensity change, for example, the Short Increment Sensitivity Index (SISI), and the use of automatic audiometry (Bekesy tracing) should help determine whether an impairment, if present, is of the middle ear, cochlear, or retrocochlear variety.

Visual Receptor. General inspection of the eyes should include whether the eyes appear in binocular balance; whether the eyes enjoy a full range of motion; and whether there are any indications of involuntary movements.

Whenever possible, appropriate information from the ophthalmologist and optometrist on visual acuity, visual fields, eyeg rounds, and eye movements should be available to the clinician.

Visual acuity, fields, and eye movements for purposes of speech reception can be roughly evaluated by the speech clinician at (a) the person-to-person communisphere distance, about 3 to 6 feet; and (b) the person-to-small-group distance, about 6 to 12 feet. Visual acuity for articulatory postures can be judged by asking the child to assume the following postures of the examiner: lip round, lip spread, bilabial, labiodental, linguadental and tongue tip-to-corner or up-or-down postures. The visual field for articulatory postures can be estimated by having the client fixate at the center of the examiner's forehead while being asked to assume again the various articulatory postures. Visual tracking of articulatory movements can be sampled by asking the child to follow with his eyes various movements of the articulators, for example, tracking of the examiner's articulators while he counts in an exaggerated fashion or tracking of rapid open-close mandibular movements, rapid pucker-spread lip movements, and side-to-side and rotatory movements of the tongue.

Specific contributions of problems in acuity and fields for articulatory postures and tracking of articulatory movements to cases of malarticulation are not known at this time. That such visual problems may be contributory to any one particular case of malarticulation should be accepted. More research is needed in this neglected area.

SPEECH EFFECTOR

The speech effector system is composed of respiratory, phonatory, resonatory, and articulatory components and is responsible for producing the speech airstream, for creating and modifying laryngeal tone, and for creating exolaryngeal speech sounds. Since the end-product of speech formulation and transmission activities is dependent on intact effectors, the effectors are critical to the completion of the speech act.

Historical and Normative Data

History on the respiratory effector that should be gathered includes problems with inspiratory or expiratory muscles, with the skeletal framework for breathing, and with the respiratory passage. Lung and bronchial conditions and hypertrophied tonsillar tissue are also worthy of note.

History on the phonatory effector should include information on the laryngeal cartilages and the extrinsic and intrinsic laryngeal musculature. For example, is there a history of congenital laryngeal webbing or irregularities of the glottal edges? Have there been or are there difficulties in creating and maintaining intrathoracic air pressure?

History on the resonatory effector should include information on the velopharyngeal closure mechanism (velum, laryngopharynx, oropharynx, nasopharynx, and related musculature); the fauces; the nasal, buccal, and oral cavities. For example, is there history of: cleft palate, irregularly-shaped pharyngeal cavities, hypertrophied tonsillar tissue, chronic upper respiratory infections, nasal allergy, asthma, nasal polyps, deviated septum, hypertrophied nasal turbinates, or irregularly-sized nasal choanae?

History on the articulatory effector should include information on congenital or acquired problems of the mandible, lips, dentition, occlusion, alveolar ridge, hard and soft palates, and the tongue. For example, is there history of: cleft lip, lateness in growth and exfoliation of deciduous teeth and in development of permanent teeth, malocclusion of first and second teeth, irregularly-shaped palatal vault, atypically small or large tongue, or tongue-tie? In terms of nonspeech function of the articulatory effector, did the individual ever have problems in sucking, chewing, or swallowing?

Pre-speech phonatory, articulatory, and resonatory functioning is also of interest. A pre-speech phonatory history of easy initiation and sustentation of crying or noncrying vocalization is important. Pre-speech articulatory functioning of interest includes: production of infantile glottal fricatives and plosives and linguavelar sounds during the first 4 to 6 weeks; production of bilabial glides and nasals, and plosive sounds up to the first 6 months; production of lateral sounds and lingua-alveolar nasals and plosive sounds up to 9 months; and production of linguapalatal and lingua-alveolar fricative sounds up to 12 months. Pre-speech resonatory function of interest would include the observation that the child was able to create adequate intraoral breath pressure for vocal play and was able to direct the speech airstream orally or nasally.

Speaking fundamental frequency is another reflection of normal functioning of the phonatory effector. The author presented pitch central tendency data for males and females at various developmental stages gathered from various sources (Mysak, 1966, pp. 152–153). Pitch central tendency data for males are: at 8 years, 297 Hz; at 10 years, 270 Hz; at 14 years, 242 Hz; at 18 years, 137 Hz; at 25 years, 119 Hz; and at 48 years, 110 Hz. Pitch central tendency data for females are: at 8 years, 287 Hz; 13 years, 238 Hz, and for the young adult, 200 Hz.

Adequate speech sound maturation is another reflection of the adequate development of the articulatory effector. "Normally all of the sounds of speech are developed by the time the child is 7 years old" (West and Ansberry, 1968, p. 54). However, some children may reflect continuing speech sound development even through age 9 or 10.

Wide variations in the order of development of the phonetic units of the language were pointed out by West and Ansberry (1968, p. 54).

It is only among the consonants and semivowels that any consistency of order can be demonstrated. The vowels and diphthongs are usually learned early, emerging gradually—and for the most part simultaneously—from the infant's random and undifferentiated vocalization. Since there are so many variants for each vowel . . . it is difficult to say much that is definite about the evolution of the vowel or diphthongal sounds of the child's speech, other than the differentiation between and among these sounds begins to take place as one of the first phenomena of speech genesis... These sounds appear before many of the consonants but continue to develop after the consonants have become well stereotyped as speech form. The history of the develoment of the consonant and semivowel sounds is that of the acquisition of a series of skilled acts of increasing difficulty of performance while the development of the vowels is largely that of the standardization of erstwhile undifferentiated vocalizations" (p. 52).

Using the semivowels as a time key for grouping speech sounds according to expected time (upper limits) of emergence, four groups may be identified: (a) *the w group*: [h, m, n, p, b] by 3 years of age; (b) the *j group:* [t, d, ŋ, k, g] by 5 years; (c) the *l group:* [f, v, θ, ð, ʃ] by 7 years; and (d) the *r group*: [s, z, dʒ, tʃ] by 9 years. Among the most frequently misarticulated sounds are those found in the l- and r-groups.

Examination Procedures

Examination of the effectors is concerned with judging: (a) the anatomical adequacy, with special reference to speech function, of respiratory, phonatory, resonatory, and articulatory mechanisms; and (b) whether, properly innervated, the coordinated action of the effectors is capable of producing efficient verbomotor code. Since emphasis in the examination is placed on effector function, overlap exists in the examination of the effector and efferent speech transmitter systems.

Respiratory Effector. Adequacy of the skeletal framework of the breathing mechanism (rib cage, spinal column, pelvic and pectoral girdles) should be determined.

The patency of the observable respiratory passage (nasal and oral cavities, nasopharynx, oropharynx, laryngopharynx, glottis) should be evaluated.

Respiratory movements may be assessed by bimanual palpation of the surface of the lower thorax and abdomen. Hands should be placed at either side of the thoracic-abdominal junction with the fingers held extended and abducted. Vegetative breathing is characterized by a relatively synchronous rise and fall of the anterior abdominal wall and of the thorax. The rate of vegetative breaths per minute (vbpm) in the mature individual is approximately 12 to 18; in children 5 to 15 years, ranges of about 15 to 30 with a mean of about 20 are reported. (Bpm of 30 and above may interfere with speech function.) Speech breathing is marked by at least three features: (a) a shift from medullary to cortical control of breathing mechanisms, (b) a transition from basically nasal to oral respiration, and (c) a transition from relatively regular inspiratory-expiratory phases to a rapid inspiratory phase followed by a prolonged expiratory phase. The speech breathing inspiratory-expiratory ratio (sb-i/e ratio) is approximately 1:6 and may vary during conversation from 1:3 to 1:10. Speech air volume (sav) is about 600 to 750 cc. (Zemlin,

1968, p. 107), the amount usually inhaled during quiet breathing, and may range up to 1500 cc.

Vegetative breaths per minute and the speech breathing inspiratory-expiratory ratio may be evaluated by pneumography; speech air volume may be measured by wet or dry spirometry. The automaticity of the transition from vegetative breathing (nasal-symmetrical pattern) to speech breathing (oral-asymmetrical pattern) may be clinically observed as well as visualized by pneumographic recording. The phenomenon may be referred to as vegetative breathing-speech breathing transition (vb-sb transition).

Phonatory Effector. The anatomical integrity of the vocal folds should be judged at the rest position and during phonation. Also, whether voicing is accompanied by an increase in extrinsic laryngeal muscle tension and a change in speech breathing pattern should be noted.

In terms of the functioning of the phonatory effector, the ability of the client to modify pitch, loudness, and time aspects of voicing should be assessed. For example, the clinician may first identify these vocal dimensions for the client and then demonstrate how they may be varied. The client may then be asked to speak at his lowest pitch level, a middle pitch level, and then a high pitch level. Similar requests may be made for varying loudness levels, that is, have him speak at his softest level, at a middle level, and then at his loudest level. Variability of vocal time may be assessed by having the client speak in his usual manner and then attempt to speak shortening the duration time of vowels and then lengthening them. A display of vocal variability by a voice client is one indicator of a favorable prognosis for vocal rehabilitation.

At the end of the examination, the important question a clinician should ask is: Is the client getting the "most" voice for the least effort? Whether the overall phonatory pattern is as euphonious as one might like is of secondary importance. From the standpoint of vocal hygiene, clinicians should be interested in phonatory effectors that produce automatic and effortless voicing.

Resonatory Effector. The major concern of the clinician with respect to the resonatory effector is the velopharyngeal closure mechanism, or that mechanism which allows for non-nasal and nasal speech-sound distinctions. Mechanisms that contribute to the resonatory effector's function of amplifying and modifying the laryngeal tone should also be inspected.

The clinician may begin by examining the nasal chambers for obstructions to the speech airstream: a deviated septum, edematous turbinates, or polyps. The presence and condition of the adenoids should also be evaluated. The oral chamber should be checked for any disproportion in size with respect to the tongue and for irregular palatal vault configurations. Then the faucial area should be examined for adequacy of size of the passageway into the oral chamber and for the presence and condition of the palatine tonsils. Finally, the velopharyngeal closure mechanism should be evaluated for adequacy of velar length and pres-ence of the velar raphe; intactness of the uvula; intactness of the hori-zontal palatine bones; and the size and shape of the oropharynx.

The function of velopharyngeal closure should also be tested. The client is asked to phonate [ɑ] while the examiner looks for symmetrical elevation of the velum and a mesial movement of the lateral pharyngeal walls (ah-test). Oral pressure is determined by having the client blow into a wet or dry spirometer first with nostrils open and then with nostrils occluded. By dividing the latter measure into the former an oral pressure index (opi) of one or less will result. Indices of 0.8 to 0.9 and above should be considered adequate. A nasal pressure index (npi) can be obtained by having the client repeat non-nasal, consonant-vowel syllables or non-nasal words or phrases while his nares are connected by nasal olives and a tube to a pressure-sensitive gauge. Requesting the client to send an airstream alternately through the nose and then through the mouth is another simple test for closure adequacy.

Articulatory Effector. The articulatory effector is responsible for modifying laryngeal tone and for creating exolaryngeal speech sounds.

The anatomical adequacy of the articulatory effector should be in-spected first, including the adequacy of the structure and mobility of the tongue, lips, and mandible; the normalcy of dentition and occlusion; and the intactness of the alveolar ridge and palatal structures.

The lips and face are required to provide appropriate speech-associ-ated facial expressions, the various labial movements for vowel produc-tion (rounding, spreading, neutral), and labial movements necessary for the production of [p, b, m, w, f, v]. To test labial articulatory ability have the client assume, three or four times in an exaggerated fashion, bilabial and then labiodental postures and movements.

Mandibular movements contribute to the production of vowels and consonants requiring narrow or wide mouth openings, for example, [i, ɑ] or [s, k]. Mandibular movements may also serve a compensatory func-tion in cases of restriction of lingual movement. The capacity for the mandible to assume necessary speech postures and movements is tested by having the client move a few times from the [i] to the [ɑ] position and from the [s] to the [k] position.

Lingual movements contribute to articulation by altering the reso-nance characteristics of the vocal tract for the production of vowels; by acting as a valve in the production of linguadental [θ, ð] and lingua-alveolar fricative sounds [s, z] and linguapalatal fricative and affricate sounds [ʃ, ʒ, tʃ, dʒ]; by redirecting the speech airstream in production of lateral [l] and retroflex sounds [r]; and by occluding the oral exit in lingua-alveolar [t, d] and linguavelar plosive sounds [k, g]. To test lingual articulatory ability have the client assume, three or four times in an exaggerated fashion, linguadental, lingua-alveolar, linguapalatal, and linguavelar postures and movements.

Teeth and dental arches contribute to articulation by serving to impede the oral exit of the speech airstream as in the production of [s, f, ʃ, θ]; by serving as tactile clues as in [s, ʃ]; and by serving as an articulatory base for the lips as in [b, p]. Palatal structures contribute to articulatory function by separating oral and nasal chambers and thereby allowing for the creation of intraoral breath pressure; by selective coupling of oral and nasal chambers in the production of nasal sounds; and by providing lingual contact points for lingua-alveolar, linguapalatal, and linguavelar sounds. The clinician needs to determine whether or not these structures are serving their speech purposes adequately.

A *phonetic inventory* completes the examination of the functional adequacy of the articulatory effector. Observation of vowel and consonant production during conversation is the approach of choice for evaluating whether the effectors are adequate for articulation, since spontaneous articulation is mediated by different neurodynamics than nonspontaneous articulation. The nonspontaneous approach toward developing the phonetic inventory is made by having the individual repeat words after the examiner, name pictures, or read words containing the phonemes under study.

SPEECH TRANSMITTER

The primary role of afferent speech transmission is to convey audiovisual nerve impulses generated by the auditory and visual receptors over lower and upper sensory neurons to higher speech centers. The primary role of efferent speech transmission is to convey patterns of motor impulses generated within the central speech system over upper and lower motor neurons to the speech effectors. Transmission processes differ from lower-order integration processes since only cerebripetal or cerebrifugal transmission of nerve impulses is involved and not transmutation of these input or output signals.

Historical and Normative Data

Historical and normative data collected under the lower-order speech integrator (input processes) and the speech receptor sections should provide pertinent background information in the area of afferent speech transmission. Specific areas of concern in the history are conditions that may affect the neural auditory pathway and its relay stations such as neoplasms, infections, anoxia, Rh factor, vascular lesions, and degenerative diseases. Data collected under the lower-order speech integrator (output patterning) and the speech effector sections should provide pertinent background information in the area of efferent speech transmission. Specific areas of concern in the history are conditions that may affect the central and peripheral divisions of the thoracic, cervical, and cranial motor nerves such as infection, trauma, neoplasms, progressive and nonprogressive diseases, and cerebrovascular accidents (CVA's).

Examination Procedures

At least three factors complicate the evaluation of the afferent transmission system: (a) the quality of the afferent inflow conducted over the lower sensory neurons depends on the integrity of the speech receptors that convert the audiovisual stimuli into the nervous inflow; (b) as the afferent inflow is conveyed over upper sensory neurons it may be selectively "filtered" and "routed" at the different levels of ascent and hence transmuted (lower-order afferent integration); and (c) the actual value of the arriving afferent inflow is in proportion to the integrity of the higher-order speech integrator.

Similarly, at least three factors complicate the evaluation of the efferent transmission system: (a) the quality of the efferent outflow conducted over the upper motor neurons is in proportion to the integrity of the higher-order speech integrator that generates and organizes the outflow; (b) as the efferent outflow is conveyed over upper motor neurons, it may be influenced by various centers in the descent pathway and hence transmuted (lower-order efferent integration); and (c) the actual value of the efferent outflow is in proportion to the integrity of the speech effectors.

Afferent Transmission. Certain audiometric tests may be used to good advantage in helping to determine whether an auditory involvement is central to the organ of Corti. For example, site-of-lesion audiometry that collects data such as configuration of the pure tone audiogram, correspondence between pure tone findings and speech discrimination scores, presence or absence of recruitment, type of Bekesy audiogram, and findings on tests of speech intelligibility under difficult listening conditions should prove helpful in determining whether retrocochlear auditory pathways are involved.

Reports of various types of visual field defects would implicate the visual transmission system for processing verbovisual code (articulatory movements) and visual paralanguage (facial expressions, hand gestures, and body postures and movements). For example, a lesion of the right optic nerve in front of the optic chiasm may produce total blindness in the right eye; a lesion of the right optic tract behind the chiasm may cause blindness in the left half of each field of vision or left homonymous hemianopia; and lesions of the middle part of the optic chiasm may cause defects in the temporal field of each eye or bitemporal hemianopia. Tests of visual fields for articulatory postures and of visual tracking of articulatory movements, described under "The Visual Receptor," are appropriately given here as well.

Efferent Transmission. The integrity of central and peripheral motor neurons supplying respiratory, phonatory, resonatory, and articulatory effectors are evaluated by testing the effectors for appropriate muscle tonus and for reflex and voluntary movements. In general, lower motor neuron involvement is reflected by muscle weakness, flaccidity, reduced or lack of voluntary movements of specific muscle groups, muscle fasciculations and atrophy, and, depending on muscle groups involved, deficits in vegetative reflex and emotional response movements. Upper motor neuron involvement is reflected by muscle weakness, more generalized involvement of muscle movements, hypertonic muscles, and no muscle fasciculations or atrophy.

The respiratory transmitter (cervical nerves I to VIII and thoracic nerves I to XII) is tested by first evaluating the tonus of thoracic and abdominal musculature during vegetative and speech breathing. Reflexive changes in breathing may be checked by fanning the air in front of the nostrils of the client or by having him hold his breath for as long as possible. In both instances, breathing should be reflexively deepened and hastened. Voluntary respiratory patterns may be assessed by having the client voluntarily alter vegetative breathing by breathing more rapidly or more slowly than usual. Evaluating the ability of the client to alternate quickly between vegetative and speech breathing (vb-sb shift) is an important test of the efficiency and condition of respiratory transmission function. Vb-sb shift may be tested by periodically directing short questions at the client during intervals of silence.

The phonatory transmitter (cranial nerve X) is judged by evaluating the tonus of the vocal folds by visual inspection and by testing certain laryngeal reflexive and voluntary movements. The glottic closing reflex may be tested by having the client lift, push, or pull in rhythmic fashion with his hands while sustaining a vowel. A "fluttering" of the vowel is a positive response. Voluntary on-off voicing should also be checked. Voicing and unvoicing behaviors should be alternated at about one shift per second.

The resonatory transmitter (branches of cranial nerves X, V, XI) is inspected by assessing the efficiency of the velopharyngeal closure mechanism. Tonus of the velum and oro- and nasopharynx should be estimated. Palatal and pharyngeal reflexes should be checked. The ability to direct an airstream orally and then nasally in alternating fashion and the ability to alternate [m] and [b], [n] and [d], and [ŋ] and [g] sounds should also be evaluated.

The articulatory transmitter (cranial nerves V, VII, IX, X, XI, XII) is evaluated by testing the function of mandibular, labial, and lingual musculature.

West and Ansberry (1968, pp. 180–181) discussed ways of distinguishing between central and peripheral motor involvement of the articulators. Six factors to consider are: (a) articulatory lapses, (b) vegetative reflexes of swallowing and gagging, (c) emotional responses (e.g., smiling, sneering, crying, sobbing), (d) specific, voluntary movements (e.g., spreading the lips, protruding the tongue, protruding the mandible), (e) .degree of muscle involvement, and (f) muscle tonus.

Muscles affected in peripheral dysarthrias are not only involved in producing specific speech sounds but are also involved in vegetative reflexes, emotional responses, and specific voluntary movements. Further, peripheral involvements are circumscribed and involved musculature is usually hypotonic. In cases of upper motor neuron involvement, vegetative reflexes and emotional responses associated with the affected muscles are generally unimpaired (however, vegetative reflexes are sometimes exaggerated and there may be a limited repertoire of emotional responses), and articulatory muscle failures and muscle failures for specific voluntary movements are in agreement. Further, central dysarthrias are usually more generalized and the musculature is hypertonic.

For more details on the testing of the efferent speech transmitter, see "Efferent Transmitter Disorders—Diagnosis" in Chapter 7.

SPEECH SENSOR

The final system to be evaluated is the complex sensor system. It is responsible for automatically controlling and monitoring spoken symbols, as well as their phonatory, resonatory, articulatory, and time dimensions. Sensor control function is concomitant with the speech act, while sensor monitor function follows the speech act. Furthermore, sensor control activity is only possible during actual speaking, while sensor monitor activity also takes place during verbal thinking. The system is composed of the primary auditory and tactile-kinesthetic sensors and the secondary visual sensor (supplementary or compensatory function). Spoken symbols and their phonatory dimension are controlled and monitored via the auditory sensor, while the articulatory dimension of spoken symbols is usually controlled and monitored via the tactile-kinesthetic sensor.

Control and monitoring of voice and articulation may also be conscious or subconscious. That is, one is usually not aware of his own voice pattern during speech but, rather, attention is given to the verbal symbols being used; however, it is possible for an individual to become more aware of his vocal patterns. Similarly, the speaker is usually not aware of the tactile and kinesthetic sensations that are processed in order to control and monitor articulation. Again, however, speakers may be made to process more consciously these touch and movement sensations. In neuroanatomical terms, and with reference to articulation, subconscious proprioceptive sensor activity may be considered a function of the cerebellar division of the proprioceptive system, while conscious proprioceptive sensor activity may be considered a function of the cortical division.

Finally, the major function of the sensor system has been described, that is, intrapersonal speech perception, however, the system is also capable of monitoring the misspoken words and misarticulated sounds of others or interpersonal speech perception. Such interpersonal speech perception of error verbal behavior is especially important to the clinician, since he may plan to sharpen the client's ability to discriminate error performance on an interpersonal level (discrimination of client's error speech as simulated by the clinician) as a first step toward activating within the client intrapersonal sensitivity to his own error speech.

Historical and Normative Data

Historical and normative data collected under Higher-Order Integrator—Speech Perception-Comprehension, the Lower-Order Integrator—Input Processing, the Afferent Transmitter, and the Receptor Systems provide pertinent background information on the speech sensor system.

The following additional information is of interest to the examiner with respect to the development of control and monitoring functions in the child during the speech development period: (a) little attention paid to the use of misspoken words or misarticulated sounds; (b) little effort spent in attempting to approximate standard production of various sounds; and (c) rapid, casual, or quickly abandoned attempts at self-correction.

Examination Procedures

Intrapersonal and interpersonal sensor control and monitoring functions are evaluated through observation as well as through the use of testing procedures.

Auditory Sensor. Under ordinary circumstances, the auditory sensor monitors verbal thinking, and it controls and monitors the actual production of verboacoustic code as well as its voicing and time dimensions. Depending on the age of the individual, the auditory sensor also makes an important contribution to the control and monitoring of speech sound articulation. Theoretically, the more the individual's age approaches and surpasses seven or eight years, the less utilized is the auditory sensor for control and monitoring of articulation.

Internal verbal monitoring may be assessed as follows: (a) asking the individual a question, and following the response having the individual shorten, lengthen, or change his response "in his mind" before responding again; (b) giving the client a speaking situation, for example, asking the boss for a raise or asking Dad for the keys to the car, then asking him to think out a series of well-planned statements relative to the situation, and then having him utter the statements.

External verbal control and monitoring may be judged best via the conversational mode. During conversation about his job, family, friends, hobby, politics, the client may be asked to become pro on a subject and then con; use circumlocutionary language and then precise language; speak only in the present tense, or the past or future tenses.

On an interpersonal level, the client may be asked to indicate whenever the clinician digresses from the subject, uses the wrong word, and so on.

Interpersonal monitoring of vocalization is assessed by having the client listen to the clinician while, during various points in the conversation, the clinician simulates the client's dysphonia. The client is asked to signal whenever he hears the error voice.

Intrapersonal monitoring of vocalization is judged by asking the client to pay close attention to his voice while he converses with the clinician. Following such conversation, the client is asked to describe what is wrong with his voice with reference to its pitch, loudness, and quality dimensions.

Altering the function of the auditory sensor may also produce important clinical data. For example, the introduction of bilateral white noise, up to voice-masking levels, into the ears of certain individuals with voice anomalies may result in improvement of the dysphonia. At least two explanations may be offered for this phenomenon: (a) in the attempt to overcome the effects of masking, the individual alters respiratory and phonatory myodynamics and in so doing influences his voice pattern in a positive fashion; (b) by masking a poorly functioning auditory channel for voice regulation, a positive influence is manifested as a result of inducing a compensatory proprioceptive monitoring of laryngeal voice function.

Such auditory masking may also result in certain stutterers becoming more fluent. Possible explanations for this effect may be: (a) a distraction phenomenon, (b) the elimination of a hypersensitive sensor for control and monitoring of speech rhythm, and (c) a shift to a more efficient tactile-proprioceptive sensor. Some stutterers also appear to benefit from speaking under conditions of delayed speech feedback. Again, the effect may be explained on the basis of forcing a shift to a more efficient speech sensor, or it may cause the auditory sensor to be used in a different manner.

Tactile-Kinesthetic Sensor. The tactile-kinesthetic sensor cooperates in the control and monitoring of actual speech articulation. As already indicated, this sensor apparently becomes more important in this activity following the completion of speech sound maturation.

Some ways of determining the integrity of this important sensor system are: (a) by evaluating right-left touch discrimination of the client in the areas of the lips, alveolar ridge, palate, and tongue; and (b) by estimating lingual kinesthetic function by providing a touch stimulus to the corners of the mouth, middle of the upper lip, and various teeth, and asking the client to locate quickly with his tongue tip the point touched. Other oral sensory-perceptual tests such as oral form identification (Ringel *et al.*, 1968), two-point discrimination (Ringel and Ewanowski, 1965), and mandibular kinesthesia (Ringel *et al.*, 1967) may also be given.

Subconscious sensor functioning (cerebellar system) in older children and adults can be estimated by the quality of the control and monitoring of speech articulation during normal and speeded conversational patterns. When deficits in articulatory control and monitoring are suspected, the individual may be asked to alter his speech in ways that raise to a more conscious level his awareness of articulatory postures and movements; for example, he may be asked to "study" his articulatory postures and movements while he speaks; he may be asked to make firmer contacts between his articulators while he speaks; or he may be asked to overarticulate. When changes in intelligibility occur under these more conscious forms of articulation, one possible explanation to consider is that the individual is now utilizing, either completely or partially, the cortical sensor system.

Appendix B represents a suggested outline for recording a general examination of the systems. In conducting such an examination one should follow an outline so that no pertinent information is missed or forgotten. However, depending on the cooperation level of the client and the fatigue factor, the order of examining the systems, the number of systems examined, and the amount of information collected under each system may be modified. Abilities as well as disabilities should also be recorded whenever possible. Finally, it is important that the functioning of the various systems be observed during conversational activity as well as during more formal speech tests.

The last section of this chapter is devoted to a discussion of the relative powers of various approaches to the diagnosis of speech disorders.

DIAGNOSTIC APPROACHES

West and Ansberry (1968, p. 257) said, "Disorders of speech may involve so many and such diverse causes that the problem of diagnosis often astounds the beginner with its complexity. Indeed, without some orderly scheme of procedure even the experienced clinician will blunder."

Diagnosis is a word that may be translated, "through knowledge." In terms of clinical speech work it means distinguishing through knowledge one speech or hearing disorder, and its cause or causes, from another.

At least nine diagnostic approaches or combinations of approaches, are available to the speech and hearing clinician to help him get to know more about a particular speech disorder: clinical, differential, direct, by treatment, by exclusion, group, instrumental, provocative, and tentative. This section of the chapter defines these approaches and identifies their strengths and weaknesses.

Clinical Diagnosis

A clinical diagnosis is made from a study of the signs (objective symptoms of a disorder observable by the examiner) and symptoms (subjective signs of a disorder) of a disorder without necessarily knowing about the morbid changes that may be responsible for them. The majority of diagnoses made by the speech and hearing clinician are of the clinical type.

Examples. Various childhood and adult disorders of speech are often diagnosed on the basis of manifested signs and symptoms. For example, speech retardation in childhood may be attributed to autism which, in turn, may have been diagnosed on the basis of certain behavioral patterns. Similarly, speech and language retardation, associated with some form of general retardation, may be diagnosed without any direct knowledge of the possible brain dysfunction underlying the retardation. Other childhood disorders of speech that are diagnosed primarily on the basis of presenting signs and symptoms are: childhood aphasia, sensorineural hypacusis or anacusis, and stuttering.

In adults, linguistic symptoms following some form of CVA are usually attributed to presumed damage to the speech brain, and rarely is there an attempt to confirm the location of the lesion. Similarly, dysarthrias associated with various adult neuropathologies are usually not studied carefully in terms of identifying the specific morbid changes that may be causing them.

Limitations. The obvious limitation in clinical diagnosis is that the assumed cause of the symptoms may not be the cause at all.

For example, linguistic retardation, supposedly connected with autism or general retardation, may turn out to be caused by involvement of the auditory system; or stuttering, supposedly associated with certain environmental factors, may be caused by actual anomalies in the rhythm control centers of the brain. Also, language symptoms after a stroke, in some cases, may be associated with problems in the auditory system or with adjustment problems and not with damage to language centers of the brain.

However, since it is not always easy or possible to correlate presenting symptoms with assumed morbid conditions, a clinical diagnosis allows the clinician at least to hypothesize about etiology, plan a therapy approach based on the hypothesis, and test the hypothesis by evaluating the results of the management plan.

Differential Diagnosis

A differential diagnosis is made by determining which of two or more disorders with similar signs a client is manifesting by systematically comparing and contrasting his signs with those of the possible disorders.

Examples. In a given case of articulatory involvement in childhood, a clinician may compare and contrast his client's articulatory profile with one associated with hypacusis, or infantilism, or with articulatory paralysis. Or in a case of alogia (without language), the clinician may compare and contrast data on history, observation and testing with similar data often found in the congenitally anacusic, retarded, or brain-injured.

Limitations. One weakness in the application of a differential diagnostic approach is that the one or two possible disorders selected by the clinician for differential comparison may not represent the background of the case at hand. For example, a clinician may compare and contrast his diagnostic data in any given case of speech retardation with those associated with hearing loss, childhood aphasia, retardation, or emotional disorder, and, on the basis of the procedure, determine that his data are most like those associated with emotional disorder. However, other possibilities such as a genetically-based language slowness or one based on some biochemical condition may not have been considered (because of a paucity of existing information on these conditions). In short, the differential diagnostic approach is limited at least by: (a) number of known conditions that may possibly explain the case in question; and (b) the accuracy of the information possessed on each of the known conditions.

Direct Diagnosis

A direct diagnosis is one made by actually observing the structural anomaly presumed to be causing the speech disorder or one made on the basis of presenting signs that are distinctively or characteristically associated with a particular speech disorder.

Examples. A direct diagnosis of a case of hypernasality may be made when it is determined that the problem is associated with an observable short or cleft velum. Pathognomonic signs of childhood velopharyngeal incompetency may be hypernasality associated with alar constriction, facial grimacing, and glottal fricatives and plosives. Certain vocal pitch, loudness, quality, and articulatory patterns, that is, "deafy" patterns, may be considered pathognomonic of congenital or infantile anacusis.

Limitations. When making a direct diagnosis the clinician must be careful not to assume too quickly that any given speech sign is associated with an observable structural deviation or is pathognomonic.

For example, numerous cases exist of individuals with short palates, or short lingual frenulums, or malocclusions that manifest adequate speech production. Also, speech patterns that may appear pathognomonic, for example, "cleft palate speech" or "deafy speech," may turn out to be on a speech model or imitative basis.

Diagnosis by Treatment

Diagnosis by treatment is one made on the basis of the results of a specific treatment plan.

Examples. Diagnosis on the basis of results of treatment is an approach often used in hard-to-diagnose cases, or in cases when insufficient data exist; for example, in the instance of speech retardation where a suspicion of a minimal, lesional brain dysfunction exists but where socioemotional and intellectual immaturities are also present. Problems in deciding which are the primary, secondary, and tertiary signs may arise and may not be easily answerable for various reasons.

Therefore, rather than engage in long-term discussions and evaluations of the child, a treatment plan may be formed on the basis of the best estimate of the problem. Then, on the basis of progress made by the child in the treatment program, a diagnosis may be made. That is, the child may show the most progress in therapy when the management plan is psychotherapeutically oriented, and hence the diagnosis that the problem is very likely of emotional origin is made.

Limitations. Limitations to diagnosis by results of treatment include: (a) difficulty in knowing exactly what is going on in therapy or just what aspects seem most efficient; or (b) secondary symptoms may be most handicapping by the time treatment is begun and hence progress in therapy aimed at those symptoms may result in the clinician identifying a secondary socioemotional cause as the original or primary cause of the problem.

Diagnosis by Exclusion

Diagnosis by exclusion is made by eliminating all those disorders of speech to which some of the presenting signs belong and leaving only one to which apparently all of them belong.

Examples. In many instances of speech sound immaturity classified as "functional" articulation cases, diagnosis is made by the exclusion approach. A child manifests interdental sigmatism, for example. He is 8 years old, he does not appear retarded, brain-injured, or emotionally-disturbed, and he does not appear to have a serious malocclusion; hence, it must be a functional case.

Similarly, in adult dysphonia the clinician may collect information that reveals that the client is free of any laryngeal pathology, has no apparent respiratory anomalies, and has no auditory perceptual problems; hence, it must be a case of psychogenic dysphonia.

Limitations. Not being aware of all the possible backgrounds for the presenting signs in any one case is the major weakness of the diagnosis-by-exclusion approach.

Group or Team Diagnosis

A group diagnosis is made by the combined efforts of an organized group of specialists acting as a unit. Health specialists with whom the speech and hearing clinician frequently works include: otolaryngologist, pediatrician, physiatrist, psychologist, neurologist, social worker, psychiatrist, plastic surgeon, dentist, orthodontist, and prosthodontist.

Examples. The speech pathologist and audiologist are frequently involved with group diagnosis in cases of infantile anacusis, cleft palate, cerebral palsy, mental retardation, and psychogenic language disorder.

In instances of suspected anacusis, the clinician usually collects historical information on the maturation of auditory and speech behavior, and data on levels of speech sound and language functioning. The specific purpose of the examination is to determine whether the information collected is in keeping with a diagnosis of anacusis and, if so, how it compares with impressions of the pediatrician, otolaryngologist, and psychologist.

In cases of congenital cleft palate, the specialist must provide information on how many of the presenting speech signs may be attributed directly to the cleft condition, how many to malocclusion, or hearing loss, and so on.

Limitations. In this day of information explosion and microspecialization, the group diagnosis approach is often very fruitful and is an approach of choice. However, the approach also has its limitations; for example, interference in communication among members of the team due to differences in professional vernacular, professional interest, and perceived status. To state this in another way, the team approach to diagnosis is as powerful as the degree of relatedness, cooperation, mutual respect, and coordination that may exist among member specialists. Another limitation has to do with the time factor. Team evaluations mean numerous examinations and substantial time spent in conferencing and gaining a diagnostic consensus. The expense of such an approach is yet another limiting factor.

Instrumental Diagnosis

Instrumental diagnosis is one made with the assistance of clinical instruments.

Examples. Some of the kinds of cases and equipment involved in instrumental diagnosis are: (a) suspected hypacusis confirmed via audiometric evaluation; (b) hypernasality apparently related to a deficit in velopharyngeal closure confirmed by cineradiography, or by lateral x-ray; and (c) a possible respiratory base for a voice disorder confirmed by spirometry or pneumography.

Limitations. At least two factors to be wary of in instrumentally-based diagnosis are: (a) the problem of instrument and (or) operator error, and (b) the tendency to accept without too much questioning the quantitative data acquired from an instrument.

To elaborate on these two points: (a) inaccurate information may be gathered from an instrument that is functioning poorly, or has not been calibrated, or is being operated by an inexperienced individual; and (b) a positive x-ray of velopharyngeal closure, or positive spirometric findings, may not necessarily explain presenting hypernasality or dysphonia in any one case.

Provocative Diagnosis

A provocative diagnosis is one made after inducing symptoms of a suspected disorder.

Examples. A common example of a provocative diagnosis in clinical speech practice is one made in doubtful cases of stuttering. That is, the client may not manifest any signs of stuttering while being examined and the clinician may decide to attempt to provoke them by applying various forms of communicative stress. For example, he may become a disinterested or a critical listener, or he may ask the individual to speak faster or more clearly.

Also, suspected linguistic impairment in certain cases of adult neuropathology may be provoked by speaking rapidly to the client or by requesting rapid responses. Suspected cases of hypacusis for speech may also be clarified by speaking softly, rapidly, or by looking away from the client while speaking to him.

Limitations. When using a provocative diagnosis approach the clinician should keep in mind that his method of provoking signs may be artificial. That is, the individual may rarely find himself in a similar situation in his actual speaking experiences and hence the "findings" may lose some of their importance.

Tentative Diagnosis

A tentative diagnosis is one based upon information available at the time and is subject to change when additional information becomes available.

Examples. Tentative diagnoses are made frequently in complex cases of language delay. For example, a tentative diagnosis of hearing loss may be made and "firmed up" or not depending on how the child responds to amplification and speech perception training (an example of diagnosis by treatment).

Limitations. One limitation of a tentative diagnosis relates to the time it may take to gather additional information. When additional information is slow in appearing, the tentative diagnosis may evolve into a more permanent diagnosis by default. That is, a diagnostician may not pursue the case, or the client may leave a clinic and the tentative diagnosis is in danger of becoming fixed.

A list of guiding statements for the diagnostician concludes the chapter.

1. The clinician should distinguish between the identification of speech or hearing signs and symptoms and a careful description of the extent of them, and a diagnosis of the probable cause or causes of these signs and symptoms.

2. Whenever possible, the clinician should diagnose predisposing, precipitating, and maintaining causes of any speech or hearing disorder. He should also consider whether predisposing and precipitating factors are still operative in any one case.

3. The clinician should distinguish between the immediate and background causes of a disorder. It may be determined that the cause of the hypernasality is an incompetent velopharyngeal mechanism; however, the cause of the incompetent closure mechanism may not be known. Similarly, speech or hearing signs may be attributed to mental retardation, emotional disorder, or brain injury by the clinician without the clinician knowing the cause of the primary complex. In short, the clinician should be aware of the depth of the diagnosis he is making in any one case. Speech and hearing clinicians should begin to collect the kind of data that would more frequently not only identify the probable immediate cause of the signs but also the probable background cause.

4. The clinician should avoid both premature decisions and overlong evaluations. If a diagnostician ceases his examination as soon as one condition is found, which may explain the signs or symptoms, he may miss additional or possibly more important ones. On the other hand, prolonged investigations of all factors whether they appear pertinent or not is inefficient and may only confuse the diagnostician.

5. The clinician must remember that anomalous structures in one individual may actually be the basis for the presenting speech symptoms, while similar structures in another person may not result in any speech symptoms.

6. Finally, wherever appropriate and whenever possible, the clinician should distinguish among primary, secondary, and tertiary speech or hearing signs. For example, in a given case of hypacusis, are the speech signs part of the primary signs of a problem that includes hearing loss, or are some part of the speech signs secondary to the hearing loss and

some tertiary to the secondary signs? Such distinctions are very difficult to make in most speech complexes, but when they can be made they may have important treatment implications.

Each of the succeeding chapters of the book is devoted to one of the speech systems. In each chapter are found discussions of the possible anomalous bodily structures and functions that may disturb the particular system, as well as discussions of preventive measures and therapy principles related to the system.

REFERENCES

Ammons, R. B., and Ammons, H. S., The Full-Range Picture Vocabulary Test. Missoula, Mont.: Psychological Test Specialists (1948).

Carrow, E., A test using elicited imitations in assessing grammatical structure in children. J. Speech Hear. Disord., 39, 437–442 (1974).

Darley, F. L., Diagnosis and Appraisal of Communication Disorders. Englewood Cliffs, N. J.: Prentice-Hall, Inc. (1964)

Dunn, L. M., Peabody Picture Vocabulary Test. Nashville: American Guidance Service (1959).

Eisenson, J., Examining For Aphasia, Rev. Ed. New York: Psychological Corporation (1954).

Fisch, L., The functions of listening and its disorders. In Learning Problems of the Cerebrally Palsied. London: The Spastics Society (1964).

Froeschels, E., Some logopedic therapeutic suggestions. In Eleventh Congress of the International Society of Logopedics and Phoniatrics, London, August (1959).

Johnson, W., Darley, F. L., and Spriestersbach, D. C., Diagnostic Methods in Speech Pathology. New York: Harper & Row (1963).

Lee, L., and Canter, S., Developmental sentence scoring: A clinical procedure for estimating syntactic development in children's spontaneous speech. J. Speech Hear. Disord. 36, 315–340 (1971).

McCarthy, J. J., and Kirk, S. A., Illinois Test of Psycholinguistic Abilities: Examiner's Manual. Urbana, Ill.: University of Illinois Institute for Research on Exceptional Children (1961).

Mecham, M. J., Verbal Language Development Scale. Minneapolis: American Guidance Service (1959).

Mysak, E. D., Organismic development of oral language. J. Speech Hear. Disord., 26, 377–384 (1961).

Mysak, E. D., Phonatory and resonatory problems. In R. W. Rieber and R. S. Brubaker (Eds.), Speech Pathology: An International Study of the Science. Amsterdam: North-Holland Publishing Company (1966).

Mysak, E. D., Neuroevolutional Approach to Cerebral Palsy and Speech. New York: Teachers College Press, Columbia University (1968).

Paine, R. S., and Oppé, T. E., Neurological Examination of Children. London: The Spastics Society (1966).

Porch, B. Porch Index of Communicative Ability. Palo Alto, Calif.: Consulting Psychologist Press, Inc. (1967).

Ringel, R. L., Burk, K. W., and Scott, C. M., Tactile perception: Form discrimination in the mouth. Br. J. Disord. Commun., 3, 150–155 (1968).

Ringel, R. L., and Ewanowski, S. J., Oral perception. I. Two-point discrimination. J. Speech Hear. Res., 8, 389–398 (1965).

Ringel, R. L., Saxman, J. H., and Brooks, A. R., Oral perception. II. Mandibular kinesthesia. J. Speech Hear. Res., 10, 637–641 (1967).

Schuell, H., and Jenkins, J. J., The nature of language deficit in aphasia. Psychol. Rev., 66, 45–67 (1959).

Spiegel, R., Specific problems of communication in psychiatric conditions. In S. Arieti (Ed.), American Handbook of Psychiatry, Vol. 1. New York: Basic Books (1959).

Stoudt, R. J., Jr., Diadochokinesis: research and norms. J. Speech Hear. Assoc. Va., 8, 14–20 (1967).

Wepman, J. M., and Jones, L. V., Studies in Aphasia: An Approach to Testing; Manual of Administration and Scoring for the Language Modalities Test for Aphasia. Chicago: Education-Industry Service (1961).

West, R. W., and Ansberry, M., The Rehabilitation of Speech. New York: Harper & Row (1968).

Zemlin, W. R., Speech and Hearing Science: Anatomy and Physiology. Englewood Cliffs, N. J.: Prentice-Hall, Inc. (1968).

3

Speech Integrator System: Higher Order

Clinical manifestations of disorders of higher-order speech integration appear in both children and adults. Both age groups may display positive verbal symptoms, or retention or release of paleovocal and paleoverbal behavior, and negative symptoms, or disturbed, reduced, or lack of verbal behavior. Symptoms may range from subclinical aphasoid lapses to a total absence of verbal behavior. Problems may be found on word-forming, word-finding, word-arranging, and word-meaning levels. This chapter discusses genetic, neurogenic, gnosogenic, psychogenic, and sociogenic forms of language dysfunction in childhood and psychogenic and neurogenic forms of language dysfunction in adulthood.

DEVELOPMENTAL AND GENETIC LANGUAGE DISORDERS

Delayed onset of verbal behavior, the persistence of early verbal patterns, or the slower-than-expected development of verbal behavior may be manifested by children who in all other respects appear to be developing normally. Specific, developmental speech lags were described by Ingram and Barn (1961) who indicated that such disorders may involve articulation only or articulation and language. Parents frequently report that a particular child was a late talker, or used baby talk, or was difficult to understand for a long time but that the child eventually talked all right. The only finding in the history of such a child may be a family predisposition toward slow development of speech.

Other children with relatively specific problems in the development of speech communication are reported whose problems may persist and may eventually involve reading and writing abilities as well. In this regard, Ingram (1960) reported on specific, developmental dysphasia and Luchsinger and Arnold (1965, pp. 337–383) reported on congenital language disability; both sources view these problems as genetically-based.

Background

The background for simple delay of the onset or slow development of spoken language may include environmental factors such as reduced or inappropriate types of verbal stimulation or lack of reward or irregular rewards for verbal behavior. Genetically-based or other types of developmental differences in the speech brain must also be considered. Masland (1969), in offering various explanations for language disability in childhood, states that possibly ". . . these are genetically or constitutionally determined organizational defects or peculiarities of the brains of such individuals which cause it to be difficult or impossible for them to form the associations or correlations essential to the establishment of language" (p. 86).

Clinical Manifestations

Simple Language Immaturity. Simple verbal immaturity may include extended use of paleovocal or protocommunication such as lalling, echolalia, and jargon; delay in the onset of the first use of words up to 30 and 36 months (alalia, alogia, aphemia); and use of language patterns typical of a younger child or paleoverbal behavior (pedolalia) such as extended use of single-word sentences (holophrasia), repetitive speech behavior (verbal perseveration), and extended use of intraverbalizing and want-need verbalization (infantile verbotype).

Genetic Language Dysmaturity. Ingram (1960) discussed specific developmental dysphasia which he believes is genetically determined. Comprehension problems were identified as well as the following formulation problems (some of which may be secondary to the comprehension problems): slowness in acquisition of words and phrases; problems in word-forming, or syllable reversals, grammatical confusions; problems in word-finding, or omission or mistaken use of small words; circumlocutionary verbalization; problems in word arrangement, or difficulty in forming sentences and organizing sequences of sentences; and problems in word-meaning, or inappropriate utterance of words or phrases. Luchsinger and Arnold (1965, pp. 377–383) also discuss genetic influences in what they refer to as congenital language disability. Symptoms of such disability may include delayed onset of speech, articulatory disorders, dysgrammatism, and specific reading and writing disability. Cluttering (tachyphemia) has also been considered a language disability ". . . resulting in confused, hurried, and slurred diction . . ." (Arnold, p. 3). The basis for the disorder is thought to be organic, familial, and aphasiform. Spoken symptoms include paraphasic slips as well as dysgrammatisms (Arnold, p. 41).

Diagnosis

Factors that help to distinguish simple language immaturity are: (a) Speech emerges by at least 36 months of age. (b) Speech patterns are typical of or appropriate for a younger child. (c) All other developmental sequences are essentially normal. (d) Simple language immaturity may be a family characteristic.

In the case of genetic language dysmaturity, (a) a family history of listening-speaking and (or) reading-writing disorders is usually reported; (b) evidence of linguistic dysmaturity rather than immaturity is found, that is, some atypical patterns even for a younger child; and (c) all other developmental patterns are basically normal.

Prognosis

Time alone eventually resolves cases of simple language immaturity. Early identification of the case and speech counseling are necessary in families that may over-react to lateness in the emergence of speech in order to reduce the possibility of adverse psychological reactions within the child.

Little information exists on the prognosis for genetic language dysmaturity. However, with early identification, family cooperation, and appropriate linguistic stimulation, progress can be made in reducing the language handicap.

Therapy

Simple Language Immaturity. Secondary preventive measures may be necessary in instances of language immaturity. If a high-risk case is identified, programs for facilitating the development of spoken language and for reducing possible social, emotional, and educational repercussions of late onset and slow development of speech may be organized.

Many activities may be recommended to parents during the pre-speech period that may facilitate the development of spoken language. For example: (a) Maintain an active communisphere during as much of the day as possible by keeping talkative children and adults within the 3- to 12-foot range of the child. (b) Increase speech output when the child is experiencing good feelings as during periods of play, feeding, and bathing. (c) Develop situations that encourage vocal or verbal reactions from the child and reward the child for such reactions. (d) Facilitate speech sound perception by eliciting localizing responses from about 6 months on to speech produced at various points from the child; and by eliciting motor reactions from the child from 9 months on to the calling of his name. (e) Stimulate paleovocal behavior such as babbling, lalling, echolalia, and jargon.

During the speech age (12 months on) parents may: (a) expand and enrich the child's social and perceptual spheres by daily exposure to speakers outside the home, that is, to relatives and neighbors, and to things and places such as cars, buses, shops, parks, beaches, and animals; (b) reward all efforts to perceive and produce speech; (c) name aloud persons, objects, and places within the child's visual field; (d) have the child point to or show body parts, familiar persons, toys, and so on;

(e) engage in self-reporting aloud in simple phrases as you move about touching and doing things; (f) report aloud, describing what the child does and contacts; and (g) engage in verbal expansion-expatiation activities (de Hirsch, 1970), or repeat the child's telegraphic utterances in more developed form (expansion) and then enlarge on the child's utterances (expatiation).

Secondary social, emotional, and educational repercussions to late onset and slow development of speech may be minimized by family counseling that is aimed at parental understanding of the nature of the problem, by use of the facilitation of language development program just described, and by enrollment in a nursery school.

Genetic Language Dysmaturity. In addition to the activities recommended for cases of simple language immaturity, additional stimulation is suggested to develop further the verbal behavior of children suffering from language dysmaturity.

Attempts to prevent secondary problems of speech perception are important since many of these children already manifest specific difficulties related to problems in memorizing, discriminating, synthesizing, and sequencing speech sounds.

At least two factors may contribute to secondary problems in speech perception: (a) if the primary problems go undetected and speech perception is difficult, the child may eventually process progressively less speech through the auditory channel; (b) if the child's difficulty with speech comprehension elicits punishing speech (criticism and words of concern) from parents, teachers, and friends the child may begin to reject speech signals.

Attempts to increase verbal memory and to improve discrimination, sequencing, and synthesizing of speech sounds should be made. Verbal memory may be developed by having the child repeat progressively longer phrases and sentences; point to an increasing number of items named; and provide answers to progressively longer and more complicated questions. Speech sound discrimination may be aided by having the child differentiate first between similar-sounding nonsense syllables and then between similar-sounding words, phrases, and sentences. Speech sound synthesizing may be stimulated by having the child reconnect and utter words that have been broken down into their component syllables or reconnect and utter phrases or sentences with component words that have been separated by progressively longer pauses. Sequencing of sounds may be encouraged by having the child unscramble component syllables of words or words of sentences.

Verbomotor activity may be primed by having the child (a) name all things in his visual field, (b) provide missing words to sentence stubs, (c) make verbal associations to various stimulus words, (d) define words, and (e) participate in sociodramas.

NEUROGENIC LANGUAGE DISORDERS IN CHILDREN

Neurogenic language dysfunction refers to cases of relatively specific language involvement based on acquired neurological disorder. Many of these children are referred to as central nervous system (CNS)-impaired, cerebrally handicapped, brain-injured, perceptually handicapped, aphasoid, congenitally aphasic, and oligophasic or as children with cerebral dysfunction, minimal brain damage, minimal chronic brain syndrome, and brain dysfunction. Depending on the examining specialist and the particular child, the child's neurological, visual perceptual, behavioral, or linguistic symptomatology may be highlighted.

Background

From what is known about the speech brain and its plasticity in the early years of life, persisting neurogenic language dysfunction in childhood is apparently associated with bilateral disturbances to hemispheral speech areas and (or) with disturbances to thalamic coordinating centers and tracts. Possible causes of injury to the speech brain include trauma, convulsive disorders, circulatory disorders, hydrocephalus, neoplasms, and infections and parasitic invasions.

Trauma. Traumatic conditions that may contribute to cerebral birth injury are precipitate or prolonged labor, abnormal presentations of the fetus, high forceps deliveries, anomalies of the birth canal, excessively large fetal heads, premature separation of the placenta, infarction of the placenta, compression of the umbilical cord, cesarean delivery, prematurity, postmaturity, and maternal diabetes.

Postnatal traumatic lesions of the brain such as those encountered in car accidents may also be the cause of childhood linguistic disorders. Such traumatic lesions of the brain include contusions, lacerations, and hemorrhages.

Convulsive and Paroxysmal Disorders. The epilepsies, narcolepsy, and migraine conditions may be associated with various forms of transient childhood aphasia. Ford (1966) defines epilepsy "as a condition characterized by recurrent, paroxysmal discharges of cerebral neurons" (p. 1131). Primary (cause unknown) and symptomatic forms (known cause) are recognized.

Grand mal seizures may be associated with pre-ictal, ictal, or post-ictal transient aphasic symptoms. Pre-ictal symptoms described by Brain and Walton (1969, p. 926) include ". . . a strong impulse to speak associated with a feeling of inability to do so." Ingram and Barn (1961) reported symptoms of acquired aphasia in two cases of congenital hemiplegia after severe epileptic attacks.

Petit mal attacks may be described by older children as a few moments when ". . . they are unable to see, hear or talk . . ." (Ford, 1966, p. 1138).

Psychomotor attacks are manifested by different patterns. One pattern is characterized by "Purposeless behavior with fighting, running, laughing, and incoherent speech" (Ford, 1966, p. 1139). Brain and Walton (1969, p. 929) refer to these attacks as temporal lobe epilepsy and include auditory hallucinations in the symptom complex.

Pyknolepsy, a form of epilepsy similar to petit mal (Espir and Rose (1970, p. 70) consider it a subtype of petit mal.), is sometimes observed in children between the ages of 4 and 12 years. It is hypothesized by West (1958, p. 201) to be associated with stuttering or phemolepsy (speech epilepsy or partially compensated pyknolepsy), late acquisition of speech, and retention of baby talk.

Focal convulsions ". . . may be defined as a type of epilepsy in which the seizures are of such a nature that they consistently indicate a local origin in some part of the brain" (Ford, 1966, p. 1158). Frontal lobe discharges ". . . arising in the motor speech area result in the interruption of speech and are sometimes followed by transient motor aphasia."

Temporal lobe discharges have been reported to have resulted in word deafness in a child (p. 1162).

Narcolepsy is a condition ". . . in which paroxysms of irresistible somnolence are associated with transient attacks of weakness or cataplexy" (Ford, 1966, p. 1174). Sleep attacks may exist alone and in a few cases attacks of weakness may only be observed. During the cataplectic attacks the patient is always conscious ". . . although speech may be impossible for a time" (p. 1176).

Migraine, or severe recurrent headache, may be associated with various focal symptoms. "Transient disturbances of speech may occur . . . before the headache develops. The chief difficulty is in finding words. Rarely is the patient unable to speak coherently. As a rule, there is numbness of the tongue and lips at such times" (Ford, 1966, p. 1183).

Circulatory Disorders. Conditions that affect intracranial blood supply, and consequently portions of the speech brain, are considered here.

Occlusion of the left middle cerebral artery in the Sylvian fissure distal to its first ascending branch has been reported in a 7-year-old girl. The condition was caused by a dissecting aneurysm and resulted in a right hemiplegia and aphasia. A 14-year-old girl who ". . . showed a marked segmental narrowing of the distal portion of the internal carotid artery and the proximal parts of the anterior and middle arteries . . ." connected with arteritis associated with sphenoid sinusitis and meningitis also exhibited dysphasia and right hemiparesis (Jacob *et al.,* 1970).

Ford (1966) identified various vascular lesions and circulatory disorders in children and adolescents which may have aphasia as a symptom. They are: changes in cerebral blood vessels associated with acute infectious diseases, for example, pertussis, pneumonia, scarlet fever, diphtheria, measles, dysentery, influenza, typhus fever, typhoid fever, meningitis, rheumatic fever (pp. 809–811); malignant hypertension and arteriosclerosis of childhood (pp. 822–825); periarteritis nodosa (pp. 825–829); and systemic lupus erythematosus (pp. 829–831).

Hemorrhage that has been caused by rupture of an intracranial aneurysm in childhood and is affecting the left hemisphere may cause aphasia (Ford, 1966, p. 859). One of the hemorrhagic disorders, thrombotic thrombocytopenic purpura, which is more common in adolescents and young adults than in older persons, may also show neurologic disturbances including aphasia, apraxia, anesthesia, and limb paralysis (Bebin, 1968, p. 1056).

Blood dyscrasias may be accompanied by various neurologic manifestations.

Sickle-cell anemia (abnormal sickle-cell hemoglobin), an inherited disorder almost always occurring in Negroes, is frequently associated with severe neurologic complications, one of which may be aphasia (Bebin, 1968, p. 1043). Clinical manifestations usually begin in childhood.

Leukemia (generalized proliferation of leucocytes and their precursors in the bone marrow, spleen, and lymph nodes) may be associated with neurologic complications due to intracranial hemorrhages. Hemianopia or aphasia has been reported in such cases (Bebin, 1968, p. 1051).

Weller (1952), following the suggestion of Meader and Muyskens, used blood examinations in the diagnosis and therapy of speech disorders. He reported deviations in blood composition for stutterers and for children with delayed speech.

Hydrocephalus. Various forms of hydrocephalus are recognized. In general, the condition is characterized by an excessive accumulation of cerebrospinal fluid in the cranial cavity.

Hagberg (1962) reported that apparently normal children with minimal brain damage resulting from spontaneously arrested hydrocephalus reveal verbal behavior which he often sees in cases of more pronounced hydrocephalus; he called it "the cocktail party syndrome." The syndrome is marked by a propensity for the children to talk and not know what they are talking about. In a study of the verbal behavior of hydrocephalic children with minimal mental and physical involvement, Fleming (1968) reported that as a group these children ". . . produced a significantly greater amount of inappropriate verbal responses . . . Especially prominent were conversational remarks and statements totally unrelated to the situation and the intended task." Schwartz (1974) has also observed "cocktail party speech" among children with myelomeningocele and hydrocephalus.

Neoplasms. Among the types of brain neoplasms found in childhood and adolescents are astrocytomas, glioblastoma multiforme, neuroblastomas, and ganglioneuromas (Ford, 1966). Motor aphasia is reported with tumors of the left frontal lobe and sensory aphasia with tumors in the left parietal region (p. 907).

Infections and Parasitic Invasions. Ford (1966) reports aphasic symptoms in children suffering from such infections and invasions of the brain as encephalitis (p. 338), typhus fever (p. 412), brain abscess (p. 420), subdural abscess of the cranium (p. 431), brucellosis (p. 454), congenital neurosyphilis (p. 512), cysticerce (p. 539), and echinococcosis (p. 543).

Worster-Drought (1971) reported on an unusual disorder in 14 children encountered during a 10-year period in which the outstanding symptom was acquired receptive aphasia. Causation of the disorder is unknown but the symptoms suggest that it may be due to a form of low-grade selective encephalitis that affects particularly the temporal lobes. In most cases, onset of the disorder was between 4 and 6 years of age and usually followed a single or a few epileptiform attacks that did not recur. Some cases showed a degree of deafness either at or shortly after the epileptiform attacks. "Then followed, in sequence, a gradual loss of comprehension for spoken language ... and a failure of executive speech, while any deafness present gradually improved (p. 568)." In all cases, intelligence was not impaired and none showed other abnormal neurologic signs; however, all cases did show electroencephalographic (EEG) abnormalities, especially in the temporal and (or) temporoparietal regions.

Clinical Manifestations

Depending on the age when the cerebral insult is suffered, symptoms of delay in onset of verboacoustic and verbomotor behaviors (as described in the section on "Simple Language Immaturity") may be found. However, the presence of atypical verboacoustic and verbomotor behaviors rather than just simple delay or retardation in such behaviors usually distinguishes neuropathic language dysfunction from simple language immaturity. Symptoms of neurogenic language disorder are usually not distinguishable from those of genetic language dysmaturity.

Speech Perception-Comprehension Problems. "Usually, a child with aphasia has a mixed problem and shows evidence of limited expressive language and a reduced ability to understand or comprehend language symbols" (Wood, 1964, p. 31). Darley (1964, p. 26) reports that a child with a specific language disability "typically indicates that he hears but does not understand spoken language. . ." "The child with receptive aphasia can hear the speech of others but he cannot comprehend it . . . They commonly comprehend a word intermittently and unexpectedly" (Myklebust, 1954, p. 149). Verbal distractibility, in the form of drifting from the conversational topic because of the tendency to make irrelevant associations to particular words and then pursuing those irrelevant associations, has also been reported (Lewis *et al.*, 1960, p. 130). Eisenson (1968) wrote that relatively few children are truly aphasic and that such children are essentially those with involvements of auditory perception.

Other symptoms of verboacoustic disorder include (a) absence of response to speech signals, (b) confusion in processing similar-sounding words (clang phenomenon), and (c) use of compensatory speechreading.

Speech Formulation-Production Problems. Highly verbal, brain-injured children have been described who appear to have good expressive language but who exhibit a gap between their language usage and its comprehension (Lewis *et al.*, 1960, p. 60). As already mentioned, Hagberg (1962) observed apparently normal children with minimal brain damage related to spontaneously arrested hydrocephalus who "... love to chatter but usually do not know very much what they are talking about." Such symptoms may be referred to as pseudoeuphasia.

Hesitant or halting speech (stutter-like) may be exhibited by children who do not as yet possess the vocabulary to allow for automatic verbalization of perceptual and conceptual processes (asymbolic dysautomaticity). Children with actual problems in vocabulary development may also exhibit such dysautomaticity.

Other symptoms of verbomotor disorder include (a) unusual discrepancies between verbomotor and verboacoustic capacities with verboacoustic behavior being near normal in some cases; (b) marked lack of language with lack of or inconsistent meanings attached to given words, difficulty in combining and recombining known words (asyntacticism), and grammatical confusions (agrammatism) (Strauss and Kephart, 1955, p. 106); (c) repetitive perseveration (simple repetition of a response) and delayed perseveration (repetition of a response given earlier) (Strauss and Lehtinen, 1947, p. 51; Mysak, 1968, p. 31); (d) compensatory use of body language; (e) inconsistent use of correct words in receptive aphasia (Myklebust, 1954, pp. 178-179); (f) delayed language and language characterized by single words in association with gestures in receptive aphasia (Worster-Drought, 1968); and (g) word-finding (anomia) and word-forming (paraphasia) problems.

Verbal Thinking Problems. Certain childhood aphasics have been identified as having specific problems with inner language used for thinking purposes (Wood, 1964, p. 31; Myklebust, 1954, p. 151). Worster-Drought (1968) reported that children with receptive aphasia may request the frequent repetition of new words (behavior reflective of deficits in verbal retention).

Other symptoms of verbal thinking problems include difficulty in carrying out verbal instructions for a sequence of motor acts (verbal programming), compulsive use of profane language (coprolalia), invented or imaginary speech (idioglossia, glossolalia, neolalia), and circumlocutionary verbalization.

Diagnosis

Numerous factors must be considered by the clinician before the diagnosis of neurogenic language dysmaturation may be made. Some of the more important ones are:

Verbal Immaturity vs. Dysmaturity Symptoms. In cases of neurogenic language involvement, the clinician should find more than paleoverbal symptoms or verbal patterns appropriate for a younger child; he should also find atypical verbal symptoms or symptoms of verbal dysmaturation.

Verbal Development vs. Other Developmental Sequences. The concept of neurogenic language dysfunction implies that the child who has such a disorder exhibits a substantial disproportion in what he can do verbally and what he can do in general. In short, the child should be linguistically retarded but near or within the normal range in most other respects.

Elimination of Other Major Causes for Language Involvement. The diagnosis of neurogenic language dysfunction also depends on the clinician's ability to eliminate other major contributors to language disorder such as serious hearing loss, general mental retardation, and serious emotional disturbance.

Presence of Other CNS Anomalies. Support for a CNS-based language disorder in a child is also obtained from finding other symptoms of nervous system disorder. Some general symptoms of possible nervous system disturbance are positive EEG findings, uneven eyeglass correction, lack of binocular balance, eating problems (manifested by difficulty in chewing; biting of tongue, lips, and cheeks; rejection of hard or chewy foods; dysphagia), hyperreflexia (exaggerated gag, patellar, and startle reflexes), retarded dextralization, degrees of scoliosis or torticollis, general clumsiness, auditory agnosia, and lip and tongue dyspraxia.

The author reviewed the following perceptual-behavioral symptoms that may also be associated with disturbances of the nervous system and may have a bearing on language-learning capacities (Mysak, 1968, pp. 19–24): rise and lability of threshold for auditory stimuli, perseverative behavior, distractibility for external stimuli, periodic behavioral fixation or "freeze" behavior, disinhibition resulting from distraction from within the individual, over-response behavior, reduced auditory retention span, rigidity and orderliness, catastrophic response, and withdrawal behavior.

Prognosis

Generalizations on prognosis in cases of neurogenic language dysfunc-

tion cannot be made. Disagreement in the literature and among clinicians concerning the nature of the disorder has interfered with the
collection of adequate data with respect to prognosis. In general, however, prognosis for improvement is dependent on an early identification
of the problem, on an accurate assessment of its components (substantial variability exists from child to child in verbal and associated symptoms), on the development of an individualized habilitation program
and on expert home and clinical application of this program, and on the
stimulation within the child of strong motivation to improve.

Therapy

Therapy procedures recommended for cases of simple language immaturity and genetic language dysmaturity are applicable here as well.
Additional ideas will be presented under the headings of preventive,
symptom, and compensatory speech therapies.

Preventive Measures. One primary preventive measure in acquired
childhood language dysfunction is parental education. Parents should
know that head trauma, cerebral circulatory disorders, and brain infections might disturb the development of spoken language. Hence, early
identification and medical attention for such problems have implications for language development as well as for general health.

Symptom Therapy. Magoun (1967) in speaking of speech therapy
proposed ". . . that a major potential for its improvement lies in the
mobilization of all the insights that have been and are continuing to
come from a variety of fields of neurological research, in determining
how better to influence and manipulate central neural activity so as to
maximize the capacity of the cerebral cortex for processing, storing,
retrieving, and utilizing information in communication through speech
and language" (p. 217).

Magoun identified at least three possible applications of the findings
of neurological research to speech therapy.

1. The simple increase of intensity of stimulation. With respect to
speech signals, simultaneous presentation of auditory and visual signals
can be used. "Sensory feedback, in the form of afferent stimulation
generated by responses, can also be employed to promote and modulate
central excitability" (p. 218). For example, in a simple repetition task a
client first sees and hears the speech signal, and then when he attempts
to repeat the word with the use of a mirror he feels and again sees and
hears the word spoken.

2. The promotion of novelty rather than of repetition of stimulation.
Provocation of the orienting reflex and the attentive state is one way of
influencing cortical excitability, and the novelty of afferent signals
plays an important role in evoking the orienting reflex. Magoun states
that ". . . repetition is the first law, not of learning, but of habituation,

whose influence upon learning is a negative, rather than a promoting one. Obviously, the promotion of novelty, rather than of repetition, should become a primary law of learning" (p. 219).

For example, when one is repeatedly presenting an object with its associated verbal symbol in a speech-learning situation he should attempt to make each presentation adequately distinctive from the preceding presentation. The associated verbal symbol may be made distinctive, for instance, by varying its loudness, pitch, quality, or durational aspects.

3. The use of reinforcement in learned behavior. "The powerful expedition of learning, either by positive or negative reinforcement, is attributable in considerable part to the marked facilitation and generalization of afferent signals, which such reward or punishment promotes" (Magoun, p. 221). Food reward, "pat-on-the-back" reward, and so on, could be important reinforcements in speech-learning. Magoun believes that ". . . learning should be initiated by orientation and then followed up to criterion and maintained by reinforcement . . ." (p. 221).

Habilitation programs for neurogenic language dysfunction in childhood may be based on developmental theories, learning theories, neurologic theories, and speech-system theories.

Following are symptom therapy techniques that are based on neurologic and developmental theories. The author has referred to some of these ideas elsewhere (Mysak, 1961; Mysak, 1968; Mysak, 1971). Furthermore, some of the techniques suggested here overlap (see "Therapy—Simple Language Immaturity" and "Genetic Language Dysmaturity").

Emotional reactions that tend to facilitate spontaneous perceptual-vocal activity stimulated. Experiences such as hunger, pain, fear, happiness, or pleasant movements are frequently accompanied by speech. Hence, the clinician should carefully stimulate certain needs, wants, and desires in the child that can be fulfilled by the child only when he attempts some form of verbomotor behavior. Depending on the child's level of intercommunication, body language alone or body language plus onomatopoetic vocalization should also be encouraged.

Amplification of perceptual experiences that tend to facilitate verbomotor behavior in the child, in turn, may increase the chances of the child's learning associated verboacoustic and verbomotor code. First, the clinician should plan in-therapy-room or out-of-therapy-room experiences that reflect strong interests of the child. Second, experiences should be planned that stimulate more than one sensory channel; for example, the use of materials that have visual, tactual, and auditory dimensions. Third, perceptual experiences may be intensified by manipulating size, form, and color aspects of visual stimuli, and by manipulating loudness, pitch, quality, and time factors of auditory stimuli.

Development and expansion of the perception and comprehension of spoken language initially concentrated on. Initial efforts at stimulating verbomotor behavior should be directed at speech perception-comprehension mechanisms. Verbal play involving "give me . . .", "put the . . .", "bring me . . .", "show me . . .", "where is . . ." activities should be emphasized.

Speech span and sequencing exercises should also be planned. Span may be developed by having the child point to or touch a progressively increasing number of objects as they are named by the clinician or by carrying out a progressively longer series of instructions. Proper sequencing behavior may be encouraged by placing emphasis on identification of objects in the right order or the carrying out of instructions in the right order.

Formulation and expression of spoken language (specific verbomotor behavior) may be stimulated in various ways. For example, the child may be asked to complete sentence stubs, take part in sociodramas, answer yes-no questions, define various words, continue stories begun by the clinician, and engage in various verbal association activities.

Verbal thinking processes are recognized in at least two forms, the external form and the internal form. The external form may be stimulated by the clinician accompanying his own behavior with out-loud self-reporting and by his reporting aloud the activities of the child. Hopefully, the child will eventually engage in such self-talk or intraverbalizing behavior that is a precursor of internal verbal thinking.

Mature verbal thinking may be stimulated through a procedure called imagery association. For example, the clinician may present an apple to the child and then ask the child to study it with his eyes, his hands, his nose (smell), and his mouth (taste buds). He then utters the word "apple." Next, the clinician removes the apple and asks the child to "see" the apple with his mind's eye, to "feel" the apple with his mind's fingers, to "smell" the apple with his mind's nose, to "taste" the apple with his mind's mouth, and to "hear" the word "apple" with his mind's ear. Finally, the child is asked to "hear" the word and then to "see" the apple, to "hear" the word and then to "feel" the apple, to "hear" the word and then to "smell" the apple, and to "hear" the word and then to "taste" the apple. Such techniques should contribute to the association of speech areas in the brain with areas that subserve visual, tactual, olfactory, and gustatory imagery.

Compensatory Therapy. The speech clinician must be ready to use compensatory therapy in cases ". . . where 1. there is little hope of attaining speech communication, or 2. the development of such communication is limited, or 3. the development of such communication is proceeding slowly and the child is well into the early language learning period" (Mysak, 1971, p. 712).

Speech compensatory activities may take the form of: (a) the use of gesture-pantomime or body language (including hand gestures, facial expressions, and body postures); (b) the use of body language in association with onomatopoesis such as gr-r-r or bang, splash; (c) the use of pictures or objects representing important wants and needs of the child, for example, food, family members, clothing; and (d) the use of some yes or no signal system in response to expressed alternatives.

General Suggestions to the Clinician. In order to facilitate verbal communication between clinician and client, the clinician should consider the following.

The speech field should be studied. The value of quiet background or a soft musical background should be explored.

Orientation to the speech signal should be facilitated by preceding each verbal message with the calling of the child's name until the child begins to scan the clinician visually and auditorially. Preceding verbal messages with tapping, or the presentation of appropriate pictures, might also be tried. Whatever technique is used, the clinician should precede his verbalizations with stimuli that will ensure the orientation of the child's speech system to the speech signals. Varying the loudness, pitch, rate, and quality of the voice may also stimulate the desired orientation.

Words and sentences should be chosen with care. Wherever possible, words that readily evoke images should be used. Sentences should be short, simple, and descriptive.

Integration time should be long enough to allow the child to make appropriate associations. Having the child echo statements or questions before making desired verbal or motor responses is one way of giving the child more time to associate words and ideas.

Modification of verbalizations should be tried by the clinician when he experiences difficulty in communicating with the child. Repeating the message, restructuring it, or saying the same thing in various ways are methods of modifying the spoken message.

Verbal assists or aids should be used when the child is having difficulty in comprehension. Verbal assists may take the form of supportive gestures, facial expressions, body postures, onomatopoetic utterances, and the use of representative objects and pictures.

"GNOSOGENIC" LANGUAGE DISORDERS IN CHILDREN

Delay in onset and slow and limited development of verbal behavior secondary to conditions that also affect motor, perceptual-conceptual, and socioemotional developments is classified here as a gnosogenic language dysfunction (language deficit based on mental deficiency). Wood (1964, p. 36) defined the mentally retarded child as one with ". . . a reduced ability to learn adequately from any experience within his environment, whereas children with aphasia, hearing loss, or emotional disturbance are able to learn from certain types of experience, depending upon their individual problems." Matthews (1971, p. 802) and Morley (1965, p. 76) believe that mental retardation is one of the most common backgrounds for speech retardation. Lillywhite and Bradley (1969, p. 1) state, ". . . communication disorders arising from various kinds of mental retardation far outnumber disorders resulting from any other single problem."

Background

Backgrounds for the various brain dysfunctions found among the mentally retarded include familial tendencies, chromosomal abnormalities, cerebral infections and intoxications, perinatal cerebral trauma, intracranial neoplasms, and various metabolic disorders. (Pseudoretardation may also result from factors such as emotional disturbance and experiential deprivation.) Those familial- and chromosomal-based varieties with characteristics likely to be seen by the speech clinician, such as anomalies of the head, face, ear, eye, nose, mouth, tongue, and teeth, are described here.

Familial Tendencies. Gellis and Feingold (1968) describe numerous conditions associated with mental retardation in which heritable factors are apparently present. Descriptions of the more prominent features of some of these conditions follow.

Albright's hereditary osteodystrophy, where intellectual functioning may vary from normal to severe retardation, is characterized by short stature and stocky build, rounded facies, occasional microcephaly, adherent ear lobes (decreased hearing), delayed dentition and (or) dental aplasia, and blue sclerae and strabismus.

Ataxia telangiectasia (Louis-Bar syndrome), in which about one-third of the patients become retarded as a result of the neurologic involvement, is manifested by dull and expressionless facies, telangiectasia (dilation of capillary vessels and minute arteries) mainly of the face, ears, neck, hands, wrists, knees, and cerebellar and extrapyramidal neurologic signs.

Bird-headed dwarf (Virchow-Seckel dwarf), in which mild to moderate retardation is frequently found, is manifested by proportional dwarfism and slender body build, hypoplasia of the malar bones (bird-like eyes and facial structure), microcephaly, prominent eyes, low-set and lobeless ears, prominent and sometimes beaked nose, micrognathia and high-arched or cleft palate, and absent or atrophic teeth.

de Lange's syndrome, in which severe retardation is found, is characterized by reduced height and weight, low-pitched growling cry (often present), microbrachycephaly (abnormally small and short head), eye anomalies (antimongoloid slant, ptosis and nystagmus, bushy and confluent eyebrows), upturned nose, "fish-like" mouth, narrow, high-arched palate, and extreme hirsutism.

Generalized gangliosidosis, marked by profound retardation, is manifested by dolichocephaly (abnormally long head), coarse-features facies, hypertelorism and strabismus, large and low-set ears, broad bridge and flaring nasal alae, hypertrophy of the alveolar ridge and maxillary process, and a large tongue.

Hyperuricemia (Lesch-Nyhan syndrome), marked by severe mental retardation, exhibits the following physical features: self-mutilation symptoms due to lip biting, finger chewing, teeth grinding, and symptoms of spasticity and choreoathetosis; and muscular hypertrophy secondary to almost constant torsion spasms.

Laurence-Moon-Biedl syndrome, in which retardation may vary from minimal to severe, is characterized by generalized obesity, acrocephaly (pointed head), polydactyly, eye anomalies (esotropia, cataracts, blindness, mongoloid slant), broad-bridged nose, and thinning or lack of hair.

Marinesco-Sjögren syndrome, marked by severe mental retardation, displays the following physical features: short stature, frequent microcephaly, bilateral cataracts and strabismus, hair anomalies (short, fine, sparse, and blond, resembling lanugo or fetal hair), kyphosis (humpback), talipes equinovarus (form of clubfoot), seizures, cerebellar ataxia, and dysarthria.

Familial microcephaly, marked by moderate to profound retardation, exhibits the following physical features: microcephaly, relatively large and protruding ears, narrow or flat-bridged nose, and high-arched palate.

Hunter's syndrome (gargoylism), in which retardation is present, is manifested by a short stature and an enlarged head, coarse-features facies, thickened eyelids and coarse eyebrows and lashes, progressive nerve deafness, wide flattened nose with broad bridge, large tongue, spade or claw-like hands with short stubby fingers, and hirsutism.

Hurler's syndrome (gargoylism), marked by severe retardation, is manifested by short stature; prominent forehead; coarse-features facies; hypertelorism; low-set ears (and hearing loss); flattened nose with broad bridge; open-mouth posture with large protruding tongue; high and narrow palate; small, peg-shaped and widely-spaced teeth; spade or claw-like hands with short, stubby fingers; hirsutism; and harsh voice.

Sanfilippo's syndrome is characterized by physical findings similar to Hurler's syndrome but not as severe.

Myotonic dystrophy, characterized by mild to moderate retardation, is manifested by hypotonia and muscle wasting, diplegia, expressionless and asymmetrical facies, ptosis and cataracts, high-arched palate, early baldness, myotonic tongue, nasal speech, and dysarthria.

Oculocerebrorenal syndrome, marked by severe retardation, and characterized by hyperextensible extremities with hypotonia and decreased muscle mass, bizarre positions, frontal bossing of the head, bilateral congenital cataracts, and rickets.

Oral-facial-digital (OFD) syndrome, in which retardation is present but usually not in severe form, is manifested by frontal bossing of the head, brachydactyly (abnormal shortness of fingers or toes), syndactyly (webbed fingers or toes), clinodactyly (abnormal deflection of fingers), camptodactyly (abnormal flexion of fingers), polydactyly (supernumerary fingers or toes), hypertelorism, cleft palate and lip or a midline notch of the upper lip, dental abnormalities, and lobulated tongue.

Otopalatodigital (OPD) syndrome, marked by mild retardation, is characterized by frontal bossing of the head and prominent occiput; hypertelorism and antimongoloid slant; abnormal ossicles and conductive loss; broad-bridged nose; small, fish-like mouth with cleft palate; and digital abnormalities.

Phenylketonuria, in which untreated patients have moderate to severe retardation, is manifested by fair hair and skin (eczema); blue eyes; microcephaly; hypotonia; fine rapid tremors; athetoid or jerky, aimless movements; and seizures.

Prader-Willi syndrome, in which retardation varies from severe to mild, is characterized by obesity and short stature, hypotonia, microcephaly, brachycephaly, dolichocephaly, "fat" facies (cheeks, under chin), almond-shaped eyes and strabismus, and fish-like mouth with micrognathia.

Sjögren-Larsson syndrome, in which mental retardation is usually severe, is manifested by congenital spastic diplegia and ichthyosis prominent in the flexural areas of the extremities.

Smith-Lemli-Opitz syndrome, marked by moderate to severe retardation, and characterized by short stature, microcephaly, epicanthal folds and ptosis and strabismus, low-set ears, increased nasolabial distance, cleft uvula and high-arched palate, micrognathia, broad-bridged nose with upturned nares, and polydactyly, syndactyly, brachydactyly.

Tuberous sclerosis, in which the degree of retardation varies, is manifested by facies that are characterized by pink to reddish-orange nodules which are generally located in a butterfly pattern on the cheeks, pupils that may be unequal secondary to brain involvement, and seizures.

Wilson's disease, in which the degree of retardation varies in severity, is characterized by a set expression facies with open, drooling mouth and teeth exposed in grimacing smile, greenish-brown Kayser-Fleischer rings of the eyes, flexion contractures especially of the wrist, abnormal posturing, extrapyramidal signs including tremor at rest or with movement, rigidity, and clumsiness.

Chromosomal Anomalies. Chromosome abnormalities may be divided into those involving the sex chromosomes, which result primarily in abnormal sex development, and those involving the autosomes, which result primarily in abnormal somatic growth and development (Smithells, p. 1). Those that reflect mental retardation and, consequently, the chance of associated language retardation will be described here. Descriptions will emphasize features that are more easily seen by the speech clinician and, consequently, will contribute to "visual diagnosis" of the condition.

Sex chromosome anomalies with associated mental retardation (Gellis and Feingold, 1968; Hamerton) include:

Klinefelter's syndrome, in which retardation is mild when present, is manifested by the following physical features: tall and slender stature, although obesity is also found; diminished facial and body hair; frontal hyperostosis of the head; myopia and astigmatism; and cleft palate and mandibular overgrowth.

Turner's syndrome (female), in which learning problems may appear secondary to cognitive and hearing difficulties, is manifested by the following physical features: short stature, webbing and(or) shortening of the neck, typical facial appearance including epicanthal folds, ptosis, strabismus and broad-bridged nose, low-set ears and nerve deafness, and high-arched palate and micrognathia.

Turner's syndrome (male), in which retardation may be mild to moderate, is reflected by the following physical characteristics: short stature, neck-webbing, ocular abnormalities (ptosis, epicanthal folds, antimongoloid slant, hypertelorism, myopia, strabismus), low-set ears and nerve deafness, broad-bridged nose, high-arched palate, and malocclusions.

Triplo-X and tetra-X females (superfemales and meta females) have also been identified (Polani, pp. 100–102). Recognizable somatic traits are not usually present in triplo-X females; however, severe intellectual subnormality appears common. No physical anomalies are reported in tetra-X females either, but severe intellectual impairment is.

Autosomal chromosome anomalies with associated mental retardation may be divided into two groups, those with numerical aberrations in which there are deviations in the number of chromosomes and those with structural aberrations in which there are deviations in the morphological appearance of the chromosomes.

Included among those with numerical aberrations are:

Down's syndrome (mongolism trisomy 21), where intellectual impairment varies considerably but where retardation is usually moderate, is manifested by the following physical features: brachycephaly and flattened occiput, ocular anomalies (epicanthal folds, oblique palpebral fissures, Brushfield spots, strabismus and nystagmus), malformed ear, broad-bridged nose, mouth abnormalities (open-mouthed posture, protruding tongue, small teeth, high-arched palate, fissured lips, furrowed tongue), simian finger line, muscular hypotonia.

Trisomy syndrome 16–18, or an extra chromosome among the chromosomes of group 16–18, has been reported (Fraccaro, Ch. 9) and appears to be associated with mental retardation. Some of the physical features include low-set and malformed ears, micrognathia, abnormal feet, flexion deformities of the fingers, and spasticity.

Trisomy 22 has been reflected by gross mental retardation with hyperkinesis, a "port-wine" nevus covering the distribution of the ophthalmic and maxillary division of the right trigeminal nerve, and buphthalmos of the right eye.

Included among the autosomal chromosome anomalies with structural aberrations (Gellis and Feingold, 1968) are:

Cri du chat, or cry of the cat syndrome (deletion of part of one of the short arms of the 4–5 group) is marked by severe retardation and characterized by cat-like cry (from birth to 5 months or more), rounded facies, microcephaly, ocular anomalies (hypertelorism, antimongoloid slant, epicanthal folds, strabismus), low-set ears, and micrognathia and occasionally cleft palate.

Deletion 18 (partial deletion of the long arm), in which retardation varies from moderate to profound, is characterized by the following physical features: short stature, microcephaly, mid-face retraction facies, ocular anomalies (epicanthal folds, hypertelorism, nystagmus), ear anomalies (low-set, atretic canals, deafness), deep voice, fish-like mouth, cleft lip and palate, hypotonia, and unsteadiness of gait.

Ring 18 (breakage from both arms with refusion to produce ring), in which retardation is usually severe, is marked by microcephaly, ocular abnormalities (epicanthal folds, hypertelorism, antimongoloid slant, strabismus, ptosis), ear irregularities (low-set, deafness, atresia of middle ear), cleft palate and micrognathia, brachydactyly, and seizures.

Gellis and Feingold (1968) have identified conditions that may include mental retardation and in which genetic involvement and chromosomal abnormalities are apparently not operative: cerebral gigantism (p. 17), Hallerman-Streiff syndrome (p. 47), happy puppet syndrome (p. 49), Sturge-Weber disease (p. 147), congenital rubella (p. 135), congenital syphilis (p. 149), congenital toxoplasmosis (p. 151), congenital hypothyroidism (p. 63), and kernicterus (p. 65).

Ford (1966) has identified the following additional conditions that may reflect mental retardation and in which genetic involvement and chromosomal abnormalities are apparently not operative: acute toxic encephalopathy (resulting from acute and severe infections such as diphtheria, pneumonia, erysipelas, scarlet fever, influenza, yellow fever, dysentery, cholera, as well as from various drugs and poisons) (pp. 593–596), toxoplasmic encephalitis (pp. 525–528), congenital heart disease (pp. 844–

848), congenital hemiplegia (pp. 26–30), Schüller-Christian disease (pp. 738–742), congenital spastic diplegia (pp. 16–24), and hemihypertrophy (pp. 150–151).

Clinical Manifestations

In a review of the literature on the speech of the mentally retarded, Matthews (1971, pp. 805–806) states (a) on the average, the mentally retarded child acquires language considerably later than the normal child; (b) when speech does emerge, the incidence of disorders is considerably higher than in the·general population; and (c) no evidence exists that disorders differ in kind from those disorders of nonretarded children. Morley (1965, Ch. 7), in a study of individuals with severe mental retardation, revealed that onset of speech was severely delayed, that the outstanding feature was the absence or poverty of speech, and that speech comprehension was better than expression.

Delay in onset of verbomotor behavior is a recognized feature of gnosogenic language dysfunction. Time of appearance of the first word among the retarded ranges from approximately 30 to 60 months (Darley and Winitz, 1961). Children classified as very severely retarded or custodial may remain nonverbal or learn only a few monosyllabic words; those classified as severely retarded or trainable may begin to use words at approximately 3 years of age; and those classified as moderately retarded or educable may begin to use words at approximately 2 years of age. Brown (1967), in a clinical observation on the first use of words by seriously retarded children reported that some may develop a few words at a nearly normal time but they disappear after a few days or after several months and never return (p. 337).

Variability in verbal behavior was described by Lillywhite and Bradley (1969) who state that "... there will be some with rather marked retardation who are more verbal than would be expected ... and there are some with mild retardation who present ... markedly deficient speech and language" (p. 115).

Verbal perseveration and the use of stereotyped phrases, frequently inappropriately, were also reported as language symptoms found among the retarded (Lillywhite and Bradley, 1969, p. 104).

Stutter-like speech may be manifested by many retarded children who suffer from a "paucity of ideas" (gnosogenic dysautomaticity). When such children are encouraged to speak about something of which they have little, if any, ideas they may lose whatever speech automaticity they may possess.

Diagnosis

Differential, direct, treatment, exclusion, and group diagnostic approaches may all be used in helping to determine gnosogenic language dysfunction.

Verbal immaturity is the outstanding gnosogenic verbal symptom. Retarded mental development is regarded as one of the most common backgrounds for retarded speech development (Matthews, 1971, p. 802; Morley, 1965, p. 76).

Verbal development and other developmental sequences are frequently correlated. Motor, intellectual, and social developments are depressed in keeping with the verbal immaturity.

Other major contributors to serious speech retardation must be eliminated. Serious hearing and visual problems should be ruled out as well as more specific brain dysfunction, emotional disorder, and experiential deprivation.

Prognosis

The prognosis for improvement in cases of gnosogenic language dysfunction is dependent on early identification; degree of severity of retardation; presence of complicating factors such as hearing and visual impairments, motor involvement, emotional disturbance; level of understanding, acceptance, and cooperation in the home; availability and quality of special schooling; and potential for medical relief of symptoms.

Therapy

At least five questions should be asked by the speech clinician planning a habilitation program for the retarded. Is the level of speech functioning in accordance with other developments, that is, does the child appear to be actualizing his full speech potential; and hence, should he be a candidate for speech therapy? How much unactualized speech potential may exist as a consequence of associated hearing problems and various adverse environmental factors? Is the retardation so severe that speech therapy is not advisable, except in the form of home stimulation carried out by the parents? Does the degree of involvement warrant special school placement and until the arrangements are made should interim speech therapy and home suggestions be offered? Even after special school placement should supplementary speech therapy and home programs be continued?

When a therapy plan is being formulated the clinician should consider appropriate activities within the full range of treatment approaches. Working with the retarded allows the clinician to use certain preventive measures as well as speech causal, symptom, compensatory, and supportive techniques.

Primary Preventive Measures. One way of reducing the incidence of gnosogenic language dysfunction is through genetic counseling. Couples in the child-bearing stage should be given information on those familial and chromosomal conditions that are associated with general as well as with speech retardation. The role of inadequate nutrition in retarding learning ability has also received an increasing amount of attention (Abelson, 1969, p. 17). To avoid nutritional brain damage, good nutrition is especially important during the first three years of life. Although no data exist on nutritionally-based language dysfunction the concept is worthy of consideration, especially in cases of children reared in poor environments.

Secondary Preventive Measures. A secondary preventive measure for the retarded includes providing optimal speech conditions for the infant to ensure that he utilizes his maximum potential for speech communication. Pre-speech-age and speech-age home programs that were recommended previously (see "Simple Language Immaturity— Therapy") are also applicable here.

Symptom and Compensatory Therapies. For ideas on symptom and compensatory therapy techniques, the reader is referred to "Genetic Language Dysmaturity—Therapy" and "Neurogenic Language Disorders in Children—Therapy." Lillywhite and Bradley (1969, Ch. 7 and 8) offer additional ideas in their two chapters devoted to management.

Supportive Procedures. The speech clinician must also accept his responsibility in those cases where little hope exists of the child's making any progress in verbal communication (Mysak, 1971). In those cases, the clinician helps the parents to adjust to their child's limitations in verbal or compensatory communication. Also, the parents should be helped to understand whatever body language or nonverbal affective communication (screams, smiles, whines, and other nonspeech signals) of which the child is capable.

PSYCHOGENIC LANGUAGE DISORDERS IN CHILDREN

Serious disturbance in socioemotional development may result in delay or retardation in verboacoustic and verbomotor behaviors. In fact, speech and language problems are considered key symptoms of childhood psychoses (Shervanian, 1967). An increasing amount of interest has grown among speech and hearing clinicians relative to their role in the evaluation and management of language dysfunction in the child with emotional disorder.

Background

Major subtypes of childhood psychosis identified by Shervanian (1967) include the nuclear schizophrenic child, early infantile autism, symbiotic psychotic child, the very young severely disturbed child with unusual sensitivities, and schizophrenic adjustment to neurological dysfunction. Kessler (1966, Ch. 11) divided the terminology used in childhood psychosis into general terms and specific categories. General terms include schizophrenia, atypical, infantile psychosis; specific categories include autism, symbiosis, organic, and nonorganic. Symptoms of schizophrenia, autism, and symbiosis are described here.

Childhood Schizophrenia. Some authorities believe that it is necessary to distinguish between childhood schizophrenia and infantile autism (Kessler, 1966, p. 267). Distinctive symptoms that are mentioned in childhood schizophrenia include: apparent signs and pathologic processes begin after five years; disordered behavior appears after an initial period of normal development; extreme anxiety, and presence of more physical and neurological symptoms such as disturbance in vasovegetative functioning, unevenness in somatic growth, EEG dysrhythmia, motor awkwardness, and perceptual problems.

Infantile Autism. Kessler (1966, pp. 265–273) reported on the following symptoms observed in autism in early infancy: no social smile, no evidence of pleasure in the mother's company, no physical reaching out to be lifted, no particular reaction to strangers, no imitation of gestures such as waving bye-bye, and no interest in social games like peekaboo and pattycake. Autistic children are described as looking normal and their motor coordination also seems normal; however, they lack eye-to-eye contact and appear "deaf" and "blind" to people. Playthings that can be manipulated, rolled, spun, juggled, fitted together, and clutched hold special interest for the autistic child. If preoccupation with special objects is the first major characteristic of such children, a second major characteristic is an obsessive desire to maintain sameness in, for example, routine or room arrangement.

Symbiosis. In contrast to autism, clinical symptoms of symbiotic psychosis are manifested between the ages of 2^1/$_2$ and 5 years (Kessler, 1966, pp. 273–275). Reported clinical features include a maternal relationship that allows no separation and abnormally low threshold for frustration. These children are described as manifesting intense and diffuse anxiety reactions, conflict between a desire for body contact and a shrinking from it, and catatonic-like temper tantrums and panic-stricken behavior.

Just as there is disagreement over types and subtypes of childhood psychosis there is controversy over their etiology. Theories on etiology include organic hypotheses and hypotheses of constitutional predisposition, parental psychopathology, and multiple causation. Some of the factors that appear important to prognosis in psychotic children include degree of regression or arrestment, presence of demonstrable neurological symptoms, and degree of disturbance of language function. For example, complete absence of speech after three years and absence of useful speech at age 5 were both reported as poor prognostic signs (Kessler, 1966, p. 291).

Another syndrome pertinent to this section is Heller's infantile dementia (Nelson, 1964, p. 1201). The condition is described "as a progressive dementia without other signs of organic neurologic disease." No definitive histopathologic pattern has been identified. Onset is in the second to fifth year of life. "The child, previously well or perhaps after an infection, becomes irritable and disobedient, has temper tantrums, may show perverse behavior, and then begins to regress in speech and mentation. Within a year he is mute, pays no attention to speech, often has tics, is incontinent, and may have to be fed." Despite extreme dementia an intelligent expression is said to persist.

Clinical Manifestations

Speech Perception-Comprehension Problems. Myklebust (1954, Ch. 8), in his discussion of psychic deafness (primarily childhood schizophrenia and autism), identifies the following symptoms: extreme fear of sounds in infancy and the relinquishing of hearing for speech in some schizophrenic children; ". . . parents state that he seems to hear but refuses to give attention to them," that is, he appears willfully to reject the auditory world; no direct responses to sound irrespective of intensity ("too deaf to be deaf"); and indirect responses to speech may be observed, for example, smiling in response to his name being spoken softly and changes in motor behavior in response to incidental comments. Shervanian (1967) indicated that in childhood psychoses auditory behavior may range from hypersensitivity to the simulation of anacusis.

Speech Formulation-Production Problems. Various symptoms of neurotigenic verbal inhibition (logoneurosis) have been observed. For example, Wood (1964, p. 81) speaks of ". . . children whose speech is limited to particular occasions or with particular people." West and Ansberry (1968, p. 240) report that some dysphemics ". . . exhibit marked reduction in the quantity of speech." Stuttering (psychogenic dysautomaticity) may also be observed and may be due to: a way to gain sympathy, attention, or provide an excuse for failure; a way to appear childish, dependent, and in need of help; a way to disrupt automatic speech that may result in the speaker's saying things he would rather not; a way to resolve the conflict between the desire to speak or to remain silent; and a way to self-fulfill the prediction that one cannot speak smoothly.

Psychotigenic verbomotor symptoms in childhood have also been identified. In a review of the literature on communication disorders in childhood psychoses, Shervanian (1967) reported the following symptoms: lack of speech, or cessation or regression of normally developing speech; cessation of interpersonal speech; silence except for animal sounds (zoophonia); long periods of silence interspersed with utterances of complete sentences; possession of a large, complex vocabulary which the child does not use in making meaningful sentences; and use of echolalia, delayed echolalia, and perseveration.

Attempts have also been made to associate language symptoms with types of developmental psychoses.

In schizophrenic children, de Hirsch (1967) identifies language symptoms accordingly: repetition of meaningless material such as long TV commercials; lack of use of speech in interpersonal relationships (reduced or inappropriate gestures, severely limited verbal output, echolalia); use of words as things instead of symbols for things; and investment of verbal symbols with highly personalized meanings.

In autistic children speech may be completely absent (mutism, alogia) or, when present, it may not be directed at a listener and may be characterized by repetition of stereotyped phrases, or be echolalic, or reflect neologisms.

In symbiotic children there may be repetition of phrases out of context, apparently without comprehension, and difficulty in the use of pronouns, that is, such children refer to themselves in the third person (Wood, 1964, p. 82). Mutism has also been reported and attributed to the existence of nonverbal or preverbal communication between symbiotic partners; episodic "talking tantrums" (verbal tantrums) have also been reported, that is, flighty and panic-stricken, irrelevant self-talk in response to frustration or spontaneously (Mahler *et al.,* 1959, pp. 827–828).

Verbal Thinking Problems. Fear of uttering certain words (logophobia) may be suspected in certain cases of developmental psychosis. Also, it has been reported that schizophrenic children occasionally experience auditory hallucinations (de Hirsch, 1967; Myklebust, 1954, p. 189). Some symptoms reported by de Hirsch (1967) also apply here, for example: absence of communicative intent; loss of symbolic status of words, or words are treated as things; and primary process distortion, or some words may be invested with highly personalized meanings and may symbolize fears of aggression and retaliation. Other symptoms of disorders in verbal thinking include logorrhea (excessive volubility) and the use of neologisms.

Clinical verbotypes that may be observed among emotionally-disturbed children are the inhibited verbotype who speaks only when spoken to; the manic verbotype who speaks continuously; the hostile verbotype who uses ridicule, hostile silence, and hostile paralanguage; the pseudocommunication verbotype who uses carefully monitored, guarded, and restricted communication; and the deceptive verbotype who uses distortion and fabrication.

Diagnosis

Diagnosis of psychogenic language dysfunction in childhood requires the clinician to rule out language dysfunction secondary to hearing loss, brain damage, mental retardation, or combinations of these. Attempts should also be made to identify linguistic patterns whenever possible and to correlate them with subtypes of developmental psychoses.

Prognosis

The prognosis for improvement in childhood psychosis is relatively poor and, hence, so is improvement in language function. Lack of progress in the resolution of the psychosis has been connected in one case with the absence of speech after three years and in another with the absence of useful speech at the age of 5. This emphasizes the potential importance of the speech clinician in the event that he could effectively apply language symptom therapy.

Therapy

The application of language symptom therapy in developmental psychoses is a relatively new area for most speech clinicians. However, an increasing number of such children are being referred to speech and hearing centers by psychiatrists and psychologists. The reason for these referrals is in part related to: (a) a major symptom of childhood psychosis is the absence of or severely disturbed language, and (b) the major healing tool of psychiatry-psychology is language. Hence, if a specialist in speech communication could stimulate or organize the language of the psychotic child, solid psychotherapy could begin. In most instances, speech therapy and psychotherapy for these children are interrelated and interdependent; and both specialists should work closely together. Following are some principles to be considered by the speech clinician who may be developing a plan of therapy for the psychotic child. The principles are based on psychologic, neurologic, and communicologic theories of language development.

Psychologic Orientation. The autism theory of speech development (Mowrer, 1958) may serve as a basis for the formulation of language symptom work with psychotic children. Briefly, the theory is applied as follows: (a) a speaker should become a positive emotional stimulus for the child by providing pleasurable sensations, for example, by feeding or sharing desired food with the child, by accompanying the child to places that apparently bring pleasure to the child, or by engaging in either parallel or cooperative play; (b) after a period of time, and after the clinician believes that the child looks forward to his visits, the clinician may begin to use a certain goal word or goal phrase during the time he engages in the various pleasure-producing situations. After the successful application of the first two steps, it is hoped that: (a) the clinician's utterances alone will evoke positive emotional feelings within the child; (b) the child will begin to approximate the clinician's word or phrase because he will self-stimulate the positive emotional feeling by his attempt; and (c) the child will continue to refine his verbal approximation because more accurate versions should evoke greater degrees of satisfaction. When the child shows behaviors b and c he should be immediately rewarded for the attempts.

The successful application of this theory by the speech clinician depends on his ability to become a positive emotional experience for the child, his ability to judge when his presence begins to elicit good feelings within the child, and his ability to judge when the goal word or goal phrase itself begins to elicit good feelings.

Neurologic Orientation. A neurophysiologic orientation to the explanation of oral language development (Penfield and Roberts, 1959) may also be utilized in formulating language symptom techniques. The theory may be applied as follows: (a) a neuronal pattern representing the object of a goal word or phrase is established in both hemispheres by having the child experience all sensory dimensions of the object over a period of time; (b) a neuronal pattern representing the heard goal word or phrase that symbolizes the object is established in the corticothalamic speech areas in the left hemisphere by the consistent association by the clinician of the uttered goal word with the object; (c) automatic and reciprocal connections between the two neuronal patterns are established by the frequency of their association; (d) the neuronal pattern representing the spoken goal word or phrase that symbolizes the object is established in the corticothalamic speech areas in the left hemisphere by virtue of establishing the object pattern, the heard word pattern, and the reflexive and reciprocal connection between the two.

The successful application of this theory by the speech clinician depends on his ability to get the "feel" of creating neuronal patterns. For example, how much and what kind of stimulation is needed before a perceptual pattern representing a given object is established? How often must the oral symbol representing the object be uttered before the auditory pattern is established?

Communicologic Orientation. Finally, a speech-system-based orientation to the explanation of oral language development (Mysak, 1966, Ch. 3) may also be used as a guide in developing language symptom techniques. At least three guiding principles may be utilized.

Primacy of perception of paralanguage and oral language may be regarded as the first guide. Comprehension of kinetic paralanguage such as body postures, facial expressions, hand gestures, and tonal paralanguage are comprehended by children before they comprehend verboacoustic code. Similarly, verboacoustic code is comprehended before children can formulate and express verbomotor code. Hence, early work in stimulating language function in psychotic children might involve simple "give me," "show me" verbal interactions, first with appropriate paralanguage and then with combinations of paralanguage and actual language. This procedure presents a simple comprehension task for the child and allows the child to respond with simple movements of the body.

Primacy of intravocalizing and intraverbalizing may be considered as a second guide. In the normal child the first six months of life are characterized by the babbling stage of speech-sound rehearsal. Babbling is basically intravocalizing behavior engaged in by the child during contented moments such as after feeding and on awakening. During the next few months, intravocalizing may be characterized by the child's repetition of self-produced sounds or sound combinations or the lalling stage of speech-sound rehearsal. At about 10 to 12 months, the child may be noted to imitate sounds and sound combinations made by others and this marks the beginning of the intervocalizing stage, or developmental echolalia.

Similarly, from about 12 to 18 months the first recognizable words may emerge and rapid development of words and speech occurs up to 3 years. During this period the child also accompanies his activities with the words he is acquiring. Apparently, one important reason for speech during this time is to verbalize perceptual processes. Intraverbalizing behavior apparently is a precursor to verbal thinking. After 3 years, a steady increase occurs in the amount of interverbalizing behavior over intraverbalizing.

The discussion should suggest various practical applications of the ideas expressed, depending on the child's level of communication. For example, the clinician might accompany parallel play activities with strings of syllables and syllable combinations. Next, he may exhibit an interest in his vocalizations by periodically repeating certain syllables and syllable combinations and by assuming a self-listening attitude while doing so. If the child begins to intravocalize, the clinician should echo the child's sounds in the hopes of triggering an organized intervocalization activity. Following this development, the clinician may then engage in intraverbalizing behavior or self-talking while he moves about the therapy room, while he plays with the child, or while he looks at or handles objects. He should use simple, short descriptive phrases to describe his activities. Hopefully, the child may begin to accompany his activities with self-talk. If there is a lag in this development, the clinician could provide a running commentary of the child's activities in the hopes of eliciting this desired intraverbalizing behavior. If all goes well in these activities, the child should exhibit a greater inclination toward interverbalizing.

Primacy of expression of kinetic and tonal paralanguage may be considered a third guide in working with developmental psychoses. Just as children first come to understand the accompanying body postures, hand gestures, facial expressions, and tonal aspects of speech communication, so too children first express themselves in this form. Hence, the clinician should reward all attempts by the child to communicate first with paralanguage. For example, the child may use body language and random vocalization or body language and accompanying onomatopoetic vocalization.

SOCIOGENIC LANGUAGE DISORDERS IN CHILDREN

Sociogenic language disorders describe those cases of delayed onset or retarded development of speech resulting from evironmental conditions. The environmental conditions referred to are usually not of the magnitude to cause important emotional disturbance.

Background

A review of the literature (Mysak, 1971) reveals reports of various socioemotional factors that may cause language retardation in childhood.

Insufficient stimulation is one factor in language dysmaturation. Such reduced stimulation may be related to absence of either parent in the home (e.g., both working), and "quiet" or relatively nonspeaking parents or parent surrogates.

Inappropriate stimulation is a possible second factor. Such stimulation may take the form of exposure to excessive amounts of verbal discipline or "angry" talk and poor language models.

Reduced motivation is a possible third factor. For example, the child may have parents or siblings who anticipate his needs and desires and make it less necessary for him to communicate.

Inappropriate rewards for speech is a possible fourth factor. Problems may arise as a result of rewards for "baby talk" or lack of rewards for progress in language development.

Other possible factors are birth of a sibling, accident, shock, and parental rejection.

Clinical Manifestations

No specific verbal symptoms of sociogenic origin are recognized. Depending on the background and severity of reaction, the problem may range from a lack of language to mild grammatical and syntactical immaturities.

Diagnosis

The diagnosis of sociogenic language dysfunction is based mainly on the ruling out of the major backgrounds for language involvement or diagnosis by exclusion.

Prognosis

If the underlying cause for the sociogenic language problem is identified and if the clinician can elicit cooperation from significant adults the prognosis is favorable.

Therapy

Depending on the diagnosis, the major approach to therapy for sociogenic language dysfunction is speech counseling for the parents plus a home program. In some cases, supplemental speech therapy by the clinician may also be necessary.

Speech counseling includes informing the parents of the apparent background of the problem and providing information on language hygiene. Language hygiene counseling may be based on the ideas of West and Ansberry (1968, p. 50) on speech development referred to in Chapter 2. "That child will develop speech earliest and best whose environment is one that provides . . . (a) rich experience with good speakers, both children and adults, (b) real need for, and pleasure to be derived from, oral communication on the part of the child, and (c) rewards for, and encouragement of, day-by-day improvement in his speech."

Home programs include instructions on the practical application of the comments of West and Ansberry on the facilitation of speech development.

Clinical programs include selected procedures and techniques found under the therapy portions of the sections on gnosogenic, neurogenic, and psychogenic language dysfunctions.

NEUROGENIC LANGUAGE DISORDERS IN ADULTS

Damage to the speech brain may result in two kinds of verbal symptoms: (a) positive symptoms or the release of paleovocal activity such as echolalia and jargon, and (or) paleoverbal activity such as excessive self-talk and perseveration; and (b) negative symptoms or the loss, reduction, or disturbance of verbal behavior.

Backgrounds

Bases for involvement of the speech brain and hence language function in the adult are numerous. Categories of conditions to be described here are trauma, vascular disorders, degenerative diseases, infections, and neoplasms.

Trauma. Brain injuries may result from automobile accidents, industrial accidents, falls, and penetrating wounds.

Concussion, cerebral contusion, cerebral laceration, and cerebral compression may follow injury to the head (Brain and Walton, 1969, pp. 336–340. Concussion results from direct injury to nerve cells, which is reversible in milder cases but may be permanent, and is not associated with the grosser changes found in cerebral contusion and laceration. Cerebral contusion is a focal or diffuse brain disturbance characterized by edema and capillary hemorrhages and chromatolysis (solution and disintegration of the chromatin of cell nuclei) of cortical nerve cells; aphasia may follow a contusion involving the cortex. Cerebral laceration describes a cerebral contusion severe enough to cause a visible separation in the brain substance. Such a tear may occur immediately beneath the site of the blow or on the opposite side of the brain (by contrecoup). Cerebral compression results when the head injury is followed by intracranial hemorrhage.

Traumatic pneumocephalus (Brain and Walton, 1969, pp. 344–346), or the presence of air within the skull resulting from head injury, is usually due to a fracture of the skull allowing communication between the air-containing cranial cavity and the interior of the skull. Focal cerebral symptoms including aphasia may be present when air invades one cerebral hemisphere.

Traumatic subdural hematoma (Brain and Walton, 1969, pp. 346–348), or an encysted collection of blood between the dura mater and the arachnoid resulting from injury, may reflect focal cerebral symptoms, among them aphasia, when the lesion is left-sided.

Vascular Disorders. Cerebrovascular disease is frequently associated with aphasia. Various forms of the disease are recognized (Minckler, 1971, p. xvii; Brain and Walton, 1969, Ch. 2).

Cerebral arteriosclerosis, or arterial thickening, may be due to degeneration of the intima (innermost of the three coats of an artery) in the form of atheroma, degeneration secondary to high blood pressure, and endarteritis (inflammation of the intima of an artery).

Cerebral thrombosis, or a clot in a cerebral blood vessel, may, for example, be due to cerebral arteriosclerosis, syphilitic endarteritis, atheroma, trauma, acute infections, or profound anemia.

Cerebral embolism, or the sudden blocking of a cerebral artery by a clot or other material brought to the place by the blood circulation, may, for example, result from clots from internal and common carotid arteries, clots from aneurysm of the innominate artery, clots following coronary thrombosis, and clots from the lung.

Hypertensive encephalopathy, a form of cerebral disturbance occurring in disorders with different pathologies but with a common tendency to cause arterial hypertension, may include aphasia as one of its focal cerebral disturbances.

Cerebral hemorrhage, or the escape of blood from cerebral blood vessels, may result from the rupturing of an aneurysm, and from toxic and infective conditions, acute encephalitis, severe anemia, leukemia, and severe trauma.

Degenerative Diseases. Various degenerative diseases may also cause language dysfunction.

Facial hemiatrophy, a disorder of early life, is characterized by progressive wasting of some or all of the tissues of one side of the face and has been known also to reflect aphasia (Brain and Walton, 1969, p. 618).

Alzheimer's disease is a progressive cerebral degeneration occurring in middle life (Brain and Walton, 1969, pp. 991–992). Symptoms include progressive dementia with speech disturbances and apraxia.

Pick's disease is marked by circumscribed atrophy of the cerebral cortex usually involving the frontal and temporal regions (Brain and Walton, 1969, p. 992). Progressive dementia and aphasia characterize the disease.

Infections. Numerous types of cerebral infections may affect speech areas and consequently language function.

Cerebral abscess may result from an infection which reaches the brain by the direct spread of otitis media or sinusitis, or via the blood stream from pneumonia or pulmonary abscess (Espir and Rose, 1970, p. 97). Cerebral abscess acts as an intracranial space-occupying lesion and, depending on its location, may result in focal neurological symptoms including aphasia.

Meningovascular syphilis is a form of neurosyphilis that particularly involves the cerebral vessels and meninges (Espir and Rose, 1970, pp. 100–101). Aphasia may be a symptom if speech areas are involved.

Nervous complications including aphasia have also been reported in whooping cough, typhoid fever, malaria, and mumps.

Neoplasms. "Primary intracranial tumours originate from the structures within the skull, e.g. the meninges (meningioma) or within the brain (e.g. glioma). The secondary intracranial tumours (metastases) originate from a primary growth elsewhere in the body, usually a carcinoma of the lung or breast" (Espir and Rose, 1970, p. 78). Involvement of speech areas by such tumors may result in aphasic symptomatology.

Clinical Manifestations

Neurogenic language symptoms in adults are discussed under the categories of disorders of speech perception-comprehension, speech formulation-production, and verbal thinking.

Speech Perception-Comprehension Problems. Numerous symptoms of verboacoustic involvement have been reported.

1. Difficulty in understanding first complex sentences and then simple elementary ones in the second stage of Alzheimer's disease (Ferraro, 1959a, p. 1047). Also in demented speech, "difficulty in understanding quick or noisy speech" (Espir and Rose, 1970, p. 65).

2. Problems in understanding speech with continued ability to speak (transcortical sensory aphasia) may follow problems with recall of names and objects in certain cases of Pick's disease (Ferraro, 1959a, p. 1058). Paraphasia leading to jargonaphasia may then develop.

3. Varieties of aphasic syndromes including verboacoustic symptoms have been reported. Among them are: (a) loss of ability to comprehend spoken words, impaired reading and writing, associated syllable and word paraphasias, and tendency toward perseveration and echolalia, with preservation of spontaneous speech (Wernicke's or sensory aphasia); (b) almost total inability to comprehend spoken words, a tendency to paraphasia, perseveration, jargonaphasia, and retention memory impairment, with ability to read, write, and to speak spontaneously (transcortical sensory aphasia); (c) inability to associate a spoken word with visual stimulus objects, but retained ability to repeat spoken words and to name objects seen or at least to demonstrate knowledge of their significance (auditory-visual aphasia; Konorski, 1967, p. 227); (d) comprehension of names of visual objects, but disturbance in comprehension of names representing parts of the body, without body scheme disturbance, and names representing textures such as rough, smooth, soft, and hard without disturbance of touch and stereognosis (auditory-somesthetic aphasia; Konorski, 1967, p. 238); (e) impaired comprehension of words based on perceptual alterations, on confusion of referential meaning, or semantic errors, and on reduction of retention span (Schuell, 1969, pp. 110–126); and (f) reduced duration of sensory impressions causing disturbance of speech perception and association as in acute diseases and brain concussion (Grashey's aphasia).

Speech Formulation-Production Problems. Verbomotor symptoms may reflect various kinds of damage to speech areas.

1. Sudden arrest of speech or difficulty in speaking correctly characterize *speech seizures,* a category of circumscribed motor seizures described by Strauss (1959, pp. 1117–1118). The symptoms are associated with abnormal discharges in the speech areas. Pre-ictal, ictal, and post-ictal dysphasia are terms used to describe speech difficulty before, during, or after seizures. Transient interference with verbomotor function may also be observed in migraine conditions (migrainous dysphasia).

2. Aphasia, a sudden convulsion, or a transient hemiplegia may herald the onset of neurosyphilis (Bruetsch, 1959). As the *syphilogenic speech disturbance* progresses, the individual is unable to form sentences (syntactic aphasia) and in the terminal phase of neurosyphilis, speech may be completely unintelligible (p. 1008).

3. Various types of *degenerative speech symptoms* have been recognized in association with forms of progressive neuropathologies. Ferraro (1959a, pp. 1047–1048) described the following forms of language dysfunction in the second stage of Alzheimer's disease: echolalia; iterative, explosive expression of words or syllables; and gradually a senseless, paraphasic jargon may be observed. With prompting, some patients may succeed in temporarily producing comprehensive language. Verbaliza-

tion ceases during the terminal stage of the disease. Difficulty in recalling words in the early stages of Alzheimer's disease, followed by paraphasic talkativeness and then a reduction to isolated words and phrases has been reported (Brain and Walton, 1969, p. 992).

More frequent occurrence of paleovocal and paleoverbal manifestations (i.e., echolalia, perseveration, palilalia, logoclony) in comparison to that in Alzheimer's disease has been described in Pick's disease by Ferraro (1959a, p. 1058). Lack of spontaneous speech, dysbulic aphasia (involvement of will to speak), reluctance to engage in conversations, and answering in monosyllables are other symptoms observed in Pick's disease. Brain and Walton (1969, p. 992) report that in the early stages of Pick's disease the patient "is often voluble and tends to make jokes and puns." As the disease progresses, speech may be reduced to a few stereotyped phrases.

Echolalia has been reported in diffuse sclerosis (Mulder, 1959, p. 1157).

In describing demented speech (related to intellectual deterioration) in adults, Rose and Espir (1970, p. 65) identify the following symptoms: incompletion of sentences begun (apotheosis), use of unnecessary additional words (paralogisms), perseveration, and echolalia.

4. Various patterns of verbomotor symptoms are: (a) loss of spontaneous speech and the ability to repeat words with relatively intact comprehension, reading, and writing (Broca's aphasia); (b) loss of spontaneous speech and the ability to repeat words, and loss of ability to write spontaneously or from dictation, but relatively intact speech comprehension and reading (transcortical motor aphasia); (c) gross disturbance in ability to repeat words, but relatively good comprehension, naming, and spontaneous speech. Gross disturbance in ability to repeat words, relatively good comprehension, with involvement of naming and spontaneous speech (forms of auditory-verbal aphasia; Konorski, 1967, p. 246); (d) difficulty in naming objects seen with intact comprehension and repetition ability (visual-verbal aphasia; Konorski, 1967, p. 249); (e) telegraphic speech, paucity of words, but retained words are spoken correctly (kinesthetic aphasia; Konorski, 1967, p. 50); (f) distorted and usually unintelligible speech, auditory awareness of distorted speech, repetitive attempts at correction (Luria aphasia, somesthetic aphasia; Konorski, 1967, p. 138); (g) limitations in verbal formulation and production due to problems in retrieval of available lexemes, phonemic disintegration resulting from reduced somesthetic and auditory feedbacks, and difficulty in arranging phrasal utterances (Schuell, 1969, pp. 110–126); (h) limitation in spontaneous expression due to reduction of incoming stimuli as with certain thalamic involvements, retrieval problems, dysarthria, and sensorimotor problems (Schuell, 1969, pp. 120–121).

Other symptoms of verbomotor involvement include: inability to express oneself in a connected manner (acataphasia); disturbance in speech due to passion or fright (pathematic aphasia); ability to utter words, but not sentences (ataxaphasia); slow utterance (bradyphasia); saying one thing when meaning to say something else (heterophasia); use of words without comprehension of their meaning (paramnesia); and inability to recall names of objects felt (myotactic paranomia).

Dysphatic dysautomaticity or stutter-like speech may be observed in some aphasics who attempt to speak at their premorbid levels of speech automaticity when they no longer enjoy automatic retrieval of needed vocabulary. Another form of central stuttering may occur in cases of involvement in volitional mechanisms due to damage in the frontal lobes and may be called dysbulic dysautomaticity or dysbulic aphasia. The stutter-like speech results when an individual is unable to automatically will-to-speak or suffers from an episodic inability to release the speech mechanism or indecisiveness about releasing the speech mechanism.

Verbal Thinking Problems. Verbal thinking problems are reflected in verbal denial patterns, verbal memory loss, hypomanic speech, reduced spontaneous speech, and verbal delirium.

Verbal denial patterns associated with brain injury and physical incapacity were described by Weinstein and Kahn (1959). Verbal patterns of denial, as modes of adaptation to stress, are categorized by the authors under the heading of explicit denial, confabulation, paraphasia, reduplication, and amnesia.

1. Explicit verbal denial, or anosognosia, is reported in connection with conditions such as aphasia, hemiplegia, toxic encephalopathy, self-inflicted head wounds, and following craniotomy and prefrontal lobotomy. In addition, such patients may exhibit a lack of verbal spontaneity and may speak only when spoken to.

2. Confabulation and delusions may be observed to accompany negation of illnesses such as head injury, self-inflicted head wounds, subarachnoid hemorrhage, and following craniotomy for removal of neoplasms. Confabulations, or ". . . the creation and recitation of fantastic, extravagant events, often changeable . . ." have been reported in senile psychosis of the presbyophrenic type (Ferraro, 1959b, p. 1029), in toxic-infectious polyneuritis, and in cerebral arteriosclerosis (Ferraro, 1959c, p. 1086). The prinicipal characteristics of Korsakoff's psychosis (chronic alcoholic disorder probably due to vitamin deficiencies) are extreme memory defects and confabulation (Thompson, 1959). Lack of judgment, suggestibility, and memory defect cause the patient". . . to fabricate all kinds of fanciful tales to fill in the gaps in his memory" (p. 1214).

3. Paraphasic misnaming, without apparent awareness by the patient, is another form of verbal denial. Misnamed objects are mainly those that relate to the person's illness and his hospitalization. Verbal "metonymyzing," or the patient talking about himself in terms of some

object (for example, in terms of a car if he was in a car accident), has also been observed.

4. Verbal reduplication for place, time, person, or body parts may also be found. A patient may claim that there are two hospitals like the one he is in; that an event or experience of the present has also occurred in the past; that a person of the same or similar identity to an existing person exists; and that he has an extra arm, four legs, or two heads (reduplicated body parts are the disabled ones).

5. Amnesia following head injury may be seen as ". . . a form of language in which the patient denies or otherwise represents his problems and expresses a relationship in his environment" (Weinstein and Kahn, 1959, p. 973).

Verbal memory loss is characteristic of various organic conditions. In the early stages of Alzheimer's disease (Ferraro, 1959a, p. 1047–1048) patients have difficulty in recalling names of persons or objects. As the disease progresses, memory becomes increasingly more impaired and "trains of thoughts are markedly disconnected." Verbal perseveration, first of phrases, then words, syllables, and phonemes, reaches its maximum and is viewed by Ferraro as reflecting ". . . poverty of thought and a path of least effort."

Amnesic aphasia is generally the first verbal symptom to appear in cases of Pick's disease with outstanding aphasic manifestation (about 25% of the cases according to Ferraro (1959a, p. 1058)).

In senility, first there is difficulty in recalling proper names, then names of abstract objects, and finally names of things. Instead of names, descriptions and circumlocutions may be used (Ferraro, 1959b, p. 1025).

For patients with left prefrontal lesions, carrying out a series of movements (programing of movements) in response to verbal instructions is extremely difficult (Konorski, 1967, p. 157).

First symptoms of bromide toxicity (bromism) may include slurred speech and defective memory and retention. Later, confabulations may be observed as a reaction to the individual's memory deficits (McGraw and Oliver, 1959, p. 1558).

Hypomanic speech or chemokinetic speech disorder may be induced by therapeutic doses of amphetamines. Individuals may ". . . become more talkative and anxious to express themselves." Larger doses or even average doses in some susceptible individuals may cause hypomanic speech where the ". . . push of speech may become so intense that incoherence or babbling results" (McGraw and Oliver, 1959, p. 1561).

Reduced spontaneous speech has been reported in patients with tumors in the dominant frontal lobe and after left frontal lobectomy and may be related to a pathologic paucity of ideas to express. Another possibility is a defect in volitional mechanisms in which the individual finds it difficult to will the initiation of speech (dysbulic speech disorder).

Verbal delirium may be observed in cases of chronic alcoholism, febrile illness, senility, and after severe head injury and may be viewed as an outward manifestation of abnormally stimulated inner speech. Mussitation, or articulatory movements with no utterance of sound (delirium mussitans), may also be observed.

Hallucinatory, delusional, and illusional episodes are experienced in delirium ar.d may be associated with a variety of distorted verbalization (Ebaugh and Tiffany, 1959). In a mild delirium individuals ". . . will respond to questions coherently, and spontaneous expressions are clearly expressed . . ."; in more severe reactions, ". . . speech becomes incoherent and in some instances consists of unintelligible muttering . . .," however, even in such cases ". . . rousing the patient and fixing his attention on simple concrete questions will usually result in coherent and often logical answers to simple questions" (p. 1233).

Diagnosis

Adult language dysfunction related to brain involvement must be differentiated from other problems that have similar symptoms. An attempt must also be made to determine the degree of specificity of the problem.

West and Ansberry (1968, pp. 163–168) have advised that aphasia be differentiated from primary amentia. Primary amentia is viewed as a congenital condition that reflects a generalized deficiency. Serious hearing loss as well as amnesia must also be differentiated from neurogenic language dysfunction. West and Ansberry define amnesia as ". . . a break in the continuity of the stream of experiences by which an individual recognizes his own identity." Such an individual may have difficulty with questions concerning temporal orientations, spatial orientation, and psychosocial relationships. Psychotigenic language dysfunction must also be differentiated from neurogenic language impairment.

In the hopes of better defining the pathophysiology of various types of aphasia, clinicians may routinely request radioactive isotope brain scan (Benson and Patton, 1967). Such studies should eventually add knowledge with respect to the correlation between site of lesion and clinical symptomatology.

Prognosis

Improvement in cases of neurogenic language dysfunction is related to medical, psychologic, language, and speech therapy factors.

Medical Factors. Prognosis for improvement is more favorable the younger the client, the more focalized the lesion, the more reversible the lesion, the greater the response to medical treatment, and the fewer the associated medical problems such as motor, visual, sensory, and convulsive problems.

Psychologic Factors. Prognosis for improvement is more favorable in cases where there are fewer so-called organic behavioral manifestations such as emotional lability, catastrophic response, and rigidity. Also important is a helpful and supportive family situation.

Language Factors. Prognosis for improvement is more favorable in cases of good premorbid language ability, in cases of more specific language involvement, and in cases where verboacoustic function is in relatively good condition. Of nine factors related to prognosis for individual aphasics, Keenan and Brassell (1974) reported that four had a definite relationship with eventual speech performance: initial listening performance, initial talking performance, motor speech impairment, and speech stimulability.

Therapy Factor. The earlier speech therapy is offered the better the prognosis. Also, in the case of certain stroke-aphasics, Hagen (1973) confirmed the value of speech therapy in a treatment vs. no treatment study which showed ". . . that while both groups exhibited spontaneous improvement during the first three months of the program, only the treatment group continued to progress beyond the point of spontaneous recovery to attain functional communication ability."

Therapy

Therapy procedures for neurogenic language dysfunction in adults are presented under the headings of primary and secondary preventive measures, and causal, symptom, and compensatory procedures.

Primary Preventive Measures. Speech clinicians should cooperate in all ways possible to inform the public on how to minimize stroke and its frequent sequela, aphasia. Appropriate exercise, proper diet, adequate rest, reduction of stress, and attention to hypertension conditions are factors that may be important in reducing the incidence of stroke-aphasia.

Secondary Preventive Measures. Factors that contribute to secondary language symptoms include reduced attempts at communication because of repeated communication failures, reduced stimulation for communication because of restricted hospital or home enviroments, reduced attempts at communication because of negative reactions by significant listeners (e.g., wife, husband, children), and reduced attempts at communication because of anticipation of needs by significant listeners.

The clinician must develop a program that will counteract these causes of secondary language involvement. Family, nurses, doctors, fellow patients, and friends must make every attempt to reinforce the patient's attempts at communication by giving him extra time to communicate and by making every effort to understand. The clinician helps in this process by assisting the client to develop compensatory forms of communication until more progress is made in speech communication.

Potential listeners should be impressed with the need to maintain a "talking" atmosphere around the client. The client must not be allowed to withdraw gradually from speaking situations because of his difficulties. Significant listeners must be cautioned against showing frustration, discomfort, and impatience with the individual and from anticipating needs in order to reduce communication encounters.

Causal Therapy. Causal therapy includes drugs and special surgery (e.g., arterial surgery) to relieve the underlying cause of the language problem. Causal therapy is carried out by the physician; however, the speech clinician has an important consultative role to play.

Symptom Therapy. There are six general principles in symptom therapy.

1. *Stimulation of verboacoustic behavior* should be emphasized especially in the early stages of aphasia. Patients frequently understand "almost everything" while they may not say too much. Part of this comprehension-formulation gap may be attributed to differential vulnerability to damage of tissues in the major speech brain, to the amount of tissue subserving verboacoustic as compared to verbomotor behavior, and to the role of the minor speech brain in comprehension.

The clinician should take advantage of this gap by engaging in intercommunication activities in which the client will enjoy success. Responses to "show me," "point to," series of questions; responses to instructions for a series of movements or acts; and "yes" or "no" responses to questions about short stories and newspaper articles read aloud are possible verboacoustic exercises.

2. *Stimulation of minor speech behavior* is recommended. Language-disturbed adults frequently retain their ability to count, give days of the week or months of the year, utter the alphabet, recite certain poems, and produce "social amenity" utterances such as, "Good morning," "How are you," and "I'm fine." Much of this verbomotor behavior may be mediated by the minor speech brain. Clients should be encouraged to utter as much of this minor speech as possible for at least two reasons. (a) Minor speech stimulates and keeps active certain recurrent speech loops, that is, it allows the phonoarticulatory system to produce intact, organized speech and the auditory and tactile-proprioceptive channels to monitor it; such recurrent speech loops must not be allowed to remain inactive, thereby chancing the development of secondary disorders. (b) At a time when the client may be capable of producing little or no major speech and when he may be despairing of ever being able to do so again, he finds that he can produce intelligible speech and he can hear and feel it; for many clients the confirmation that they continue to be able to produce organized speech is an important motivating factor.

3. *Stimulation of echo speech behavior* should also be planned wherever possible on a daily basis. The client might echo a series of utterances related to personal identification, for example, "What is my name—

My name is...."; "How old am I—I am ... old"; "Where do I live—I live at. . . ." Other functional speech units should be based on family members, food, clothing, personal needs, and so forth. Such work, in addition to serving the purposes mentioned in the previous section, serves to restimulate more volitional use of such functional speech.

4. *Verbal thinking activities* should also be planned. The techniques here are similar to those described in "Neurogenic Language Disorders in Children—Therapy." Periodically, during each day inter-reporting should be carried out by significant others in the client's environment. The client should be informed about the technique. Inter-reporting is simply describing aloud and in short, simple phrases the activities of the client, for example, "You are getting out of bed . . . You are putting on your pants . . . your socks . . . your shoes . . . and your shirt." As soon as it is possible, the client should be encouraged to lead all his behavior with short, out-loud descriptions, or to intra-report. Inter-reporting and intra-reporting allow for great amounts of daily verbal stimulation and keep active verbal thinking loops.

5. *Encouragement of kinetic paralanguage support of verbomotor attempts* is also useful. The client should be encouraged to accompany speech attempts with appropriate paralanguage, for example, as he attempts to ask for a glass of water, he may reach out, grab an imaginary glass, bring it to his lips, and pretend to drink. Such supportive body language is associated with early attempts at verbalizing and may serve to facilitate the production of the desired utterance.

6. *Expansion of verbal association time* is another helpful technique. A common problem in aphasia is the need for increased time before various verbal associations may take place. Two techniques designed to counter this association-time problem are: (a) A client may be asked to refrain from attempting to respond to a question until he has formulated a response in his mind and checked it for accuracy. (b) A client may be asked not to respond to a question or instruction until he has repeated the utterance aloud as well as in his mind.

Compensatory Therapy. When language recovery is proceeding slowly, appears limited, or is not possible at all, compensatory techniques should be used. Such techniques include developing paralanguage communication, using objects and pictures to indicate needs, and using a language board. These techniques may be used very early in cases where there is great frustration in communication and where the client is reacting negatively to his limited ability to communicate via speech.

PSYCHOGENIC LANGUAGE DISORDERS IN ADULTS

Psychogenic language disorders in adults describe the various disturbances of language function that may accompany emotional disturbance.

Background

Some of the more common psychoses and psychoneuroses that reflect language disintegration are schizophrenia, manic-depressive states, hysteria, and obsessive behavior.

Schizophrenia. Arieti (1959a, Ch. 23) offers the following general description of schizophrenia. Anomalous behavior usually begins between the time of puberty and the early thirties. The symptoms may appear in a gradual fashion or in some cases in a more or less acute fashion. Categories of possible symptoms include content-of-thought symptoms, general behavior symptoms, mood and affective symptoms, and speech and language symptoms.

Content-of-thought symptoms include ideas of reference where the person thinks "certain things are related to him or have a special meaning," delusions or false beliefs (generally negative), illusions or misperceptions, and hallucinations or false perceptions (usually auditory).

General behavior symptoms include odd "mannerisms, grimaces, purposeless acts, stereotyped motions, impulsive gestures."

Mood and affective symptoms are reflected by the individual appearing ". . . angry, highly emotional, suspicious, cynical, etc. . . ." Frequently the emotional tone is inappropriate ". . . ranging from a relative coldness to complete apathy . . . ." The patient may appear withdrawn and to have lost interest in his surroundings.

Speech and language symptoms include evasive responses to questions, unrelated word sequences (word-salad), perseveration, neologisms, blocking, and mutism.

Paranoid, hebephrenic, catatonic, and simple types are specific forms of schizophrenia described by Arieti (1959a).

The paranoid type reflects, in general, the symptomatology just described. Characteristic features include slightly later onset of disorder and suspiciousness and bitterness from the beginning; ideas of reference symptoms and delusions (persecutory) are more prominent, and hallucinations (especially auditory) are common.

The hebephrenic type is considered the most difficult to define. Some characteristic features include: grandiose delusions are more common than in the paranoid type; hypochondriacal ideas, preoccupations with body image and kinesthetic delusions are more common; hallucinations are common; mood is often characterized by apathy and detachment; and language disorders are prominent (word-salad, clang associations (confusing words that sound alike), and neologisms are common).

The catatonic type is more characteristic than the other types and its symptoms include: after a period of agitated and apparently aimless behavior, the patient gradually slows down to almost complete immobility; in the catatonic stupor the individual cannot dress himself, feed himself, or talk; the individual suffers a disturbance in his faculty to will and hence cannot will to move; the body may be placed in awkward positions that are maintained, or the patient himself may assume unusual positions and maintain them; mannerisms, grimaces, and bizarre acts are found; and echolalia and neologisms are also observed.

The simple type begins slowly and symptoms generally occur before puberty; however, major symptoms occur after puberty. Characteristics of this type include gradual restriction of activities (he may refuse to go out, to go to school, or to go to work) and ability to talk about only a few concrete things (poverty-of-thought symptom). Hallucinations, delusions, ideas of reference, and other symptoms are absent.

Mild or oligosymptomatic forms of the various types of schizophrenia also occur.

Manic-Depressive Psychosis. "Manic-depressive psychosis manifests itself with recurring attacks of depression and of manic elation in various forms and cycles" (Arieti, 1959b, p. 424). Some of the fundamental symptoms of depression include prominent mood of melancholia, gloomy morbid ideas, hypochondriasis, delusions of poverty, ideas of guilt, difficulty in concentration, reduction in general activity, reduction in sleep, and decrease in appetite and weight loss. The main types of depression are simple, acute, and paranoid depressions and depressive stupor.

Major characteristics of the manic attack are: "(1) a change in mood, which is one of elation; (2) a disorder of thought processes, characterized by flight of ideas and happy content; and (3) an increased mobility" (Arieti, 1959b, p. 428). Many forms of manic states have been described, namely, hypomania, acute mania, delirious mania, and mixed states.

Hysteria. "Conversion hysteria and dissociative reactions display dramatic somatic symptoms and personality disturbances: gross paralytic, spasmodic, and convulsive motor disturbances; exaggeration, diminution, or perversion of sensation; dumbness, deafness, or blindness. Amnesias, fugues, and somnambulisms may attract first attention" (Abse, 1959, p. 272).

Obsessive Behavior. Rado (1959, p. 324) uses the term obsessive behavior to describe individuals who have obsessive attacks and obsessive traits. He divides obsessive attacks into " . . . spells of doubting and brooding, bouts of ritual making, and fits of horrific temptation."

Examples of spells of doubting and brooding may include repetitive checking of lights, doors, gas jets. Bouts of ritual making are characterized by repetitive execution of a sequence of motor acts such as a certain way to take a bath, get dressed, or go to bed. Ritual making also includes obsessive hand washing and obsession to count, to touch, to avoid, or to step on certain spots. Fits of horrific temptation may be characterized by a sudden urge or idea to kill someone. Obsessive traits include overconcern with minutiae and excessive and inappropriate orderliness.

Clinical Manifestations

West and Ansberry (1968, pp. 250–251) described speech disturbances due to profound psychopathology in this way " . . . the acoustic envelope of words may be poorly formed, resulting in the omission of initial and final sounds or in elisions and transpositions of sounds; the relation of a word to others may be disturbed by the omission of prefixes, suffixes, prepositions, and copulatives; a word may lose its precise function in the sentence by reason of agrammatisms, with a loss of inflections of gender, case, mode, person, tense, and numbers, and a misuse of auxiliary verbs; a word may lose its relation to the idea expressed, resulting in the substitution of one word for another, in the repetitious use of certain words, and in the invention of new words (neologisms)." West and Ansberry (1968) pointed out that the verbal disturbances described are very similar to those found in aphasia.

In their description of psychotigenic dyslogia, West and Ansberry (1968) identified symptoms on the speech sound and word level, word and sentence-relational level, and the word-meaning level. In linguistic terms, they described a full-range of phonemic, morphemic, lexemic, grammatic, syntactic, and semantic symptoms.

Specific psychogenic language symptoms in adults are discussed under the categories of disorders of speech perception-comprehension, speech formulation-production, and verbal thinking.

Speech Perception-Comprehension Problems. Psychogenic deafness and mutism (surdomutism) has been described as a verbal conversion hysteria (Luchsinger and Arnold, 1965, pp. 779–784). Spiegel (1959) describes a problem in perception communication, or disturbed empathic communication, in the obsessional character. By attempting to alienate himself from affects, the interpersonal communication of the client is disturbed since, "One by-product of the flight from having emotional experiences is very often a repudiation of awareness of emotion and mood experiences of others, indeed a flight from empathy . . . " (p. 929). In contrast, the schizophrenic patient " . . . is often extremely sensitive to affects [enhanced empathic communication], emotions, and personality qualities in those about him . . . . He is particularly alert to the other person's pseudocommunication, cliches, or disproportionate reassurances" (p. 937). Perceptual changes in depressive states have also been observed; for example, a patient may report that all became dull and toned down, " . . . the radio voices remote, everything hushed . . . " (p. 941).

Speech Formulation-Production Problems. Verbomotor problems have been recognized in schizophrenia, depressive states, hysterical character, and obsessional individuals. Some of the symptoms reported here overlap with those presented under "Verbal Thinking Problems."

In schizophrenia two forms of dysphrasia have been recognized by Luchsinger and Arnold (1965, pp. 785–791): aphrasia, or the refusal to speak, and schizophrasia, or " . . . fantastic, senseless, or disjointed speech. . . ." Symptoms of dysphrasia are: singsong speech, senseless rhyming, stereotyped phraseology, paragrammatisms, problems in syntax (acataphasia), automatic repetition of expressions in meaningless sequence after using them correctly (catalogia, verbigeration), neologisms, echophrasia, and various combinations of these disorders or verbal salad (schizophrasia).

According to Spiegel (1959), in schizophrenia, fantasied communication prevails and verbal and nonverbal messages " . . . may be incomprehensible to their receiver and to the sender . . . ." Such unintelligible speech may be intentional, consciously or subconsciously, or unintentional. Messages may be intended to be understood but are not so perceived because they are garbled or because the listener is unable to decode them. "They range from utter confusion, to skillful distortion, to exquisite subtlety, perceptiveness, and accuracy" (p. 932). " . . . In the autistic state, language may be fixated at any station from unformed phonemal utterances to well-phrased, recognizable thought and fantasy. It may be in the form of neologisms, of word-salads, or expressions that are prophetically intoned and oracular in import" (p. 935). Various forms of body language may be used by the schizophrenic after he abandons the use of words.

Patterns of disturbed communication in the four classic varieties of schizophrenia are (Spiegel, 1959): (a) In the paranoid state, communication is distorted (paranoid dyslogia) and, "Verbal communication may function competently as language but not as thought," or it may be abandoned and replaced by noncommunicative autistic signs. (b) In hebephrenic reaction, the individual has set up " . . . disjunctive operations in pseudocommunication, verbal language fragments, gesture and expressive utterance" or verbal noise (hebephrenic dyslogia). (c) In the catatonic state, verbal communication, in general, is abandoned and residual communication is empathic and in the form of body language (catatonic alogia). (d) In simple schizophrenia " . . . communication is very much reduced and constricted." (pp. 938–939).

In depressive states, in contrast to the schizophrenic's involvement with his disturbed communication, the person experiences " . . . a diminished impulse toward communication and despairs of attaining it, though he longs for it" (Spiegel, 1959). Some patterns of verbal communication among the depressions are: (a) In classical retardation depression, language style is intact, although content is restricted and unimaginative and the ". . . voice is heavy, inert, of narrow range in pitch, monotonous, and hesitant." (b) In agitated depression, language content reflects the kind of agitation and " . . . the voice may be rasping and low-pitched, but articulation is brisk and fairly rapid, tense, with considerable range of pitch." (c) In the hypomanic state, "Voice and verbal content are diversified, with the familiar flight of ideas, which seem to be quite well related to the communication situation, especially at the beginning of the response, and then depart from the other communicator" (p. 946).

The hysterical character " . . . is remarkable for the use of emotionality and histrionics in interpersonal communication, and for the highhanded bending of fact and truth to her own purposes and to the distortion of meaning and significance for the other person . . . " (Spiegel, 1959, p. 928). Hysterical loss of speech and even of whispering has been termed apsithyria.

The obsessional individual's communication, in contrast to the hysterical character, " . . . is often experienced by the listener as dry and brittle, as though only the steel structure of thought remained" (Spiegel, 1959, p. 929). He does not necessarily lack affect, but he often lacks affect language and respect for affect.

These are some other symptoms of verbomotor disorder. Incoherent speech (agrammalogia), insane repetition of meaningless words and sentences (verbigeration, cataphasia, catalogia), and sluggish speech (bradylogia) are some symptoms of psychotigenic dyslogia identified by Travis (1931, Ch. 2). Self-repetition of words and phrases (autoecholalia or palilalia), repetition of words or sentences spoken by others (interpersonal echophrasia or echolalia), and uncontrollable use of obscene or curse words (coprolalia, coprolalomania) have been identified as symptoms in the rare latah syndrome (Arieti and Meth, 1959, p. 556). Rapid, distorted speech (agitophasia) and the use of series of words containing the same consonant sounds (dysphrastic alliteration) may also be observed.

Verbal Thinking Problems. Primary attention will be given here to problems in verbal thinking in schizophrenia and in obsessive and manic states.

According to Kaplan (1966) the major components of well-articulated symbol situations are the addressor (communicator), the addressee (communicant), the intention (that which the addressor wants to communicate), the referent (object or state of affairs to which the addressor directs the addressee's attention), the context (situation in which communication takes place), the scene (locus of referent if different from context), and the medium (the means by which the addressor communicates his intentions and(or) represents his referents).

In schizophrenia and related disorders, psychopathologic symbol situations may be characterized by (Kaplan, 1966, pp. 670–681):

(a) A fusion between the patient and his momentary addressee, or lack of differentiation among addressees. (b) The patient's intentions are invariably fused, ambivalent, unknown to him. " . . . Rarely is he oriented toward an impersonal, factual communication . . . his posture is egocentric-affective . . . ." (c) The patient's relations to his actual and potential referents (i.e., his world of objects and events) undergo dissolution; he exhibits tendencies to construe impersonal events in personal-emotional terms. (d) The " . . . patient often cannot exclude the context, even when it is irrelevant to the communication situation . . . or . . . he frequently takes no cognizance of the socially defined context in expressing himself." (e) The patient may fuse his current context with the scene or locus of the referent. (f) The relationships between addressor and medium are altered, he endows symbol system with idiosyncratic-emotional significance, he may experience words and gestures as " . . . incarnate objects and efficacious actions . . . ." Such interpretation sometimes results in the patient's refusal to use symbols, " . . . or to dismember words as he would things that threaten him . . . or to construct his own forms and to imbue these with significance that they have for him alone . . . hence, in part, the emergence of neologisms, neomorphisms, glossolalias, and the like." (g) The patient may eventually exhibit a dissociation between thought-feelings and his utterances; his utterances may become dystaxic or agrammatic, or may verge on verbigeration, the final result being word-salad.

Hallucinatory thoughts-out-loud have been discussed as part of the autistic behavior of the schizophrenic individual (Spiegel, 1959). Such pathologic intraverbalization is reminiscent of the physiologic intraverbalization of childhood, which may be viewed as verbal thinking in the making. "This overwhelming immersion in verbal communication with the self obliterates verbal communication with others" (p. 931).

In obsessional states there appears to be rather general agreement ". . . that there is retreat from feeling to thinking" (Spiegel, 1959, p. 928). Fear of emotions and things that arouse them causes the compulsion neurotic to flee " . . . from the macrocosm of things to the microcosm of words" (Fenichel, 1945). By means of manipulating intrapsychic communication, the obsessional character can escape from direct experience of feeling states.

In the manic attack, "The thinking disorder is prominent and reveals itself in the verbal productions of the patient." (Arieti, 1959b). Verbal behavior is marked by rapid speech, and rapid shifting from one topic to another. The " . . . talk as a whole is verbose, circumstantial, not directed toward any goal or toward the logical demonstration of any point which is discussed. The ensemble of these thoughts and language alterations is what we call 'flight of ideas'" (p. 427). Verbosity accompanying the manic state may be termed logorrhea, verbomania, polylogia, or panglossia.

Oneiric verbalization (sleep talk) and its possible similarities to the speech of severely disturbed schizophrenics, and hypnagogic verbalization (drowsy talk) and the possibility that such verbalization represents in slow motion the manner in which thoughts are transformed into verbal forms are discussed by Kaplan (1966, pp. 681–682) and warrant further study.

More specific symptoms of disorder in verbal thinking are: use of a poor approximation of a desired term (metonymy); absence of speech due to a paucity of ideas for utterance (alogia); speech into which many neologisms are incorporated (neolalia); incoherent, illogical or delusional speech (paralogia, lingual delirium, allophasis); reduced will to speak (verbal dysbulia); fear of speaking (laliophobia or logophobia); excessive self-talk (release of paleoverbal behavior); morbid dread of hearing a certain name or word (onomatophobia); undue dwelling on one subject (thematic paralogia); voluntary refraining from speech (aphrasia, Kussmaul's aphasia); increased use of verbal metaphors, prayers, vows, proverbs, humor, slang, and profanity in individuals under stress (Weinstein and Kahn, 1959, p. 965); silent reproduction of a word or words (endophasia); insertion of meaningless words into speech (embolophrasia); use of unknown or imaginary language (glossolalia); and use of female linguistic patterns and styles by males (gynoglossia, gynologia) and of male linguistic patterns and styles by females (androglossia, andrologia).

Clinical verbotypes that have been recognized among adults include emotionally-charged, histrionic patterns (hyperaffective verbotype); neutral, bland patterns (hypoaffective verbotype); alloplastic and autoplastic verbotypes; authoritarian and hostile verbotypes; and pseudo-communication and noncommunication verbotypes.

Diagnosis

The speech specialist has at least two diagnostic goals when examining adults who are apparently reflecting psychogenic language dysfunction.

(a) The clinician should attempt to determine whether any components of the language complex appear secondary to end-organ hearing loss or neurogenic language involvement; (b) the clinician should attempt to identify the language profile as accurately as possible, that is, does it suggest schizophrenic reaction or manic, depressive, hysterical, or obsessional states. As speech pathologists become more experienced in identifying language profiles of various psychological states, they should make important contributions to the diagnosis of primary or secondary psychologic disorders.

Prognosis

Since so little language-symptom therapy has been applied by speech pathologists to adult psychogenic disorders, nothing of substance can be said with respect to prognosis. The best indicator of a favorable prognosis for the language dissolution is a positive reaction of the patient to psychiatric-psychologic treatment. Hopefully, as speech clinicians develop language-symptom techniques such treatment programs will become important factors in prognosis for the fundamental psychologic disorder.

Therapy

Language-symptom therapy for psychogenic language dissolution in adults is still experimental at this time. The speech clinician has not usually been involved with such patients in the past. However, just as the speech specialist is doing more work with children with psychogenic disorders, it is anticipated that he will in the future be working with much greater frequency with these adult patients in team therapy programs. Spiegel (1959) states, " . . . Not only is the psychiatric patient's communication with others seriously impaired; so also is his relatedness to himself—his intrapsychic communication. As part of therapeutic achievement, he is to be helped to communicate better with himself and with others . . . " (p. 909).

In developing language-symptom programs for adults, speech clinicians might consider the following principles:

The Clinician as a Positive Emotional Stimulus. Early contacts with the patient should be devoted to becoming a supportive, nonthreatening communicator. Interaction should be such that it will result in the patient looking forward to the visit of the clinician.

Establishing a Mode of Intercommunication. Depending on the severity of the dissolution in speech communication, the clinician might develop a paralanguage mode of intercommunication. The use of body postures, facial expressions, hand gestures, and pleasant vocal tone might very well serve as a beginning for the re-establishment of speech communication.

Re-establishment of Audioverbal Monitoring. A good portion of the verbomotor disorganization in psychogenic language dysfunction appears to be based on changes in intrapersonal speech perception. (One of the six characteristics of schizophrenic language identified by Chaika (1974) was " . . . failure to self-monitor, e.g., not noting errors when they occur"). Helping the patient to perceive his disorganized speech may restimulate self-correcting processes. Some suggested techniques are:

The disorganized speech of the patient may be amplified and fed directly back to him via headsets and an amplifier. Such a unit may be used during conversational interaction between clinician and patient. The clinician may echo the disorganized speech directed at him. Recordings of the disorganized speech may also be played for the patient. (Additional ideas on the stimulation of the sensor system in language rehabilitation are found in Chapter 8.)

Maintaining a Meaningful Conversational Situation. In terms of major components of symbol situations (Kaplan, 1966), the clinician should assist the patient to keep separate and distinct the speaker from the listener, to understand his speech intentions, and to be clear about the context in which the communication is taking place. The clinician should provide assistance basically through verbal clarification of the patient's conversational confusions.

All language-symptom techniques should be planned in conjunction with psychiatric-psychologic team members.

REFERENCES

Abelson, P. H., Malnutrition, learning, and behavior. Science, 164, 17 (1969).

Abse, D. W., Hysteria. In S. Arieti (Ed.), American Handbook of Psychiatry, Vol. 1. New York: Basic Books (1959).

Arieti, S., Schizophrenia: The manifest symptomatology, the psychodynamic and formal mechanisms. In S. Arieti (Ed.), American Handbook of Psychiatry, Vol. 1. New York: Basic Books (1959a).

Arieti, S., Manic-depressive psychosis. In S. Arieti (Ed.), American Handbook of Psychiatry, Vol. 1. New York: Basic Books (1959b).

Arieti, S., and Meth, J., Rare, unclassifiable, collective, and exotic psychotic syndromes. In S. Arieti (Ed.), American Handbook of Psychiatry, Vol. 1. New York: Basic Books (1959).

Arnold, G. E., I. Present concepts of etiologic factors. III. Signs and symptoms. In Studies in Tachyphemia: An Investigation of Cluttering and General Language Disability. New York: Speech Rehabilitation Institute.

Bebin, J., Blood dyscrasias. In J. Minckler (Ed.), Pathology of the Nervous System, Vol. 1. New York: McGraw-Hill (1968).

Benson, D. F., and Patten, D. H., The use of radioactive isotopes in the localization of aphasia producing lesions. Cortex, 3, 258–271 (1967).

Brain, W. R., and Walton J. N., Diseases of the Nervous System. London: Oxford University Press (1969).

Brown, S. F., Retarded speech development. In W. Johnson and D. Moehler (Eds.), Speech Handicapped School Children. New York: Harper & Row (1967).

Bruetsch, W. L., Neurosyphilitic conditions. In S. Arieti (Ed.), American Handbook of Psychiatry, Vol. 2. New York: Basic Books (1959).

Chaika, E., A linguist looks at "schizophrenic" language. Brain Lang., 1, 257–276 (1974).

Darley, F. L., Diagnosis and Appraisal of Communication Disorders. Englewood Cliffs, N. J.: Prentice-Hall, Inc. (1964).

Darley, F. L., and Winitz, H., Age of first word: Review of research. J. Speech Hear. Disord., 26, 272–290 (1961).

de Hirsch, K., Differential diagnosis between aphasic and schizophrenic language in children. J. Speech Hear. Disord., 32, 3–10 (1967).

de Hirsch, K., A review of early language development. Dev. Med. Child Neurol., 12, 87–97 (1970).

Ebaugh, F. G., and Tiffany, W. J., Jr., Infective-exhaustive psychoses. In S. Arieti (Ed.), American Handbook of Psychiatry, Vol. 2. New York: Basic Books (1959).

Eisenson, J., Development aphasia: A speculative view with therapeutic implications. J. Speech Hear. Disord., 33, 3–13 (1968).

Espir, M. L. E., and Rose, F. C., The Basic Neurology of Speech. Philadelphia: F. A. Davis Company (1970).

Fenichel, O., The Psychoanalytic Theory of Neurosis. New York: W. W. Norton & Company, Inc. (1945).

Ferraro, A., Presenile psychoses. In S. Arieti (Ed.), American Handbook of Psychiatry, Vol. 2. New York: Basic Books (1959a).

Ferraro, A., Senile psychoses. In S. Arieti (Ed.), American Handbook of Psychiatry, Vol. 2. New York: Basic Books (1959b).

Ferraro, A., Psychoses with cerebral arteriosclerosis. In S. Arieti (Ed.), American Handbook of Psychiatry, Vol. 2. New York: Basic Books (1959c).

Fleming, C. P., The verbal behavior of hydrocephalic children. In Studies in Hydrocephalus and Spina Bifida. London: Spastics International Medical Publications (1968).

Ford, F. R., Diseases of the Nervous System. Springfield, Ill.: Charles C Thomas (1966).

Fraccaro, M., Autosomal chromosome abnormalities. In J. L. Hamerton (Ed.), Chromosomes in Medicine. London: The Spastics Society.

Gellis, S. S., and Feingold, M., Atlas of Mental Retardation Syndromes. Washington, D. C.: U. S. Department of Health, Education, and Welfare (1968).

Hagberg, B., The sequelae of spontaneously arrested infantile hydrocephalus. Dev. Med. Child Neurol., 4, 583–587 (1962).

Hagen, C., Communication abilities in hemiplegia: effect of speech therapy. Arch. Phys. Med. Rehabil., 54, 454–463 (1973).

Hamerton, J. L. (Ed.), Chromosomes in Medicine. London: The Spastics Society.

Ingram, T. T. S., Pediatric aspects of specific development dysphasia, dyslexia, and dysgraphia. Cerebral Palsy Bull., 2, 254–277 (1960).

Ingram, T. T. S., and Barn, J., A description and classification of common speech disorders associated with cerebral palsy. Cerebral Palsy Bull., 3, 57–59 (1961).

Jacob, J. C., Maroun, F. B., Heneghan, W. D., and House, A. M., Uncommon cerebrovascular lesions in children. Dev. Med. Child Neurol., 12, 446–453 (1970).

Kaplan, B., The study of language in psychiatry. In S. Arieti (Ed.), American Handbook of Psychiatry, Vol. 3. New York: Basic Books (1966).

Keenan, J. S., and Brassell, E. G., A study of factors related to prognosis for individual aphasic patients. J. Speech Hear. Disord., 39, 257–269 (1974).

Kessler, J. W., Psychopathology of Childhood. Englewood Cliffs, N. J.: Prentice-Hall, Inc. (1966).

Konorski, J., Integrative Activity of the Brain. Chicago: The University of Chicago Press (1967).

Lewis, R. S., Strauss, A. A., and Lehtinen, L. E., The Other Child. New York: Grune and Stratton (1960).

Lillywhite, H. S., and Bradley, D. P., Communication Problems in Mental Retardation: Diagnosis and Management. New York: Harper & Row (1969).

Luchsinger, R., and Arnold, G., Voice-Speech-Language. Belmont, Calif.: Wadsworth Publishing Co. (1965).

Magoun, H. W., Lacunae and research approaches to them. II. In F. L. Darley and C. H. Millikan (Eds.), Brain Mechanisms Underlying Speech and Language. New York: Grune and Stratton (1967).

Mahler, M. S., Furer, M., and Settlage, C. F., Severe emotional disturbances in childhood: psychosis. In S. Arieti (Ed.), American Handbook of Psychiatry, Vol. 1. New York: Basic Books (1959).

Masland, R. L., Brain mechanisms underlying the language function. In Human Communication and its Disorders—an Overview. Report of the National Institute of Neurological Diseases and Stroke. Washington, D. C.: U. S. Dept. of Health, Education, and Welfare (1969).

Matthews, J., Communication disorders in the mentally retarded. In L. E. Travis (Ed.), Handbook of Speech Pathology and Audiology. New York: Appleton-Century-Crofts (1971).

McGraw, R. B., and Oliver, J. F., Miscellaneous therapies. In S. Arieti (Ed.), American Handbook of Psychiatry, Vol. 2. New York: Basic Books (1959).

Minckler, J. (Ed.), Pathology of the Nervous System, Vol. 2. New York: McGraw-Hill (1971).

Morley, M. E., The Development and Disorders of Speech in Childhood. Baltimore: The Williams & Wilkins Co. (1965).

Mowrer, O. H., Hearing and speaking: An analysis of language learning. J. Speech Hear. Disord., 23, 143–152 (1958).

Mulder, D. W., Psychoses with brain tumors and other chronic neurologic disorders. In

S. Arieti (Ed.), American Handbook of Psychiatry, Vol. 2. New York: Basic Books (1959).

Myklebust, H. R., Auditory Problems in Children: A Manual for Differential Diagnosis. New York: Grune and Stratton (1954).

Mysak, E. D., Organismic development of oral language. J. Speech Hear. Disord., 26, 377–384 (1961).

Mysak, E. D., Speech Pathology and Feedback Theory. Springfield, Ill.: Charles C Thomas (1966).

Mysak, E. D., Disorders of oral communication. In M. Bortner (Ed.), Evaluation and Education of Children with Brain Damage. Springfield, Ill.: Charles C Thomas (1968).

Mysak, E. D., Cerebral palsy speech habilitation. In L. E. Travis (Ed.), Handbook of Speech Pathology and Audiology. New York: Appleton-Century-Crofts (1971).

Nelson, W. E. (Ed.), Textbook of Pediatrics. Philadelphia: W. B. Saunders Co. (1964).

Penfield, W., and Roberts, L., Speech and Brain Mechanisms. Princeton, N. J.: Princeton University Press (1959).

Polani, P. E., Sex chromosome anomalies in man. In J. L. Hamerton (Ed.), Chromosomes in Medicine. London: The Spastics Society.

Rado, S., Obsessive behavior: So-called obsessive-compulsive neurosis. In S. Arieti (Ed.), American Handbook of Psychiatry, Vol. 1. New York: Basic Books (1959).

Schuell, H., Aphasia in adults. In Human Communication and Its Disorders—An Overview. Report of the National Institute of Neurological Diseases and Stroke. Washington, D. C.: U. S. Dept. of Health, Education, and Welfare (1969).

Schwartz, E. R., Characteristics of speech and language development in the child with myelomeningocele and hydrocephalus. J. Speech Hear. Disord., 39, 465–468 (1974).

Shervanian, C. C., Speech, thought, and communication disorders in childhood psychoses: Theoretical implications. J. Speech Hear. Disord., 32, 303–314 (1967).

Smithells, R. W., Chromosomes and the clinician. In J. L. Hamerton (Ed.), Chromosomes in Medicine. London: The Spastics Society.

Spiegel, R., Specific problems of communication in psychiatric conditions. In S. Arieti (Ed.), American Handbook of Psychiatry, Vol. 1. New York: Basic Books (1959).

Strauss, A. A., and Kephart, N. C., Psychopathology and Education of the Brain-Injured Child, Vol. 2. Progress in Theory and Clinic. New York: Grune and Stratton (1955).

Strauss, A. A., and Lehtinen, L. E., Psychopathology and Education of the Brain-Injured Child. New York: Grune and Stratton (1947).

Strauss, H., Epileptic disorders. In S. Arieti (Ed.), American Handbook of Psychiatry, Vol. 2. New York: Basic Books (1959).

Thompson, G. N., Acute and chronic alcoholic conditions. In S. Arieti (Ed.), American Handbook of Psychiatry, Vol. 2. New York: Basic Books (1959).

Travis, L. E., Speech Pathology. New York: Appleton-Century-Crofts (1931).

Weinstein, E. A., and Kahn, R. L., Symbolic reorganization in brain injuries. In S. Arieti (Ed.), American Handbook of Psychiatry, Vol. 1. New York: Basic Books (1959).

Weller, H. C., Blood examinations in the diagnosis and treatment of speech disorders. Central States Speech J., March, 1–4 (1952).

West, R., An agnostic's speculations about stuttering. In J. Eisenson (Ed.), Stuttering: A Symposium. New York: Harper & Row (1958).

West, R. W., and Ansberry, M., The Rehabilitation of Speech. New York: Harper & Row (1968).

Wood, N. E., Delayed Speech and Language Development. Englewood Cliffs, N. J.: Prentice-Hall, Inc. (1964).

Worster-Drought, C., Speech disorders in children. Dev. Med. Child Neurol., 10, 427–440 (1968).

Worster-Drought, C., An unusual form of acquired aphasia in children. Dev. Med. Child Neurol., 13, 563–571 (1971).

4

Speech Integrator System: Lower Order

Lower-order speech integration is described in Chapter 1 as an automatic and subconscious "doing" operation, in contrast with the less automatic and more conscious "thinking" operation of higher-order speech integration. Disturbances in function of the lower-order integrator are observed in children and adults and, in general, are manifested by: (a) problems in arousal and selective attention to speech input signals, including audiovisual paralanguage; and (b) problems in coordinating and refining speech output signals, including tonal-kinetic paralanguage. Problems in lower-order speech integration are discussed in terms of difficulties with input processing and with output patterning.

INPUT PROCESSING DISORDERS

Lower-order input processing involves the integration of verboacoustic and verbovisual (speech-associated articulatory movements) signals and audiovisual paralanguage, including speech-associated body postures, facial expressions, hand gestures, and tonal components. The function may be described as the automatic "turning on," "tuning in," and "fine tuning" of the speech-receiving system. This automatic process includes arousal to, and fixing and tracking of, all aspects of the speech signal and the maintenance of selective attention to the signal even under conditions of competing environmental stimuli.

Background

Problems in audiovisual localization of the speech signal, of arousal and sensitization of the audiovisual system, and of audiovisual tracking may be related to disorders of the colliculi, the ascending reticular activating system, and the thalamic centers. Lesions involving these areas may be associated with congenital brain involvements such as in the cerebral palsies, and with cerebrovascular accidents (CVA's), cerebral neoplasms, and encephalitis.

Clinical Manifestations

The clinical behavior of individuals with lower-order processing problems may be manifested in various ways. Audiovisual attention may be effected only after repeated utterance of the individual's name; the individual may appear to have trouble in fixing and tracking speech-associated audiovisual stimuli, or he may find it difficult to sustain attention to the speech signals, depending on the length of utterance and the amount of competing signals in the environment. It may be difficult in any one case to determine the contribution to problems in initial and sustained speech tracking, of problems in retinal localization of the speaker's face and its expressions, and of problems in optokinetic tracking of speech articulatory movements.

In general, problems of lower-order afferent integration are manifested in at least two ways. (a) There may be difficulty in obtaining or maintaining auditory and visual attention to speech events. Wepman (1969, p. 139) advanced the concept that children with primary autism may have an impairment for processing audiovisual events that may be based on a reticular system involvement. (b) There may be easy loss of listener contact under conditions of competing speech and environmental noise. Such difficulty may be observed in the aged, in older, brain-involved individuals, and in so-called hyperkinetic children suspected of thalamic dysfunction.

Diagnosis

Problems of lower-order input processing may be determined by a combination of diagnostic approaches. Clinical diagnosis of the involvement is based on signs of problems in arousal to speech events and in the fixing and initial and sustained tracking of them. These signs should be compared and contrasted with those that may be associated with end-organ auditory and visual problems and with involvements of higher-order speech integration (differential diagnosis). Support by other specialists of organic involvement of neural mechanisms associated with lower-order input processing is also essential (group diagnosis). Responses to certain treatment techniques are also useful in contributing to a diagnosis (diagnosis by treatment).

Prognosis

Since so little organized information is available in clinical and research literature in the area of lower-order input processing, it is not possible to make meaningful statements on prognosis. Hopefully, in the future more clinicians will be aware of the problem, will diagnose it earlier, will attempt various remedial procedures, and will, thereby, contribute to information on the conditions amenable to rehabilitation procedures.

Therapy

Symptomatic techniques to counter problems in arousal and in orienting, fixing, and tracking of speech signals may be grouped under the headings of amplification of stimulation, novelty of stimulation, maintenance of the attentive state, and competing-signal stimulation.

Amplification of Stimulation. Orienting to and fixing of the source of audiovisual speech stimuli may be facilitated by increasing the intensity of the stimulation. Increase in intensity of stimulation may be effected by actually increasing sound pressure energy (auditory stimuli) or radiant energy (visual stimuli) and by exciting additional sensory channels. For example, the use of a hearing aid (irrespective of whether there is an actual acuity loss) set to amplify speech signals even to a slight degree may facilitate orienting to and fixing of speech events. Exaggeration of speech-associated hand gestures, facial expressions, and articulatory movements and decreasing the speaker-listener distance are ways of intensifying important visual stimuli. A further increase in the intensity of speech stimulation may be achieved by having the client repeat aloud the question or direction uttered by the clinician and, consequently, having the client self-generate additional auditory as well as tactile-kinesthetic stimulation.

Novelty of Stimulation. The orienting reflex and the attentive state may be facilitated by the use of novel afferent stimulation. Application of this concept with respect to speech signals may be carried out by having the speaker vary the pitch, quality, or time aspects of his voice. Varying accompanying visual speech stimuli could also be tried. Changing speaking positions, that is, speaking while seated, standing, or walking, should also be helpful in stimulating orienting and fixing processes.

Maintenance of the Attentive State. Attempts at increasing auditory and visual tracking time should also be made. Speaking comprehension tasks may be planned so that the clinician speaks progressively longer speech units and follows them with simple questions to determine whether the client has successfully maintained attention. Similar speaking comprehension tasks requiring progressively longer amounts of attention could also be planned, such as listening to television newscasts, speeches, and short dramas.

Competing-Signal Stimulation. Developing an individual's capacity for speech tracking under competing-signal conditions may be done by progressively raising his tolerance for such conditions. Tracking may first be done in an environment free of competing auditory and visual stimuli, then in one where general background room noise is introduced, and then in environments where increasing amounts of competing stimuli are introduced.

OUTPUT PATTERNING DISORDERS

Lower-order output patterning is responsible for various forms of verbal stereotypy as well as for refining and coordinating motor speech. More specifically, the system appears capable of producing minor speech such as emotional utterances (e.g., curse words and stereotyped phrases associated with shock, surprise, terror, fear, passion), social gesture phrases (e.g., "Good morning," "Goodbye," "How are you," "I'm fine," etc.), and memorized speech (e.g., songs, poems, alphabet, counting, days of the week, etc.). The system is also responsible for: (a) speech-associated affect and muscle tonus; (b) fine, smooth, and accurate speech movements; (c) coordinating respiratory, phonatory, resonatory, and articulatory movements; and (d) compensatory speech movements in response to concomitant motor behavior such as bending or turning of the head or walking.

Background

Brain regions that cooperate in lower-order output patterning are the cerebellum, basal ganglia, and the minor speech hemisphere. Numerous diseases and disorders may affect these brain regions.

Disorders of the Minor Speech Hemisphere. Conditions that affect the minor speech hemisphere are those that may also involve the major speech hemisphere, that is, trauma, vascular disorders, degenerative diseases, infections, and neoplasms. These conditions have already been discussed in Chapter 3. Involvement of the minor speech brain may have implications for the use of minor speech behavior such as emotional utterances, social-gesture speech, and memorized speech.

Basal Ganglia Disorders. The basal ganglia are the nuclei of the extrapyramidal system and include the corpus striatum (globus pallidus, putamen, and caudate nuclei), substantia nigra, subthalamic nucleus, and the red nucleus. These nuclei contribute to control of tone, posture, and movement (Espir and Rose, 1970, p. 49). Among the conditions that involve these nuclei are Parkinson's disease, Sydenham's chorea, Huntington's chorea, congenital chorea, congenital athetosis, congenital rigidity, hemiballismus, torsion dystonia, and Wilson's disease.

Parkinson's disease may be divided into two categories, primary parkinsonism and symptomatic parkinsonism. Primary parkinsonism (idiopathic, paralysis agitans), a degenerative disease of middle age of unknown etiology, is characterized by mask-like facies (reduced, slow, and stiff movements of face), excessive salivation and drooling, "at rest" hand tremor (course and rhythmical), cogwheel rigidity of the limbs, stooped posture, and a festinant gait. Symptomatic parkinsonism describes parkinsonian symptoms that are secondary to encephalitis, arteriosclerosis, and various toxicities (carbon monoxide, manganese, drugs). Parkinsonism may be associated with phonatory, articulatory, and speech rhythm symptoms. Espir and Rose (1970, p. 52) describe parkinsonian speech as monotonous and weak, as reflecting articulatory deficits and festinant rate, and also as showing a tendency toward phrasal repetitions. Darley *et al.* (1969) reported that parkinsonian speech was characterized by one cluster of speech symptoms (correlated symptoms) and four uncorrelated ones. The prosodic insufficiency cluster is composed of monopitch, monoloudness, reduced stress, short phrases, short rushes of speech, variable rate, and imprecise consonants. Uncorrelated symptoms include inappropriate silences, breathy voice, harsh voice, and low pitch.

Sydenham's chorea, possibly associated with rheumatic fever, is characterized by choreiform movements (jerky movements of peripheral parts of limbs), grimacing, and "fidgeting and dropping things" (Espir and Rose, 1970, p. 50). Ford (1966, pp. 583–588) states that Sydenham's chorea is usually viewed as another symptom of rheumatic fever; that it occurs most often between the ages of six and nine and is more common among girls; that the typical symptoms include involuntary movements (jerky, twitching movements), incoordination, hypotonus, and weakness; that the face, tongue, neck, and trunk may be involved; that there are no disturbances of sensibility; that there may be marked emotional instability; and that mild cases may recover in two or three months and severe cases may last for a year. Espir and Rose (1970, p. 50) state that the speech is hesitant and jerky and due to jerky movements of articulatory and respiratory muscles. Ford (1966, p. 585) indicates that speech is characterized first by irregular rhythm and later by indistinct articulation. Ford also indicated that some individuals may not attempt speech when tongue control is very difficult.

Huntington's chorea, an inherited and progressive disease, appears between the ages of 30 to 50 years and is characterized by choreiform movements and dementia. The associated dysarthria eventually leads to unintelligible speech (Espir and Rose, 1970, p. 50). The disease involves the cerebral cortex as well as the corpus striatum (Brain and Walton, 1969, p. 551).

Congenital chorea is characterized by sudden, jerky, and irregular movements beginning after six months or more. Speech and swallowing difficulties and facial grimacing may be observed (Ford, 1966, p. 46). Darley *et al.* (1969) identified at least five clusters of speech deficits in choreic speech, prosodic excess, prosodic insufficiency, articulatory-resonatory incompetence, phonatory stenosis, and resonatory incompetence. Prosodic excess is composed of slow rate, excess and equal stress, phonemes prolonged, intervals prolonged, and inappropriate silences. Prosodic insufficiency is composed of monopitch, monoloudness, reduced stress, and short phrases. Articulatory-resonatory incompetence is composed of imprecise consonants, distorted vowels, and hypernasality. Phonatory stenosis is composed of low pitch, harsh voice, strained-strangled voice, pitch breaks, and voice stoppages. Resonatory incompetence is composed of hypernasality, nasal emission, imprecise consonants, and short phrases. Other speech dimensions found in choreic speech include inappropriate silences, variable rate, and irregular articulatory breakdown.

Congenital athetosis, where agenesis or dysgenesis, anoxia, or kernicterus may be causative agents, is characterized by "writhing, purposeless, involuntary movements" (Espir and Rose, 1970, p. 51). Involuntary movements of the tongue, lips, and face may result in severe articulatory anomalies and facial grimacing, and irregular contractions of the respiratory muscles may be reflected by irregular and "jerky" vocalization.

Congenital rigidity, where excessive muscular rigidity may be present from very early in the child's life, tends to worsen during the first two years. Various stimuli such as noises or lights may increase the symptoms. Bulbar symptoms are present in the majority of cases (Ford, 1966, p. 46).

Hemiballismus, an uncommon disease apparently caused by damage to the subthalamic nucleus, is manifested by "continued wild, flail-like movements of one arm" (Gatz, 1966, p. 172). The affected arm is opposite the site of the lesion. Brain and Walton (1969, p. 554) indicate that, while involuntary movements may affect the limbs unilaterally, the face may be involved on both sides.

Torsion dystonia (dystonia musculorum deformans) is frequently familial, and when it is familial the onset usually occurs in childhood or adolescence. Symptoms may begin with spasmodic plantar-flexion of the feet. Involuntary movements in upper limbs "consist of rotation or torsion round the long axes and are associated with similar torsion movements of the vertebral column, especially in the lumbar region." Lordosis and scoliosis may be apparent when the individual walks. Tremor and myoclonic muscular contractions have also been described. Muscular wasting is not present and sensibility is unimpaired (Brain and Walton, 1969, p. 539).

In a review of the medical literature, Jones (1968) found reports of no speech disturbance in dystonia to reports that speech disturbance may herald the disease. Descriptive terms used to identify the speech symptoms of dystonic patients included: slurred, thick, clumsy, indistinct, choppy, freezing, and explosive. Jones studied six speech characteristics (clarity of articulation, normalcy of vocal quality, appropriateness of the time factor, vocal pitch flexibility, loudness control, overall speech adequacy) of 18 patients with dystonia. During both spontaneous speech and oral reading the six speech characteristics were judged moderately defective; defectiveness ranged from essentially normal to severely impaired.

Darley *et al.* (1969) identified at least three clusters of speech symptoms in dystonia, articulatory inaccuracy, phonatory stenosis, and prosodic insufficiency. Articulatory inaccuracy is composed of imprecise consonants, irregular articulatory breakdowns, and distorted vowels. Phonatory stenosis is composed of low pitch, harsh voice, strain-strangled voice, pitch breaks, short phrases, and slow rate. Prosodic insufficiency is composed of monopitch, monoloudness, reduced stress, and short phrases.

Wilson's disease (hepatalenticular degeneration), a progressive disease of early life, is often familial. Symptoms in younger individuals are characterized by general plastic rigidity followed by tremor or athetoid movements; in individuals in which onset occurs over the age of 20, tremor precedes rigidity. Voluntary movement and deglutition are affected early and severely. Other symptoms that may be present are mask-like facies, loss of emotional control, and mild dementia. "Speech may become unintelligible or the patient may even lose entirely the power of articulation" (Brain and Walton, 1969, p. 536).

Cerebellar Disorders. The cerebellum is composed of a right and a left hemisphere joined by a structure called the vermis. Three cerebellar peduncles (superior, middle, and inferior) join each hemisphere to the corresponding side of the brain stem. Important connections exist with vestibular mechanisms and with cranial nerve nuclei involved with movements of the eyes and neck. Coordination of movements and maintenance of balance and muscle tonus are dependent on the cerebellum and its connections. Speech muscles, as well as muscles of the eyes, neck, trunk, and limbs, are affected by cerebellar dysfunctioning. Specific clinical manifestations of cerebellar deficiency include: (a) *dyssynergy*, or the inability to coordinate one muscle system with another (e.g., the phonatory with the articulatory); (b) *dysmetria*, or movements that are out of proportion to acts performed; (c) *disintegration*, or the failure of movements that were once acquired; (d) *dysdiadochocinesis*, or disturbed ability to engage in serial repetitive movements; (e) intention tremor; (f) mask-like facies; (g) disturbance of stance and gait; (h) ocular and head nystagmus; (i) vertigo; (j) headache; (k) dysarthria; and (l) possible associated involvement of nuclei of cranial nerves V, VI, VII, VIII, IX, X, and XI.

Terms used by Espir and Rose (1970, pp. 53–54) to describe ataxic dysarthria include "slurring," "slow and thick," "slurring and jerkiness," "scanning," "staccato," "explosive and unintelligible," and anarthric. Brain and Walton (1969, p. 63) indicate that lesions of the vermis are more likely to cause articulatory and phonatory disturbances than are lesions of one lobe. Articulation is described as jerky, explosive, and slurred, and phonation is described as often too loud with irregular separation between syllables. In cases of unilateral lesions, considerable recovery of speech usually occurs.

Luchsinger and Arnold (1965, p. 251) state that the cerebellum is responsible for the eurhythmy, eumetria, eutaxy, and diadochocinesia of all phonatory and articulatory movements and hence cerebellar disease may produce the following speech signs: "exaggerated movements of respiration, overloud or interrupted phonation with nystagmic ataxia of the vocal cords, iterative articulation, as well as disturbances of the rhythm and fluency of diction."

Worster-Drought (1968) described articulatory and phonatory repercussions of cerebellar disorders in children resulting from trauma, cerebellar dysgenesis, cerebellar encephalitis, and Friedreich's hereditary ataxia. The ". . . articulation is slow, laboured and monotonous together with a jerky irregularity. Phonation is sometimes even more affected than articulation and the utterance may be curiously explosive with pronounced separation of syllables."

Darley *et al.* (1969) found three distinct clusters of speech deficits among their cerebellar patients, articulatory inaccuracy, prosodic excess, and phonatory-prosodic insufficiency clusters. The articulatory inaccuracy cluster is composed of imprecise consonants, irregular articulatory breakdowns, and distorted vowels. The prosodic excess cluster is composed of excess and equal stress, prolonged phonemes, prolonged intervals, and slow speech rate. The phonatory-prosodic insufficiency cluster is composed of harsh voice, monopitch, and monoloudness.

Among the conditions and diseases that may affect the cerebellum are congenital disorders, familial tendencies, degenerations, neoplasms, infections, vascular lesions, and metabolic and toxic disorders.

Neoplasms of the cerebellum may be of the median variety, or midline cerebellar tumors, or of the lateral variety, or tumors of the cerebellar hemisphere. Among the symptoms of median lesions are: giddiness, unsteadiness on standing, ataxic gait, and muscular hypotonia. Included in the symptoms of lateral lesions are: clumsiness of the ipsilateral hand, a tendency to stagger to the side of the lesion, giddiness in shaking or turning of the head, marked nystagmus, hypotonia, wide-based gait, and abnormal attitude of the head (Brain and Walton, 1969, pp. 252–254).

Congenital malformations of the cerebellum may be reflected by defects (ageneses, dysgeneses) in which the vermis and hemispheres may be absent, the vermis may be absent without gross defect of the hemispheres, one hemisphere and part of the vermis may be absent, and the cerebellum may be very small but symmetrically formed. Head balance, sitting up, standing, and walking are late. Reaching may be associated with an intention tremor of the hands. Walking is associated with side-to-side sway and frequent falls. Speech rhythm is frequently affected and characterized by scanning or staccato-type patterns; articulation is usually distinct, however (Ford, 1966, p. 48). Espir and Rose (1970, p. 57) report underdevelopment of orofacial muscles, grimacing, drooling, delayed speech development, and slurred and jerky speech.

Hereditary forms of cerebellar ataxia include at least four types (Ford, 1966, pp. 260–266).

Hereditary cerebellar ataxia of Freidreich is familial and characterized by progressive degeneration of the spinocerebellar tracts, the corticospinal tracts, and the posterior columns of the cord. First symptoms usually occur during childhood. It is not unusual for the child to experience normal early development; however, slowness in learning to walk or clumsiness may be reported. Gait symptoms are usually the first to be noticed. Learning to write and to handle a fork or spoon may also present difficulties. Later, speech may become "jerky" and "indistinct." Therefore, the most obvious early symptoms are ". . . unsteadiness of gait, ataxia of the arms and disturbances in speech."

Hereditary cerebellar ataxia with spasticity and optic atrophy (Behr's syndrome) is familial and characterized by degeneration of the spinocerebellar tracts, the pyramidal tracts, and the optic nerves. Symptoms begin in early childhood. Gait disturbance is the first symptom, followed by ataxia of the arms, visual disturbances with optic atrophy, and spasticity of the legs. Dysphagia and bulbar disturbances may also develop.

Familial degeneration of the cerebellar cortex with mental deficiency in childhood is characterized by early childhood symptoms of variable mental deficiency, cerebellar ataxia, and nystagmus. No other symptoms are observed.

Familial cerebello-olivary degeneration in childhood is characterized by late childhood symptoms of gait disturbance, ataxia, tremors, and speech difficulty. The disease is progressive, and generalized muscular rigidity and mental deterioration characterize the late stages of the disease.

Other diseases of the cerebellum mentioned by Espir and Rose (1970, pp. 55–56) include: (a) multiple sclerosis manifesting "slurred, scanning, staccato" speech; (b) idiopathic, cerebellar atrophy beginning after 40 or 50 years; and (c) metabolic and toxic disorders such as hypothyroidism and alcoholism.

Clinical Manifestations

Speech manifestations of problems in lower-order output patterning may be categorized with respect to brain regions that are thought to be most contributory to the presenting symptoms, or they may be categorized under speech descriptive terms. Since it is difficult to ascribe specific symptoms to any one region responsible for lower-order efferent integration, the latter plan for presenting clinical manifestations was selected. However, whenever possible, the suspected brain region will be identified.

Reduced or Exaggerated Minor Speech. The use of emotional utterances, social-gesture speech, and memorized speech may be reduced or exaggerated in cases of bilateral hemispheral damage to speech centers. Since both major and minor speech brains are considered capable of mediating such verbal behavior, bilateral damage to speech centers may reduce the use of both complex and simple verbal behaviors; whereas damage to the major speech brain only may lead to reduced use of complex verbal behavior and an exaggerated use of minor speech as a result of the loss of inhibitory control by the major speech brain over the minor speech brain. For example, senseless rhyming or repetition (verbal release phenomena), partially on an involuntary basis, may be observed in certain cases of generalized and progressive cortical atrophy (e.g., Alzheimer's disease).

Persistence of Paleoverbal Behavior. The extended or excessive use by children of paleoverbal speech utterances such as single-word sentences, repetitive speech, and emotional utterances, already discussed in the previous chapter, may be related to: (a) the slow assumption of inhibitory control by the major speech brain over the minor speech brain, or (b) the slow development within the major speech brain of the capacity for more complex verbomotor behavior.

Reduced or Exaggerated Nonverbal Affective Communication. Speech-associated facial and tonal expressions are complementary to verbomotor behavior. Hence, in cases of basal ganglia or cerebellar lesions associated with mask-like facies and reduced speech melody (e.g., parkinsonism, cerebellar ataxia), the effectiveness of speech communication is decreased by virtue of depressed faciovocal affective communication. Midbrain lesions may also depress faciovocal affective communication; or, in cases of brain damage that releases the midbrain from inhibition by higher centers, attempts at speech communication may be associated with exaggerated facial expressions and reflexive crying and laughing.

Reflexogenic Articulatory Disorders. Reflexogenic articulatory disorders may be of three varieties. (a) Children are found who are equal in all ways but who manifest persisting residuals of infantile feeding reflexes such as the suckle-swallow, mouth-opening, lip, rooting, biting, and chewing reflexes. If articulatory attempts concomitantly elicit some of these involuntary movements, articulation and speech rhythm may suffer. (b) In cases of frank brain injury, such as cerebral palsy, these reflexes may persist and compound the dysarthria of cerebral palsy. (c) In certain cases of adult neurologic disorder, some of these reflexes may be released and also compound any speech involvement. Reflexogenic articulatory problems have been discussed by the author in another place (Mysak, 1968, pp. 91–92).

Problems in Programing of Articulatory Movements. Articulatory dypraxia (also aphemia, Broca's aphasia, motor aphasia, speech apraxia, oral dyspraxia, apraxic dysarthria, cortical dysarthria) describes a neurogenic articulatory disorder, due to a lesion of the anterior left cerebral hemisphere, in which limitations in direction and range of articulatory movements or significant weakness, slowness, or incoordination of articulatory movements are not major contributory factors. Johns and Darley (1970) studied the articulatory characteristics of individuals with apraxia of speech. They summarized their findings as follows:

"Initial consonant production in speech apraxia is characterized by a high degree of inconsistency of articulation errors; predominance of substitution, repetition, and addition errors as opposed to distortion errors of dysarthria; marked prosodic disturbance without phonatory and resonatory changes; increase of difficulty from spontaneous to oral reading to imitative speech conditions; facilitation of correct articulation by visual monitoring in the auditory-visual stimulus mode in contrast to the auditory (repeating tape-recorded stimuli) or visual (reading words) modes; deterioration of articulation with increase in length of word; and improvement when the patient is allowed to make several consecutive attempts to produce a desired response."

In contrast to the more familiar view of apraxia as a motor or output speech disorder is the finding of Rosenbek *et al.* (1973), "As a group [but not all] patients with apraxia of speech show significant oral sensory-perceptual deficit as measured by tests of oral form identification, two-point discrimination, and mandibular kinesthesia."

Skelly *et al.* (1974) reported on the use of American Indian Sign as a facilitator of verbalization in adults with articulatory apraxia.

Speech Dyscoordination. Problems in coordination of speech muscles (ataxophemia, ataxic dysarthria), specifically in the coordination of respiratory, phonatory, resonatory, and articulatory mechanisms or in coordinating movements within such mechanisms, may be an indication of cerebellar involvement. For example, individuals experiencing difficulty in coordinating phonatory and articulatory mechanisms may manifest voicing-unvoicing confusions. Those presenting problems in performing rapidly repetitive or alternating articulatory movements (articulatory dysdiadochocinesis) may manifest speech slowing (bradylalia), and those displaying poor control in range and precision of articulatory movements (articulatory dysmetria) may show speech slurring.

Speech Disintegration. A deterioration in speech ability while attempting simultaneous activities such as walking or writing may also implicate cerebellar mechanisms.

Speech Dyskinesias. Interference with respiratory, phonatory, resonatory, and articulatory movements by involuntary tremor and athetotic and choreiform movements may be associated with various types of lesions of the basal ganglia (athetotic dysarthria, choreic dysarthria).

Speech Dysrhythmias. Lesions of the basal ganglia, thalamus, and cerebellum may be reflected by various types of speech-time disorders (neuromotor dysautomaticity) such as problems in controlling rate and rhythm, use of pause time, and the ease of initiating and arresting speech. Specific symptoms of cerebellar speech dysrhythmia include: uttering each syllable of a word as though it were a separate word, or scanning speech, and misplaced and inappropriate loudness emphasis on syllables of words, or staccato speech (Espir and Rose, 1970, p. 54). Canter (1971) describes disfluency symptoms in certain cases of acquired cerebellar lesions that apply here. These symptoms may be marked by unusually severe tonic blocks that the individual finds difficult to break as well as by accelerating tonic blocks that may terminate in tense prolongations or in sudden speech stoppages.

Specific symptoms of basal ganglia speech dysrhythmia as found in parkinsonism were also discussed by Canter (1971) and include: "articulatory freezing" or consonantal prolongation upon attempts to articulate at normal or above-normal rates; palilalia, or articulatory attempts characterized by rapid syllable, word, and phrasal repetitions; and episodic long silent blocks in cases of advanced postencephalitic parkinsonism and similar problems in patients who have undergone unsuccessful bilateral thalamic surgery. Another symptom found in parkinsonism is articulatory festination, or the involuntary tendency to increase progressively the rate of articulation, sometimes to the point of unintelligibility. Other symptoms of speech dysrhythmia include spasmodic repetition of the end syllables of words (logoklony), choreic stiffening of lips with stuttering (labiochorea), and cluttering.

Wyke (1970) has hypothesized about neurological mechanisms in stammering. He proposes that stammering could be regarded ". . . as a manifestation of phonatory ataxia, resulting from temporal dysfunction in the operations of the voluntary and/or reflex mechanisms that continuously regulate the tone of the phonatory musculature during speech. . . ." He postulates two clinical types of stammering, voluntary, or cortical stammering, and reflex stammering. Cortical stuttering ". . . could arise from genetic, acquired or emotional inability to produce accurate voluntary presetting of the phonatory musculature for the utterance of particular sounds . . .;" while reflex stammering might describe a condition where the voluntary presetting of the musculature occurred but where ". . . the intrinsic laryngeal reflex systems failed to maintain the musculature in the desired preset phonatory posture."

Emotiomotor Speech Disorder. Emotiomotor speech disorders are those speech repercussions resulting from emotional release of the inhibitory control by the hypothalamus over the autonomic nervous system. The physical expression of emotions such as anxiety, guilt, frustration, and hostility may take the form of increased heart rate and elevation of blood pressure and sweating, as well as increased speech rate, elevated speaking fundamental frequency, and speech disfluency. More specifically, problems in speech output related to disturbances in glandular, muscular, or vascular functioning caused by certain memories, thoughts, or ideas may be described as ideoglandular, ideokinetic, or ideovascular speech disorders.

Diagnosis

Language symptoms of disorders of lower-order output patterning, that is, exaggerated use of minor speech and persistence of paleoverbal behavior, must be distinguished from gnosogenic and psychogenic language dysfunction. Articulatory deficiencies associated with released or retained infantile feeding reflexes, failure of intra-articulatory system coordination, and involuntary movements of the articulators must be distinguished from other forms of neurogenic articulatory problems, for example, those that impose consistent limitations on the direction and range of articulatory movements and those associated with problems of sensory feedback. Finally, rhythm symptoms of disorders of lower-order output patterning must be distinguished from various environmentally-based speech dysrhythmias.

Prognosis

Prognosis for speech therapy for output patterning disorders is dependent on the nature of the background disease. Answers to various questions will contribute to the clinician's estimate of what to expect from speech therapy in any one case. Is the disease chronic? Is it degenerative and progressive? Is it amenable to medical intervention? For example, in cases where symptoms are expected to disappear, such as in Sydenham's chorea, the role of the clinician may be to wait until the medical problem is resolved and to see whether any of the speech symptoms has been habituated. Prognosis for elimination of such habituated speech symptoms is good. In cases of relatively static disease involvement, such as in cases of congenital athetosis or ataxia, the prognosis of at least some speech improvement following speech therapy is also supportable. However, in cases where degeneration is usually irreversible but where the rate of degeneration is variable, such as in parkinsonism, Huntington's chorea, torsion dystonia, and hereditary cerebellar ataxia, prognostic statements with respect to the usefulness of speech therapy are made in different terms; that is, not in terms of improving speech, although this may be seen for short periods in those cases not actualizing full potential at various stages of disease progression, but rather in terms of maintaining the level of the person's speech communication for as long as possible or in slowing down the rate of speech deterioration.

Therapy

Planning therapy for output patterning disorders depends on whether the background condition is congenital or acquired and whether it is resolving, static, or progressive. For example, if we are dealing with problems resulting from congenital and early acquired cerebral palsy, wide-spectrum speech techniques may be applied, including work under categories of speech preventive measures and speech causal and speech symptom procedures. The author (Mysak, 1971, Ch. 27) has already devoted an entire chapter to this area.

The present therapy discussion is limited to specific suggestions to counter some of the symptoms cited in the section on clinical manifestations.

Stimulating Faciovocal Affective Communication. Symptoms of reduced facial expression and vocal variability (loudness, pitch, time) can be attacked in direct fashion. Sessions devoted to "face talk" and "voice talk" are the major techniques here. For example, a client may be asked to express with his face the contrasting feelings of happiness-sadness, surprise-boredom, and comfort-pain. Demonstrations by the clinician may be necessary. The client should be asked to "remember" the muscle sensations associated with the various facial movements. Similarly, the client may practice communicating calmness, anger, joy, and so on via the manipulation of the vocal variables of loudness, pitch, and rate.

Suppressing Persisting Infantile Oral Reflexes. Oral reflexes that may be observed to persist in children with various neuropathologies are the rooting, mouth-opening, lip, biting, suckling, and chewing reflexes (Mysak, 1968, p. 97). As already stated, in certain children speech attempts may concomitantly elicit these reflexes, which, in turn, may interfere with articulation and speech rhythm.

Suppression of these infantile feeding reflexes is done basically by providing the appropriate stimulation and resisting the expected response. Therefore, if the jaw deviates and the lower lip depresses when the angle of the mouth is stimulated (part of the rooting reflex), the clinician should apply the stimulus and physically prevent the occurrence of the response. Similar resistance maneuvers should be executed if the mouth opens reflexively in response to touch or to a visual stimulus (mouth-opening reflex), if tapping near the angle of the mouth evokes involuntary movements of the lips in addition to eventual lip closure and pouting (lip reflex), if placing an object between the dental arches elicits reflexive mouth closing and holding (biting reflex), and if stimulating the gums or teeth elicits reflexive chewing (chewing reflex). Reflex-weakening activities should be carried out two or three times a day.

The following portions of this therapy section contain suggestions for counteracting symptoms associated with irregular tonus, speech rate, range of articulatory movements, force of articulatory contacts, and speech rhythm. In general, the suggestions are aimed at improving the eurhythmy, eumetria, eutaxy, and diadochocinesia of the phonoarticulatory system.

Improving Speech System Coordination. Work that contributes to speech system coordination includes laryngopraxis, articulopraxis, and articulolaryngeal diadochocinesia activities.

Laryngopraxis exercises are used in cases in which the client exhibits difficulty in coordinating voicing-unvoicing activity with articulatory activity. In some cases, for example, voicing may continue throughout the utterance, irrespective of the need for unvoiced sounds, and ceases only during pause time. At least two forms of laryngopraxis work may be requested. (a) The client may be asked merely to initiate and cease a series of short vowel phonations (about one per second). For example, he is asked to produce an [ɑ-ɑ-ɑ] series or an [u-u-u] series. Success in the task is marked by the production of a series of clear, on-off phonatory units. (b) The client may be asked to produce accurately various voiced-unvoiced syllable combinations such as [bʌ – pʌ, vʌ – fʌ, ðʌ – θʌ, dʌ – tʌ, zʌ – sʌ, and gʌ – kʌ].

Articulopraxis exercises may be used in cases where poor control in range and accuracy of articulatory movements exists. The author (Mysak, 1968, p. 101) previously described the exercises under the heading of oroeupraxia. Well-performed and coordinated movements of the articulatory system is the goal of this work; speed of movement is not a factor. Depending on the capacity of the client, two-syllable, three-syllable, and four-syllable combinations are prepared. Two-syllable combinations are formed by a base syllable plus a progressively receding or preceding syllable. The receding or preceding syllable refers to the place of articulation. The receding sequence would be: bilabial, labiodental, linguadental, lingua-alveolar, lateral, linguapalatal, retroflex, and finally linguavelar sounds. An example of a two-syllable combination series is: [bʌ – vʌ (each combination is repeated three times), bʌ – ðʌ, bʌ – dʌ, bʌ – nʌ, bʌ – zʌ, bʌ – lʌ, bʌ – ʒʌ, bʌ – rʌ, bʌ – gʌ]. Two-syllable work should be continued until each receding syllable has served as the base syllable, for example, [vʌ – bʌ (complete preceding combinations with each new base syllable before returning to receding combinations) vʌ – ðʌ, vʌ – dʌ, vʌ – nʌ, vʌ – zʌ, vʌ – lʌ, etc.]. In preparing the series, sounds that cannot be made easily by the client may be eliminated until they can be produced. Following successful work with two-syllable series, three and four-syllable series should be prepared.

Articulolaryngeal diadochocinesia work should follow successful articulopraxis activities. Laryngodiadochocinesia is laryngopraxis work with the element of speed added. Hence, the client must not only produce clear on-off phonatory units but must do so at progressively higher speeds, until some maximum rate is reached. Similarly, articulo-diadochocinesia is articulopraxis with the element of speed added. Again, the client must not only produce well the two-syllable, three-syllable, and four-syllable series but must do so at progressively higher speeds, until maximum rates are reached.

Reducing Involuntary Movements of the Speech System. Resisted movements, sensory fencing, and differentiation activities are techniques designed to reduce involuntary speech movements.

Resisted movement techniques are applied to an oscillating speech organ in an attempt to develop muscle balance in opposing muscle groups and hence to stabilize the speech organ. In the case of alternating lip spreading and puckering movements associated with speech attempts, the clinician may resist the pucker movement by holding the corners of the mouth in the lip spread position and then resist the spread movement by holding the cheeks. The resisted movement aspect of the procedure is applied in an alternating fashion, first to prevent the spreading and then the puckering movements, and so on. Resistance is applied for different amounts of time, that is, a longer or shorter resistance of the spreading or the puckering movement, and with different degrees of force. This careful attempt at balancing or "playing" of muscle tonus in opposing muscle groups should eventually contribute to improved labial muscle stability. Similar maneuvers may be planned to counter involuntary mandibular and lingual movements.

Sensory fencing of a speech organ describes a process in which the clinician provides touch clues to the oscillating organ in the hopes of decreasing the range of its oscillation. If tongue protrusion elicits irregular lingual oscillation, for example, the clinician may encompass the range of the lingual movement with his two index fingers. The individual is asked to keep his tongue from making contact with either of the index fingers. As the individual meets with success, the clinician narrows the allowable range of oscillation by progressive approximation of his fingers until the client achieves maximum stabilization of the speech organ. Oscillations of the lips and jaw may be treated in a similar way.

Differentiation work is done to achieve or maintain the ability to move each of the speech organs in isolation. For example, the individual may be asked to extend his mandible to a half-open position and then spread and pucker his lips while keeping the mandible and tongue still. Then, with the mandible in a three-quarters-open position, he is asked to elevate the tongue tip to the alveolar ridge behind the upper incisors and to depress the tongue tip to the alveolar ridge behind the lower incisors in an alternating fashion while keeping the mandible and lips still. Finally, he is asked to flex and extend his mandible while inhibiting any lip or tongue activity. Maximum isolation of the movement of each speech organ should be sought or maintained.

Adjusting Speech Rate for Maximum Intelligibility. The author has already indicated that symptoms of pathology of central neural mechanisms for speech-rhythm control could include: scanning, staccato, or explosive speech; irregular speech acceleration-deceleration; episodic inability to initiate speech and speech arrest; and palilalia. Such forms of neurogenic speech dysrhythmia in cerebral palsy have already been described by the author (Mysak, 1971b, p. 689). Techniques described below are aimed primarily at irregular speech acceleration that interferes with speech intelligibility.

One technique is to have the client think of and use a "slow motion" form of articulation. Another is to have the client "gear down" his speech rate by requesting that he use harder contacts during articulatory efforts. Having the client use an "over-articulation" style of speaking is still another technique designed to regularize speech rate. In each of these techniques, the client is being asked to modify his speech consciously and, by so doing, the client may transform his speech patterns from the usual automatic-reflexive type, or speaking thoughts, into the voluntary-conscious type, or speaking words. Whatever benefit may be derived from these techniques may be related to the fact that different neurodynamics underlie the two types of speech. Also, the techniques tend to "amplify" the tactile-kinesthetic-pressure feedbacks associated with articulatory movements.

REFERENCES

Brain, W. R., and Walton, J. N., Diseases of the Nervous System. London: Oxford University Press (1969).

Canter, G. J., Observations on neurogenic stuttering: A contribution to differential diagnosis. Br. J. Disord. Commun., 6, 139–143 (1971).

Darley, F. L., Aronson, A. E., and Brown, J. R., Clusters of deviant speech dimensions in the dysarthrias. J. Speech Hear. Res., 12, 462–496 (1969).

Espir, M. L. E., and Rose, C. F., The Basic Neurology of Speech. Philadelphia: F. A. Davis Company (1970).

Ford, F. R., Diseases of the Nervous System in Infancy, Childhood and Adolescence. Springfield, Ill.: Charles C Thomas (1966).

Gatz, A. J., Manter's Essentials of Clinical Neuroanatomy and Neurophysiology. Philadelphia: F. A. Davis Company (1966).

Johns, D. F., and Darley, F., Phonemic variability in apraxia of speech. J. Speech Hear. Res., 13, 556–583 (1970).

Jones, W. O., Speech Disorder Associated with Dystonia Musculorum Deformans. Teachers College, Columbia University: Doctoral Dissertation (1968).

Luchsinger, R., and Arnold, G., Voice-Speech-Language. Belmont, Calif.: Wadsworth Publishing Co. (1965).

Mysak, E. D., Neuroevolutional Approach to Cerebral Palsy and Speech. New York: Teachers College Press, Columbia University (1968).

Mysak, E. D., Cerebral palsy speech habilitation. In L. E. Travis (Ed.), Handbook of Speech Pathology and Audiology. New York: Appleton-Century-Crofts (1971).

Mysak, E. D., Cerebral palsy speech syndromes. In L. E. Travis (Ed.), Handbook of Speech Pathology and Audiology. New York: Appleton-Century-Crofts (1971).

Rosenbek, J. C., Wertz, R. T., and Darley, F. L., Oral sensation and perception in apraxia of speech and aphasia. J. Speech Hear. Res., 16, 22–35 (1973).

Skelly, M., Schinsky, L., Smith, R. W., and Fust, R. S., American Indian Sign (AMER-IND) as a facilitator of verbalization for the oral verbal apraxic. J. Speech Hear. Disord., 39, 445–456 (1974).

Wepman, J. M., Approaches to the analysis of aphasia. In Human Communication and its Disorders—an Overview. Report of the National Institute of Neurological Diseases and Stroke, United States Department of Health, Education and Welfare (1969).

Worster-Drought, C., Speech disorders in children. Dev. Med. Child Neurol., 10, 427–440 (1968).

Wyke, B., Neurological mechanisms in stammering: an hypothesis. Br. J. Disord., Commun., 5, 6–15 (1970).

5

Speech Receptor System

Disorders of the speech receptor system may be found at any age; however, the effects of such disorders are significantly more serious among children. Primary and secondary speech problems associated with the speech receptor system may be identified. Primary problems are characterized by distorted, decreased, or lack of reception of speech information because of various degrees of involvement of the auditory and visual speech receptors; secondary problems are manifested by deviations in language, articulation, voice, and speech-time attributes based fundamentally on deficient models of these speech dimensions also resulting from involvement of the receptors. Symptoms may range from slight auditory and visual problems, causing little or no involvement of speech functioning, to total involvement of auditory and visual speech receptors, resulting in a complete loss of speech functioning. This chapter is oriented toward speech repercussions resulting from early and severe problems in the auditory and(or) visual speech receptors.

Although the chapter is divided, for reasons of exposition, into auditory receptor, visual receptor, and bireceptor disorders, it should be understood that intersensory collaboration exists between auditory and visual receptors, that the auditory receptor is dominant, and that disturbance in one component of the receptor system usually leads to the reduction of efficiency of the total system and compensatory functioning of the intact component.

AUDITORY RECEPTOR DISORDERS

The auditory speech receptor, as already described, is composed of those parts of the auditory system that are responsible for receiving speech-associated auditory stimuli and for converting those stimuli into appropriate codes of neural impulses (i.e., the outer, middle, and inner ears).

Background

The auditory speech receptor may be disturbed by numerous general as well as relatively localized human disorders. Categories of disorders described here include: general congenital conditions, specific congenital conditions, infections, toxins, oxygen deprivation, trauma, and Rh and other incompatibilities. This background discussion is devoted to describing the various kinds of human diseases in which hearing involvement may be found; it is not within the purpose of this chapter to describe the types of hearing loss that may be found.

General Congenital Conditions. The category of general congenital conditions is meant to cover conditions that involve more than just the ear, may be detected at birth, and may be due to heritable factors, chromosomal anomalies, infections, or to unknown causes.

Some of these conditions have already been described in Chapter 3 in the section "Gnosogenic Language Disorders in Children" and need not be discussed again. These include: "Albright's Hereditary Osteodystrophy," "Hunter's Syndrome," "Hurler's Syndrome," "Sanfilippo Syndrome," "Otopalatodigital Syndrome," "Turner's Syndrome" (male and female), and the Deletion 18 and Ring 18 chromosomal anomalies.

Following are brief descriptions of observable characteristics of other congenital conditions that may reflect hearing involvement and that have been described by Gellis and Feingold (1968).

Crouzon's disease, where mental retardation is usually not found, presents the following physical characteristics: abnormally-shaped head due to craniostenosis (usually brachycephaly); eye anomalies (exophthalmos, exotropia, nystagmus, hypertelorism); low-set ears; and prognathism secondary to hypoplasia of the maxilla.

Ectodermal dysplasia, in which retardation is not a constant feature, is manifested by the following physical characteristics: frontal bossing of the head, eye anomalies (thin, wrinkled eyelids, conjunctivitis); protruding or deformed ears; chronic rhinitis; dental anomalies (delayed or absent dentition; teeth, when present, may be small and wide-spaced with peg-shaped incisors and canines); skin anomalies (translucent, smooth, thin, dry); hypotrichosis of scalp and body; dysphagia; and hoarse voice.

Metaphysial dysplasia, in which intellection is normal, presents the following physical characteristics: macrocephaly; eye anomalies (hypertelorism, heterotropia, nystagmus, visual loss); broad nose with bony prominence of the glabella; enlarged mandible with prognathism; delayed dentition; and cranial nerve abnormalities (secondary to obstruction of the cranial foramina).

Morquio's disease, in which intellection is usually normal, is manifested by the following physical characteristics: severe dwarfism, broad mouth with prominent maxilla and widely-spaced teeth, and very short neck.

Oculoauriculovertebral dysplasia, in which intellection is normal, is characterized by the following physical characteristics: eye anomalies (epibulbar dermoids, coloboma of upper lid); ear anomalies (small, low set, abnormally shaped; stenosis or atresia of external auditory meatus; preauricular fleshy appendages); and unilateral hypoplasia of the mandible.

Osteogenesis imperfecta, in which mental retardation is infrequent, presents the following physical characteristics: triangular facies; overhanging occiput and hydrocephalus; eye anomalies (blue sclerae, corneal opacities); possibly protruding ears; and dental anomalies (caries, easily broken, translucent bluish-gray or yellowish-brown in color).

Osteopetrosis, in which retardation is usually not present, is manifested by the following physical characteristics: short stature with brittle, fragile bones; enlarged, square-shaped head; eye anomalies (prominent, progressive visual loss, muscle abnormalities, cataracts, optic atrophy); broad-bridged nose; and abnormally-developed, carious teeth.

Treacher Collins syndrome, in which retardation is usually not present, is characterized by the following physical characteristics: facial bone abnormalities (flattened facial bones, hypoplasia of maxilla and mandible); eye anomalies (antimongoloid slant, colobomas of lower lid); ear anomalies (hypoplasia or absence of auricles, stenotic or atretic meatuses); nose anomalies (beaked nose with narrow nostrils); and mouth anomalies ("fish-like," high-arched palate with infrequent cleft lip or palate, dental abnormalities).

Waardenburg Syndrome, in which retardation is not present, presents the following physical characteristics: eye anomalies (lateral displacement of medial canthi, heterochromia, hypertrichosis and graying of medial portion of eyebrows); prominent nose with flaring nasal alae; prominent mandible; full lips; and white or gray forelock.

Cerebral palsies are frequently accompanied by hearing disorders of every variety and degree, including conductive and sensorineural losses (Mysak, 1971, p. 678). Incidence figures have been reported to go as high as 30 to 40%. In terms of the major types of cerebral palsy, the highest incidence of hearing loss has been reported among the athetotics and then in decreasing figures among the ataxics and spastics.

Specific Congenital Conditions. By specific congenital conditions is meant those anomalies that involve the external, middle, and inner ears, that may or may not have a familial basis, and that are thought to be present at birth.

Included in this category of anomalies are malformations of the auricle alone that have no real significance for hearing loss (Davis, 1970, p. 101), atresias of the external auditory canal, anomalies limited to the middle ear, and combined external and middle-ear anomalies (Goodhill et al., 1971, pp. 298–302) that are significant with respect to hearing loss.

Involvements of the inner ear include cochlear aplasia, "or developmental arrest of the cochlea, spiral-ganglion, and/or neural auditory pathway . . . ;" heredodegenerative hypacuses, in which atrophy or degeneration of the organ of Corti and the sensorineural auditory pathway begins around the twelfth or fifteenth month (in some cases onset may be delayed until later childhood or adolescence); and otosclerotic sensorineural hypacusis (Goodhill et al., 1971, pp. 320–322). A specific type of hereditary deafness, noted by Davis (1970, p. 126), in which abnormalities appear only in the cochlear duct and saccule (Scheibe's type), is thought to be present in about 70% of cases of hereditary deafness.

Infections. Goodhill et al. (1971, pp. 302–308) identify the following types of infections involving the middle ear: acute otitis media, acute suppurative mastoiditis, unresolved otitis media and mastoiditis, and chronic purulent otitis media with ossicular destruction and mastoiditis. Syphilis and tuberculosis may also affect the middle ear (Davis, 1970, p. 107).

Forms of infection that may affect the inner ear include: congenital and acquired syphilis; bacterial infections such as meningitis, typhoid fever, and diphtheria; and viral infections such as rubella, mumps, measles, encephalitis, chickenpox, whooping cough, and influenza.

Toxins. Certain drugs taken during pregnancy may affect the developing hearing system. The cochlea appears susceptible to damage from the following drugs: quinine, streptomycin, dihydrostreptomycin, kanamycin, and neomycin. Alcohol and tobacco may also have indirect and direct toxic effects upon the developing cochlea (Goodhill et al., 1971, p. 323).

Oxygen Deprivation. Significant deprivation of oxygen at birth (hypoxia, anoxia) may damage irreversibly the neural epithelium of the organ of Corti (Goodhill et al., 1971, p. 326). Background factors for such oxygen deprivation include "long labors, heavy maternal sedation, obstruction of the respiratory passages with mucus, incomplete development of the lungs, and congenital circulatory and cardiac defects."

Trauma. At least two forms of physical trauma may affect the ear, indirect trauma via physical trauma to the head and direct trauma to the cochlea (acoustic trauma). Indirect natal ear damage may be caused by cephalic trauma and intracranial hemorrhage due to maternal pelvic abnormalities, injudicious use of forceps, and irregular presentations at birth (Goodhill et al., 1971, p. 326).

Rh and Other Incompatibilities. Various types of blood-group incompatibilities between mother and fetus such as the Rh factor may cause direct or indirect injury to the auditory system in the infant (Davis, 1970, p. 122).

Morley (1965, pp. 98–99) reported on 110 children with hearing loss sufficient to cause language retardation. Eighty-four of the problems were considered to be congenital and the rest had illnesses in infancy that might have caused the problem. For the greater number of congenital cases, the cause was unclear. In the history of the 24 suspected cases of acquired hearing loss, the following diseases were found: meningitis, severe measles, severe whooping cough, pneumonia, and mumps. Kendall (1966, p. 216) states, in his extensive review of the literature on auditory problems in children, "most retrospective studies have been unable to assign a definite or fairly certain etiology to more than about fifty percent of the child population with severe hearing impairment. . . ."

Clinical Manifestations

Speech problems associated with involvement of the auditory receptor may be divided into primary and secondary types. Primary speech symptoms of auditory receptor problems are those of perception of speech stimuli; secondary speech symptoms are those of production of speech stimuli.

Differences in patterns of primary and secondary symptoms among the deaf and severely hard of hearing may be attributed to time of onset of hearing loss; type and degree of hearing loss; intelligence and motivation of the client; speech environment of the client; and method used in helping the client learn speech.

Primary Problems. Primary symptoms include raised thresholds for speech reception without important distortion of the speech signal, as in middle-ear hearing losses, and raised thresholds for speech reception accompanied by degrees of distortion in the speech signal, as in cochlear losses. If the loss is great enough, little if any auditory reception of the speech signal occurs and, therefore, speech perception processes may not be possible at all. Di Carlo (1964, p. 43) states, in his review of definitions of childhood deafness, "There now seems to be a general agreement that a hearing loss of 80 dB or more in the speech range, if present prior to the acquisition of language and speech, should be accepted as a satisfactory definition of deafness."

In general, the degree of hearing involvement in early childhood affects speech perception as follows: severe hearing loss usually results in a lack of development of verboacoustic comprehension; partial loss of hearing for all frequencies may result in a delay in and restriction of verboacoustic comprehension; while specific high-frequency hearing loss may place restrictions on verboacoustic comprehension.

In one aspect of a system used by the American Academy of Ophthalmology and Otolaryngology (Silverman, 1971, p. 401), the ability to perceive speech is related to the average hearing threshold level for 500, 1000, and 2000 Hz in the better ear. When the loss is not more than 25 dB, no significant difficulty occurs with faint speech; when the loss is more than 25 dB but not more than 40 dB, difficulty is experienced only with faint speech; when the loss is more than 40 dB but not more than 55 dB, frequent difficulty occurs with normal speech; when the loss is more than 55 dB but not more than 70 dB, frequent difficulty is experienced with loud speech; when the loss is more than 70 dB but not more than 90 dB, one can understand only shouted or amplified speech; and when the loss is more than 90 dB, one usually cannot understand even amplified speech.

More specifically, children with high-frequency losses will reflect difficulty in differentiating among words that contain high-frequency consonants and are also voiceless, and hence have little phonetic power, such as [s, θ, f, k, p, ʃ, tʃ, h, hw] (Newby, 1972, p. 344). Morley (1965, p. 90), in discussing discrimination of consonants as a function of hearing for pure tones, indicated that the differentiation of the voiceless consonants [p, t, k, f, s, ʃ, θ] "depends on appreciation of the higher frequencies of sound in the range 1000 to 2000 c.p.s., with component tones extending possibly to 6000 c.p.s." Morley (pp. 90–91), reporting on the findings of Fletcher and Watson and Tolan, stated that speech intelligibility is reduced by 10% when frequencies above 3000 Hz are cut out and by 70% when frequencies above 1500 Hz are eliminated.

Finally, West and Ansberry (1968, pp. 146–147) discussed the effects of hearing losses in various frequency ranges "upon the ability to learn and understand orally." They indicated that, if an individual were insensitive only to the low-frequency range of speech sounds (about 100 to 400 Hz), he might have difficulty in distinguishing differences in pitch of voices, in distinguishing between voiced and voiceless sounds, and in perceiving the first formants of some vowels. If the problem lay with the middle-frequency range of speech sounds (about 500 to 3000 Hz), he might have difficulty in distinguishing among vowels and among voiced consonants; and if the significant problem were with the high-frequency range of speech sounds (about 3000 to 8000 Hz), his ability to recognize the difference among many consonants would be seriously affected, especially for voiceless consonants such as [f], [s], [θ].

Secondary Problems. Speech production problems secondary to hearing loss take various forms. Speech may be absent, retarded, or poorly produced because of an absence, reduction, or distortion in the reception of speech signals. Production problems are related to reproducing poorly-perceived speech signals and to a lack of or inadequate audiomonitoring of speech stimuli. Auditory control and monitoring capacities are treated more specifically in Chapter 8, which is devoted to the speech sensor system.

The following relationships exist between the severity of the primary involvement and the degree of the secondary involvement: severe hearing loss may result in an absence of speech; partial hearing loss for all frequencies may result in substantial delay in onset of speech and articulatory deficiencies; and high-frequency hearing loss may result in little delay in speech onset but substantial deficiencies in articulation (Morley, 1965, p. 97). Partial hearing loss of the conductive variety, depending on its severity and time of onset, may cause little if any difficulty with reference to the onset of the use of spoken symbols or of their articulation.

Of the 110 severely hypacusic children discussed by Morley (1965, p. 102), 29 did not say any words, and 28 of the remaining 81 children spoke their first words by four years. Di Carlo (1964, pp. 94–95) states, "Unless the deaf child has had intensive early instruction, he probably has less than twenty-five words at the age of five years." Further, he states (p. 99) that evaluation of the speech of the deaf reveals severe delay and restriction in ". . . vocalization from birth, the time at which single words appear, the use of single sentences, the proficiency of articulation of speech sounds, the general length of the speech responses in communication, the amount of speech output, and the vocabulary usage."

After a review of studies of the language of hard-of-hearing children, O'Neill (1964, pp. 109–110) does not believe that generalizations can be made yet on deficits in comprehension and usage. However, some evidence exists to indicate that children with mild to moderate hearing losses may reflect language deficits.

More specifically, Carhart (1970, p. 363) indicates that hearing loss may result in articulatory defects as well as defects in nonphonetic elements of speech such as melody, quality, time, and force. Various types of phonetic lapses have been noted in cases of serious impairment in hearing. Some of these are: (a) difficulty in producing high-frequency voiceless consonants such as [p, h, f, θ, s, $\int$, t$\int$, t, k]; (b) giving visible for nonvisible sound substitutions, for example [d/g, j/l, w/r]; (c) the tendency to omit sounds in final positions because of their lowered phonetic power; and (d) giving voiced for voiceless sound substitutions, for example [$\eth$/ θ, v/f, z/s, ʒ/ $\int$].

West and Ansberry (1968, pp. 149–150) commented on the difference in speech profiles between conductive and sensorineural hearing impairments. The audiogenic dyslalia associated with a significant conductive loss may be characterized by difficulty in discriminating between vowels and voiced consonants, distorting voiceless consonants, and a tendency toward speaking with reduced pitch variability and loudness level. Audiogenic dyslalia associated with significant sensorineural involvement may result in some consonantal distortions, omissions, or substitutions. Sounds such as [s, f, θ] and those not visible to a listener when produced are expected to be most affected.

In regard to connatal or early acquired deafness ("loss of all serviceable hearing"), Luchsinger and Arnold (1965, pp. 631–632) describe respiratory, voice, articulatory, and accentuation deviations in speech production. Speech breathing may not be coordinated with articulatory movements, rate of breathing may be high (tachypnea), and air wastage may be present. Phonatory patterns may be characterized by distorted modulation and an elevated speaking pitch. Exaggerated movements and contacts of the lips, jaw, and tongue (articulatory hyperkinesis) may accompany articulatory efforts; hence plosive sounds are made best while fricative sounds are less well made. Sibilants are severely distorted: [s] and [ʃ] are usually pronounced like [ts] and [t ʃ] (addental lisping), and palatal lisping (tongue too far back) and lateral lisping are also frequently found. Also, because of the lack of audioregulation, speech attempts may be associated with various paraphonic sounds, for example, noisy breathing, grunting, smacking, and clicking.

Luchsinger and Arnold (1965, pp. 637–638) also describe audiogenic dyslalia in cases of partial hearing loss due to conductive or sensorineural involvements. Characteristic speech symptoms in middle-ear losses include: low and weak voice, monotonous speech melody, and a tendency toward hyponasality and unvoicing of final consonants. In inner-ear losses, speech symptoms include: high and loud voice, monotonous speech melody, frequent hypernasality, and omitted or slurred sibilants.

Diagnosis

At least two factors must be determined by the diagnostician before certain speech symptoms may be attributed to problems in the auditory speech receptor: (a) the involvement of the auditory receptor must be established, and (b) the speech profile should reflect audiogenecity.

Various approaches to the collection of diagnostic information may be utilized in establishing that an early hearing impairment exists. Data on auditory maturation and prespeech vocalization should be collected whenever possible. Then, the following kinds of examinations and referrals may be made as needed: utilization of various tests such as auditory reflex testing, alerting-orienting testing, conditioning audiometry, various forms of electrophysiological audiometry (electrodermal response, electroencephalograph), and speech audiometry (instrumental diagnosis); utilization of contributions from various related specialists such as the otolaryngologist, pediatrician, and psychologist (group diagnosis); observation of reactions to amplification and visual clues (diagnosis by treatment); and distinguishing deviant auditory behavior from deviant behavior associated with brain dysfunction, emotional disorder, and mental retardation (differential diagnosis). General behavioral characteristics of the anacusic child have been described by Myklebust (1954, pp. 111–141) as follows: (a) motor development is normal, (b) he may use a shuffling gait, (c) emotional development is somewhat delayed, and (d) he is unduly sensitive to visual (including facial expressions) and tactile stimuli and unusually active with respect to touching things.

Prognosis

The prognosis for developing usable speech communication in children with early and substantial involvement of the auditory speech receptor is dependent on numerous factors. Among these are: age of onset of hearing involvement; degree and type of hearing loss; the child's intelligence, motivation, patience, tenacity, and energy level; parental and family cooperation; and the time and quality of speech, hearing, and otologic and special educational intervention. The presence of this multiplicity of prognostic factors may help explain why some children with relatively mild hearing impairments have serious speech perception and production problems, while others with relatively severe hearing impairments exhibit only minimal speech perception and production problems.

Therapy

Management of speech problems associated with involvement of the auditory speech receptor is discussed in this section.

Primary Preventive Measures. All health specialists and especially speech and hearing clinicians must make strenuous efforts toward helping to prevent disorders of the auditory speech receptor. The public should be made aware of those heritable conditions that may be accompanied by hearing involvements, and genetic counseling must be made available. Also, potential parents and new parents should be made aware of the possible dangers to the auditory speech receptor of the various infections, toxins, and so on described in the background portion of this section of the chapter. Early and periodic auditory screening should be strongly recommended.

Secondary Preventive Measures. As soon as a high-risk infant has been identified, secondary preventive measures should be applied. The measures outlined in the therapy portions of the sections devoted to simple language immaturity and genetic language immaturity in Chapter 3 also apply here. Until the hearing impairment is confirmed, speech events should be amplified by reducing the distance between speakers and infant, by having speakers raise their loudness levels, and by the use of loudspeaker units. As soon as the hearing loss is confirmed, personal hearing aids should be used. Certainly they should be introduced by 18 months.

Causal Therapy. Etiologically-oriented therapy procedures include any medical treatment for the relief or improvement of the hearing involvement that otologists or other medical specialists may be able to offer and the fitting of an appropriate hearing aid.

Symptom Therapy. Speech-symptom therapy is begun during the speech age (about 1 to 2 years) and is designed to supplement the efforts made in the application of secondary preventive measures and causal therapy. The specific goals are to expand, improve, and correct speech perception and production.

Some of the general guides to practice with respect to speech and hearing training for the deaf offered by Silverman (1971, pp. 413–424) include the following. (a) The creation by significant others (parents, siblings, friends, teachers, relatives) of a dynamic speech atmosphere where "speech is experienced as a vitally significant and successful means of communication" (p. 417). (b) Spontaneous use of speech should be encouraged, supplemented by formal instruction when appropriate. (c) In the development of articulation, Silverman identifies the two ends of the continuum in approaches: the elemental, analytical approach, where individual sounds are developed out of speech contexts, and the natural approach, where sounds are developed within words and phrases. Silverman believes in a middle approach and indicates that the "syllable is a suitable unit for the development of articulation and of desirable temporal patterns in speech" (pp. 417–418). (d) In terms of language, Silverman identifies vocabulary, multiple meanings, verbalization of abstractions, and complexity of structure as major problems for the child. He describes two major approaches to instruction in language: "the natural method, sometimes known as the synthetic, informal, or mother method; and the grammatical method, sometimes referred to as the logical, systematic, formal, analytical or artificial method" (p. 423). At this point in time, Silverman recommends a combination of the best aspects of a grammatical method with a natural method. Some of his suggested guides to practice are that "language teaching should be related to significant and meaningful experiences;" that language should always be purposeful; that language teaching be related to current ideas that are developing in children; and that homes and schools should create an active language atmosphere (speaking, listening, reading). (e) Finally, auditory training or the use of all residual hearing potential should begin in the first year of life. Formal auditory training is essential in addition to the fitting of a hearing aid; "instruction should teach children to discriminate, even though grossly, various environmental sounds, and, within the limits of their hearing, teach them to understand speech by hearing" (p. 420).

Compensatory Therapy. At the beginning of this chapter it is stated that auditory and visual speech receptors naturally collaborate in the process of speech perception. Also that disturbance in one component of the receptor system usually causes a reduction in the efficiency of the total system and, relevant to the present discussion, compensatory functioning of the intact component. The implication is that we may expect a child with severe involvement of the auditory speech receptor to compensate spontaneously with the visual speech receptor. However, to ensure maximum development of intercommunication ability among the deaf, methods of teaching compensatory verbovisual communication as well as compensatory use of other sensory channels have been developed.

Compensatory speechreading, or verbovisual communication, is one form of compensatory behavior that should be facilitated in those with serious involvement of the auditory speech receptor and should be begun as soon as hearing involvement is suspected. Body language in terms of general postures, hand gestures, and facial expressions, always in association with oral language, should be emphasized during the prespeech period; that is, whenever possible speech play with involved infants should be accompanied by enriched body language. Such speech play should take place at various distances within the child's communisphere, or within the 3- to 12-foot range. The repertoire of the child's body-language comprehension can be developed quite early. For example, he can learn to understand common, whole-body attitudes accompanying speech associated with states of excitement and sleepiness; common hand gestures associated with words and phrases such as "no," "yes," "come here," and "go away"; and common facial expressions associated with words and phrases such as "good" and "bad" and with feelings such as happiness and sadness. Normal young children naturally attend to such kinetic paralanguage, and it is reasonable to expect that hearing-involved children will have even a greater tendency to do so. The goal of speakers in the involved child's communisphere is to be sure to stimulate that tendency.

As the child enters the speech age, the emphasis in verbomotor communication should be placed on facial expressions and speech-associated articulatory movements. The child should be encouraged to watch the face of the speaker and to comprehend the expressions associated with speech that describe pleasant vs. unpleasant events, sad vs. happy events, exciting vs. dull events, and so on, and expressions that signify fatigue, disinterest, concern, and so on. Then he must learn to identify as many phonemes as possible by the articulatory movements of which they are composed.

Articulatory visual acuity, fields, and tracking exercises should also contribute to verbomotor perception. Acuity for articulatory postures can be exercised by having the child first imitate various articulatory postures at the outer limits of the person-to-person communisphere (about 6 feet) and then at the person-to-small-group distance (about 12 feet). Visual fields for articulatory postures can be stimulated by having the child fix at the center of the clinician's forehead and again assume the various articulatory postures displayed by the clinician. Visual tracking can be exercised by having the child volitionally track exaggerated nonspeech movements of the articulators as well as various speech movements.

Other forms of compensatory visual activity include the use of various systems of orthography to assist in the comprehension and use of speech units, finger spelling, and various electronic devices that transmute aspects of verboacoustic code into visual displays.

Compensatory tactile-kinesthetic communication is another form of compensatory therapy used with children with serious involvement of the auditory speech receptor.

The most common use of vibrotactile stimulation is to have the child place his fingertips or hand on key locations of the speaker's face so that he can feel the vibrations of the nasal alae when nasal sounds are produced, or the vibrations in the larynx when voiced sounds are produced, or the puffs of air or streams of air when plosive or continuant sounds are produced. When attempting to reproduce sounds, the child holds both the speaker's face and his own in the hopes of identifying a match in vibration and tactile sensations. Providing the child with touch-pressure-movement dimensions of a target sound may be accomplished by actually taking the child's articulators through the positions and movements of which the sound is composed or by the utilization of Young's moto-kinesthetic method.

Other forms of compensatory skin communication include braille reading, palm writing, and the decoding of vibratized skin language. These forms are basically used when the individual exhibits visual complications; more will be said about these compensatory techniques under "Bireceptor Speech Disorders."

Compensatory manual communication in the form of the manual alphabet and(or) manual signs is often used when oral approaches fail and when children enter the special school situation. For further discussion, see "Bireceptor Speech Disorders."

VISUAL RECEPTOR DISORDERS

The visual speech receptor is responsible for receiving stimuli connected with speech-associated body postures and movements, facial expressions, and articulatory movements. Although speech reception is acknowledged to be a bisensory function, the field of speech pathology and audiology has paid comparatively little attention to the role of the visual speech receptor in certain types of speech deficits. Hence, this section is written more with the hope of stimulating interest in this relatively neglected area of our field than with the goal of providing substantial information about visuogenic speech disorders.

Background

The visual speech receptor composed of the eyelids, eyeballs, rectus and oblique muscles, retinae, and the oculomotor, trochlear, and abducens nerves may be affected as part of general congenital conditions.

Such general conditions are discussed here as well as symptoms of certain specific visual and oculomotor problems.

General Congenital Conditions. As in the case of the auditory speech receptor, general congenital conditions include abnormalities detected at birth that may be due to heritable factors, chromosomal anomalies, infection, or unknown causes. Descriptions of conditions with refractive and oculomotor involvements already discussed under "Gnosogenic Language Disorders in Children" in Chapter 3 and in the preceding background portion on the auditory speech receptor and that need not be repeated here are: "Albright's Hereditary Osteodystrophy" (lenticular calcification, cataracts, blue sclerae, strabismus); "Ataxia Telangiectasia" (telangiectasia of the bulbar conjunctiva, nystagmus, abnormalities of conjugate movements); "Cerebrohepatorenal Syndrome" (hypertelorism, shallow supraorbital ridges, cataracts and(or) glaucoma); "Deletion 18" Syndrome (partial deletion of the long arm) (epicanthal folds, hypertelorism, nystagmus); "Cry of the Cat Syndrome" (hypertelorism, antimongoloid slant, epicanthal folds, strabismus, optic atrophy); "Crouzon's Disease" (bilateral exophthalmos, divergent strabismus, nystagmus, hypertelorism); "Klinefelter's Syndrome" (myopia, astigmatism); "Laurence-Moon-Biedl Syndrome" (esotropia, microcornea, cataracts, blindness, mongoloid slant); "Metaphysial Dysplasia" (hypertelorism, nystagmus, visual loss); "Myotonic Dystrophy" (ptosis, cataracts); "Oculoauriculovertebral Dysplasia" (epibulbar dermoids, colobomas), "Osteogenesis Imperfecta" (blue sclerae, corneal opacities, hypermetropia); "Osteopetrosis" (progressive visual loss, eye-muscle abnormalities, cataracts, optic atrophy); "Treacher Collins Syndrome" (antimongoloid slant, colobomas, absent eyelashes, occasionally microphthalmia and cataracts); and "Turner's Syndrome" (female, male) (epicanthal folds, ptosis, strabismus, blue sclerae, antimongoloid slant, hypertelorism, myopia, strabismus).

Following are brief descriptions of observable characteristics of other congenital involvements that may present eye anomalies and that have been discussed by Gellis and Feingold (1968).

Hallerman-Streiff syndrome, in which intelligence ranges from normal to severe retardation, presents the following characteristics: eye anomalies (bilateral microphthalmia, congenital cataracts, nystagmus, strabismus, blue sclerae); brachycephaly or scaphocephaly; low-set ears; thin, beaked nose; mouth anomalies (small, thin lips, high-arched palate, dental irregularities, micrognathia); and proportional dwarfism.

Mucopolysaccharidosis (Scheie's syndrome), in which intellection is usually normal, presents the following characteristics: eye anomalies (hazy or cloudy corneas, retinitis pigmentosa); broad mouth; skeletal abnormalities; and hirsutism.

Oculodentodigital dysplasia, in which mental retardation if present is usually mild, presents the following characteristics: eye anomalies (microphthalmia, hypotelorism, glaucoma, epicanthal folds, abnormal irides); narrow and elongated head; thin nose with small nasal alae; mouth anomalies (hypoplastic enamel, small incisors, occasional cleft palate); and hand anomalies (camptodactyly, syndactyly, brachydactyly).

Rieger's syndrome, in which intellection is usually normal, presents the following characteristics: eye anomalies (abnormalities of the iridies, glaucoma); mouth anomalies (hypodontia, anodontia, enamel hypoplasia, missing maxillary incisors); and broad facies with prognathism.

Congenital rubella, in which intellection ranges from normal to severe involvement, presents the following characteristics: eye anomalies (cataracts or glaucoma, strabismus, nystagmus, iris hypoplasia); open anterior fontanel and microcephaly; hearing loss; and motor retardation.

Specific Symptoms of Visual and Oculomotor Problems. Following are some symptoms of certain visual and oculomotor abnormalities. Large-scale roving eye movements are typical of blindness acquired before the age of fixation (2 or 3 months). Congenital nystagmus is usually associated with diminished visual acuity. Blindness acquired under 2 or 3 years of age is usually accompanied by a degree of nystagmus (Paine and Oppé, 1966, pp. 99–100). Paralysis of nerve III causes the affected eye to deviate laterally and slightly downward and causes ptosis of the upper lid and dilation of the pupil. Paralysis of nerve IV may cause a slight elevation of the affected eye. Paralysis of nerve III or IV is associated with tipping rather than turning of the head. Paralysis of nerve VI causes medial deviation of the affected eye and may cause the patient to turn the head slightly toward the paretic side. Forced downward deviation of the eyes at rest ("setting sun sign") is an important sign of increased intracranial pressure in newborn and young infants and is also observed in kernicterus in early infancy (Paine and Oppé, 1966, pp. 111–112).

Clinical Manifestations

As with the auditory receptor, speech problems associated with involvement of the visual receptor may be divided into primary and secondary forms.

Primary Problems. Primary problems include reduced communicative sensitivity resulting from deficits in eye-to-eye interaction during speaking and reduced or absent awareness of speech-associated body postures, hand gestures, facial expressions, and articulatory movements. Pauses and silent periods in conversation are also more difficult for the blind to decode. Reduced visual perception also affects the development of language that grows to describe and catalog visual percepts.

Secondary Problems. Secondary problems may take the form of difficulty in learning to produce accurately speech sounds that contain more obvious visual clues, for example, bilabials, labiodentals, and linguadentals. With an intact auditory receptor it would be expected that, in most cases, when all else is equal, all speech sounds would eventually develop irrespective of a serious or total problem with the visual speech receptor. However, with a serious or total involvement of the visual speech receptor, there might very well be a reduction in or limited use of speech-associated body postures, hand gestures, and facial expressions. Congenitally-blind speakers frequently speak in a rather "stiff" manner, that is, a noticeable lack in their repertoire of speech-associated body language may be apparent. Other problems include establishing proper speaker-listener head orientation (the blind speaker cannot easily and automatically orient toward the target listener) and obtaining visual feedback responses to one's utterances.

Diagnosis

A visuogenic speech disorder is based first on the determination of some form or complex of visual problems, such as problems in visual acuity (e.g., blindness, nearsightedness, farsightedness), visual fields (e.g., homonymous hemianopia, bitemporal hemianopia, homonymous quadratic defects), or in eye postures and movements (strabismus, nystagmus). This determination is made by ophthalmologists and optometrists. Next, the speech pathologist must determine whether the eye problem is of the kind that may contribute to the kinds of primary and secondary communicative problems just described; in the case of blindness or near-blindness, it is clear that such a condition exists. When it comes to various degrees of refractive involvement and(or) oculomotor abnormality, the speech clinician may not be too sure whether the problem is of such a nature as to produce speech repercussions.

To assist the clinician in determining whether the eye problem may have speech implications, the visual tests described in Chapter 2 should be utilized, that is, tests for acuity of articulatory postures, for visual fields' sensitivity for articulatory postures, and for visual tracking of articulatory movements.

Finally, speech symptoms observed should be explainable on the basis of involvement of the visual speech receptor. In terms of primary involvement, for example, the child may lack comprehension or may not be sure about comprehension of language used to name and describe objects that are visualized; in terms of secondary involvement, the child may be showing or have had difficulty in learning speech sounds with more obvious visual dimensions and(or) may be exhibiting a limited or stereotyped repertoire of speech-associated body language.

In a study of speech problems among 293 elementary school children (average age, 10.1 years) attending two schools for the blind, almost one-third were found to have some type of speech deviation (Miner, 1963). About 25% had some form of articulation problem. However, the author cautions that it should not be generalized that one-third of all blind children have speech deviations, but rather that the incidence of speech difficulty among the visually handicapped is substantially higher than most estimates of defective speech in public school surveys. A similar finding of high incidence of speech disorder among residents of a school for the blind was reported by Lezak and Starbuck (1964). A study of 173 residents (age range was from 5 to 21 years) showed that approximately 50% had some form of speech disorder; approximately 40% had articulatory problems.

Therapy

Therapy for those with visual speech receptor problems is presented in this section. Again, since the speech and hearing field has paid little if any attention to this area, little exists in the way of established information.

Secondary Preventive Measures. When partial blindness or serious acuity and(or) oculomotor problems are suspected in a child, at least two steps should be recommended to parents by the speech clinician. (a) Speakers should speak to the child within the arms-length communisphere as often as possible. The child should also be allowed and encouraged to feel the face and articulators of the speaker. (b) The auditory reception of speech sounds may be facilitated by slowing the speech flow and by producing speech sounds more precisely.

Causal Therapy. Whenever visuogenic speech repercussions are suspected by the clinician, he should make referrals to opthalmology-optometry. Medical treatment, visual training, and eyeglass corrections should be encouraged. Such referrals on the part of the clinician acknowledge the importance of the visual speech receptor for the optimum development of speech and kinetic paralanguage abilities.

Symptom Therapy. Unlike the substantial speech repercussions accompanying serious involvement of the auditory speech receptor, the possible persisting symptoms accompanying serious involvement of the visual speech receptor (when all else is equal) include articulatory deficits, reduction in the use of kinetic paralanguage, and subtle language deficits based on naming and describing objects and events that are perceived visually either poorly or not at all.

For the articulatory lapses, the self-adjusting approach to articulation therapy to be described in Chapter 8 is recommended.

To remedy the possible reduction in the use of kinetic paralanguage by the child, (a) the concept of kinetic paralanguage or body language should be introduced, (b) he should be encouraged to use his remaining vision and(or) to feel facial expressions and hand gestures accompanying the speech of his parents, and (c) he should be encouraged and reminded to accompany his speech attempts with appropriate kinetic paralanguage.

Compensatory Therapy. In the case of a child with severe involvement of the visual speech receptor, varying degrees of spontaneous compensatory use of the auditory channel for speech reception should be expected. And since the auditory channel is the major speech receptor, such spontaneous compensation may be sufficient to minimize speech symptoms. However, to ensure the maximum development of verbal intercommunication among the blind and severely visually handicapped, clinicians should be prepared to facilitate the use of compensatory sensory channels.

Compensatory verboacoustic communication can be facilitated in various ways. The child may be asked questions at various distances and at various loudness levels. He may be asked to identify tonal paralanguage in speech such as speech that sounds tense, happy, suspicious, or worried. He may be asked to repeat various sounds and sound combinations at various distances and at various loudness levels.

Compensatory tactile-kinesthetic communication has already been discussed under "Auditory Speech Receptor—Therapy."

"BIRECEPTOR" DISORDERS

The field of speech pathology and audiology has contributed little clinical research to the area of combined, severe involvement of auditory and visual speech receptors (referred to here as bireceptor problems).

Rusalem *et al*. (1966) presented the proceedings of a research seminar on the rehabilitation of deaf-blind persons held by the Industrial Home for the Blind (IHB). Four research areas were explored at the seminar: communication, learning, rehabilitation, and resettlement. "A primary goal of the IHB Research Seminar was to stimulate interest in, and thinking about expanded research activities relating to the rehabilitation of deaf-blind persons" (p. 4).

The discussion of clinical manifestations and therapy that follows is based primarily on the experiences of the IHB's Anne Sullivan Macy project while dealing with the communication problems of the deaf-blind. The following statement in the proceedings should serve as an inspiration for speech and hearing specialists to exert a greater effort in clinical services and research in this area: "Communication is the Rosetta Stone of the rehabilitation of deaf-blind persons" (p. 7).

Clinical Manifestations

Reduced Motivation and Need to Communicate. By the time many deaf-blind adults began to participate in the Anne Sullivan Macy project they had withdrawn from sociocommunicative contacts and hence had lost what communicative effectiveness they once had. They showed a limited desire to communicate, they appeared to have little to communicate about, and they seemed to have little need for communication. Some of the background for the progressive constriction in sociocommunicative activity among the deaf-blind and blind-deaf is offered below.

The deaf-blind are those individuals whose deafness preceded their blindness. In IHB's Anne Sullivan Macy project, almost 80% of the deaf-blind adults were either deaf at birth or became deaf in early life. Also, a majority of these individuals lost hearing and vision as a result of retinitis pigmentosa (Usher's syndrome); hence, deafness appeared first while blindness developed later with early symptoms appearing during puberty.

As children, most of these individuals were exposed to oral methods; however, because of their deafness and frequent associated problems they were only partially successful with the oral approach. Then, during their school years they began to rely upon manual communication (signs or signs and the manual alphabet) and their communication became limited to manual intercommunication with deaf individuals, although they possessed some speech ability. Then as vision was progressively lost, manual communication became less useful, and gradually they lost sociocommunicative contact with their deaf friends. This sequence of events was evidently the basis for the deaf-blind individual's progressive loss of the communicative ability he may have once possessed, for his apparent reduced desire to communicate, and for his paucity of things about which to communicate.

The blind-deaf are those individuals whose blindness preceded their deafness. In IHB's Anne Sullivan Macy project, about 20% of the individuals were hearing individuals during the period of language development. Therefore, this group developed speech but, when deafness came, they gradually lost their hearing-speaking partners (family, friends, etc.). And because they and their normal speaking partners were not prepared to develop compensatory manual communication they, too, slowly became communicative isolates. However, because their blindness and deafness tended to be more recently incurred, their speech and motivation problems tended to be less acute.

Expressive Characteristics. As already stated, depending upon which speech receptor was lost first and when, expressive modes vary among individuals with bireceptor problems.

The deaf-blind tended to know the manual alphabet, but because it was often learned informally it might contain idiosyncrasies such as regional and local short-cuts in manual signs that might impede reception by others. Also, their deafness-based language deficiencies were reflected in their manual communication.

The blind-deaf are individuals who usually developed speech and language before the onset of complicating deafness. (Their major problem, therefore, is in the reception of messages via manual communication.) Also, because of their relatively good predeafness language ability, they could also communicate through typewriting and, if they retained some vision, even through script-writing. They usually found communicating with other deaf-blind via manual communication unrewarding.

Receptive Characteristics. Language limitations and perceptual problems complicate the reception of messages by those with bireceptor problems. Hence, even normals who master the manual alphabet must be careful in their use of abstract words, phrases, and colloquialisms. Also prolonged social isolation may deprive those with bireceptor problems of reality-testing experiences, which may lead them to retain invalid and even bizarre ideas and behavior.

Intrapersonal Communication Characteristics. Because of the frequently-encountered tendency for those with bireceptor problems to gradually lose their sociocommunicative contacts, there is a tendency for them to withdraw within themselves, and excessive intrapersonal communication may be observed.

Communication with Normal Persons. Although manual communication, such as the manual alphabet, can be learned relatively easily by normal communicators, some normal individuals, because of the required physical contact (manual signs must be felt), may be reluctant to communicate in this way. Also, some normals who develop sociocommunicative contacts with persons with bireceptor problems may not persist in the relationship, because the involved persons may not have much of interest or much of anything about which to communicate.

Therapy

Some general ideas on communication rehabilitation for those with bireceptor disorders are offered here. The reader should be reminded that ideas presented in "Auditory Receptor Disorders—Therapy" and "Visual Receptor Disorders—Therapy" also apply here.

Secondary Preventive Measures. In both forms of bireceptor involvement, efforts should be made early by family, friends, and professional workers to prevent the gradual constriction of sociocommunicative contacts among individuals with bireceptor problems.

Such individuals must be kept informed about current events and personal interests and must be kept as active as possible each day. An active communisphere must be created so that the individual finds a need to communicate and is rewarded for doing so. Also, normal speakers must be found, in addition to handicapped associates and professional workers, who are willing to learn manual communication and who are ready to enter into long-term sociocommunicative relationships with the involved individual.

Hopefully, these activities will counter the tendency for the deaf-blind and blind-deaf to engage in excessive amounts of intrapersonal communication.

The deaf-blind should be helped to develop as much speech as possible during their preblindness period (if there is one). They should not be allowed to become dependent on manual methods of communication, and they should not be allowed to limit their relationships to other deaf persons.

The blind-deaf should be encouraged to develop their speech capacity to the fullest degree during their predeafness period. They should be helped to develop their hearing skills to the fullest also in order to take advantage of whatever hearing may eventually remain. They should be taught compensatory manual communication in preparation for the eventual dual disorder, and they should not be allowed to limit their relationships to normal speakers.

Causal Therapy. Whatever residual hearing or vision remains in individuals with bireceptor disorders should be amplified or magnified by appropriate hearing aids and lenses.

Symptom Therapy. With the *deaf-blind,* symptom work should be directed at expanding language and vocabulary and on improvement in the use of the manual alphabet. With the *blind-deaf,* emphasis should be placed on preserving their speech communication, developing typing skills, and providing familiarity with one or more methods of manual communication.

Compensatory Therapy. Compensatory communication techniques have already been discussed. However, because individuals with compound receptor disorders are most in need of compensatory work, further discussion of such therapy is warranted.

It is natural for the *deaf-blind* to compensate for their lack of verboacoustic perception during the preblind period with compensatory perception of verbovisual events (i.e., kinetic paralanguage and articulatory movements). Compensation for their limited speech ability is not as natural and is usually taught in the form of manual communication (signs, alphabet, palm writing, braille reading).

The job of the communication specialist is to facilitate the natural, compensatory increase in attention to kinetic paralanguage and articulatory movements in the hopes that the individual may possess some residual vision after the onset of his visual complication and to ensure the acquisition of manual communication in preparation for the bireceptor disorder.

It is natural for the *blind-deaf* to compensate for their lack of verbovisual perception during the predeaf period with compensatory attention to verboacoustic events (tonal paralanguage and acoustical speech stimuli). Speech communication is usually well enough developed and hence no compensatory expressive communication is usually developed.

The jobs of the communication specialist are: to facilitate the natural compensatory increase in attention to verboacoustic events in the hopes that the individual may retain some residual hearing after the onset of his hearing complication; to maintain the highest level of speech communication; and to ensure the acquisition of manual communication in preparation for the bireceptor disorder.

Electromechanical devices should also be considered to complement or supplement the communication of those with bireceptor problems. These devices include the use of the typewriter (a special typewriter where depression of the typewriter keys elevates the corresponding point pattern in braille within the touch cell, which then can be felt by the deaf-blind; Tellatouch system), tactile hearing aids, and the use of vibratized alphabetical code.

Research Needs. Participants in the IHB Research Seminar identified various research needs in the whole area of combined receptor disorders. Among the questions raised in the area of communication were: (a) What is the relevance of nonverbal communication in improving communication among those with bireceptor disorders? (b) What is the nature of the language of those with bireceptor problems, and what is the best means of influencing this language? (c) What is the nature and degree of intrapersonal communication among those with bireceptor problems? (d) What is the influence of the personality, attitudes, and perceptions of communication mediators upon the communication skills of those with bireceptor problems? (e) What is the value of teaching communication skills in reality situations, for example, during vocational training, as compared with "laboratory environments?" (f) Might other forms of tactile communication, for example, reception of messages via vibratized alphabet applied to various parts of the skin, prove of value for those with bireceptor problems? (g) What is the possible role of the perceptions of taste, smell, vibrations, and kinesthesia as supplements to touch communication with those with bireceptor problems?

REFERENCES

Carhart, R., Development and conservation of speech. In H. Davis and S. R. Silvermann (Eds.), Hearing and Deafness. New York: Holt, Rinehart and Winston (1970).

Davis, H., Abnormal hearing and deafness. In H. Davis and S. R. Silverman (Eds.), Hearing and Deafness. New York: Holt, Rinehart and Winston (1970).

DiCarlo, L. M., The Deaf. Englewood Cliffs, N. J.: Prentice-Hall (1964).

Gellis, S. S., and Feingold, M., Atlas of Mental Retardation Syndromes. Washington, D. C.: U. S. Department of Health, Education and Welfare (1968).

Goodhill, V., Guggenheim, P., Hoversten, G., and MacKay, D. Pathology, diagnosis, and therapy of deafness. In L. E. Travis (Ed.), Handbook of Speech Pathology and Audiology. New York: Appleton-Century-Crofts (1971).

Kendall, D. C., Auditory problems in children. In R. W. Rieber and R. S. Brubaker (Eds.), Speech Pathology: An International Study of the Science. Amsterdam: North-Holland Publishing Company (1966).

Lezak, R. J., and Starbuck, H. B., Identification of children with speech disorders in a residential school for the blind. Int. J. Educ. Blind, 14, 8–12 (1964).

Luchsinger, R., and Arnold, G. E., Voice-Speech-Language. Belmont, Calif.: Wadsworth Publishing Co. (1965).

Miner, L. E., A study of the incidence of speech deviations among visually handicapped children. New Outlook for the Blind, 57, 10–14 (1963).

Morley, M. E., The Development and Disorders of Speech in Childhood. Baltimore: The Williams & Wilkins Company (1965).

Myklebust, H. R., Auditory Disorders in Children: A Manual for Differential Diagnosis. New York: Grune and Stratton (1954).

Mysak, E. D., Cerebral palsy speech syndromes. In L. E. Travis (Ed.), Handbook of Speech Pathology and Audiology. New York: Appleton-Century-Crofts (1971).

Newby, H. A., Audiology. New York: Appleton-Century-Crofts (1972).

O'Neill, J. J., The Hard of Hearing. Englewood Cliffs, N. J.: Prentice-Hall (1964).

Paine, R. S., and Oppé, T. E., Neurological Examination of Children. London: The Spastics Society (1966).

Rusalem, H., Bettica, L. J., Haffly, J. E., and Parnicky, J. J., New Frontiers for Research on Deaf-Blindness. New York: Anne Sullivan Macy Service for Deaf-Blind Persons, The Industrial Home for the Blind (1966).

Silverman, S. R., The education of deaf children. In L. E. Travis (Ed.), Handbook of Speech Pathology and Audiology. New York: Appleton-Century-Crofts (1971).

West, R. W., and Ansberry, M., The Rehabilitation of Speech. New York: Harper and Row (1968).

6

Speech Effector System

The speech effector system is responsible for producing the speech airstream, creating and modifying laryngeal tone, and producing exolaryngeal sounds. Respiratory, phonatory, resonatory, and articulatory mechanisms, as well as an adjunctive endocrine system, make up the system. Disorders of speech effectors are found in children and adults; however, resonatory and articulatory disorders are more apt to be found among children, while respiratory and phonatory complications are more likely to be found among adults. Severity of symptoms may range from a relatively mild and specific dento-occlusal sigmatism to the phonatory-resonatory-articulatory complex that may characterize the speech of a child with cleft palate.

RESPIRATORY EFFECTOR DISORDERS

The major purpose of the respiratory effector is to generate and deliver the speech airstream for processing by the laryngeal, resonatory, and articulatory structures. Structures that, when defective, can interfere with the generation and delivery of the speech airstream are: the trachea, bronchi, and lungs; the skeletal framework for breathing, including the spinal column, rib cage, and pectoral and pelvic girdles; and the muscles of inhalation and exhalation.

Background

Causes of disorders of the respiratory speech effector are discussed under the headings of lung diseases and disorders, skeletal framework anomalies, and muscle afflictions. (Neurogenic backgrounds for resonatory involvements are discussed in Chapter 7.)

Lung Diseases and Disorders. Subsumed under the category of lungs are involvement of the lungs proper, the bronchi, and the trachea.

The author (Mysak, 1966), in his review of literature pertaining to infraglottal origins of dysphonia, reported the following kinds of problems that may affect the respiratory effector: infraglottic stenosis, or compression of the trachea in trauma or thyroid enlargement; constriction of the bronchi due to bronchial asthma; pneumothorax (accumulation of air or gas in the pleural cavity causing partial collapse of lung), which may also show displacement of the trachea and larynx toward the unaffected side; enlarged heart, which reduces the space in the thorax that can be used for expansion of air sacs of the lungs; subtotal or total removal of a lung; and various diseases such as tuberculosis, emphysema, and vascular disease.

Skeletal Framework Anomalies. Postural problems associated with spinal column anomalies may have indirect effects on speech breathing. Included among these spinal column abnormalities are: lordosis (exaggeration of the normal anterior curve in the lumbar region), which may be due to long convalescence, malnutrition, and rickets or may be secondary to neurological involvement of back muscles; kyphosis (exaggeration of the normal posterior curve of the upper spine), which may have a postural origin or may be due to tuberculosis of the spine; and scoliosis (s-shaped lateral curvature of the spine), which may be due to congenital defects of the vertebrae or ribs or may be secondary to neurological involvement of the back muscles.

Muscle Afflictions. Various conditions may affect the functioning of inspiratory and expiratory muscles and thus the generation of an adequate speech airstream.

Fatigue or illness may reduce the efficiency of the respiratory muscles.

Congenital absence of muscles is discussed by Ford (1966, pp. 1210–1213). Among the muscles most frequently missing is some part of the pectoralis major or minor (help to raise ribs). Other muscles that have been found missing or defective are the serratus magnus (raises ribs in inspiration) and the abdominals (cooperate in compressing abdomen in expiration). Anomalies of the diaphragm have also been described. Defects are usually unilateral and confined to single muscles or muscle groups; however, bilateral symmetrical defects are also found. Information is lacking on the exact effects, if any, of missing respiratory muscles on the ability of the respiratory effector to create an adequate speech airstream.

Muscular dystrophies describe a "common heredofamilial disease which is characterized by progressive wasting and paralysis of the skeletal muscles" (Ford, 1966, p. 1226). Several clinical types are recognized and their classifications depend on muscle groups affected, age of onset, and rate of progression. Regardless of type, there are some common clinical features: both males and females are affected; onset is insidious and may occur at any time during childhood; and frequent early symptoms reported by parents include clumsy gait, difficulty in climbing stairs, and prominent abdomen. Essential symptoms include progressive weakness and wasting of first the muscles of the shoulder and pelvic girdles and then the muscles of the upper arm and thigh. Sensory disturbances are absent, and occasionally mental deficiency may be exhibited. The symptoms are generally slowly progressive and many individuals survive for from 10 to 30 years after the onset of symptoms.

Following are some of the recognized types of muscular dystrophy and some of their symptoms. (a) The facioscapulohumeral type usually begins before the tenth year, progresses slowly, and is characterized by involvement of the facial muscles. A typical appearance includes a mask-like expression, absent nasolabial folds, and a pendulous lower lip. (b) The juvenile scapulohumeral type usually begins between the sixth and tenth years and affects the trapezius and serratus magnus first and later the pectorals, latissmus dorsi, and so on. (c) The pseudohy-pertrophic type usually begins very early (although onset is sometimes delayed until adolescence or even adulthood) and delay in walking is frequent; it is sometimes considered the most rapidly progressive. Muscles of the thighs and hips are usually affected first. Pectorals, serratus magnus, and abdominal muscles are commonly affected. Also the tongue may be hypertrophied in rare cases (Ford, 1966, pp. 1230–1231).

Mullendore and Stoudt (1961) studied the speech patterns of 31 individuals with muscular dystrophy. Among the speech patterns identified were a lack of ability to sustain phonation, a tendency toward weak voice, hypernasality, and a high incidence of malarticulation.

Clinical Manifestations

The symptoms of involvement of the respiratory speech effector result from a reduction in the amount of air available for phonation and from a lack of adequate subglottal air pressure.

Vocal weakness (phonasthenia), or quality-loudness symptoms, may range from a lack of voice or whispered voice (hypophonia), to a breathy voice (pneumophonia), to a hoarse voice (trachyphonia), to a tremulous voice (tromophonia), to just a weak voice (leptophonia), and finally to some form of unpleasant voice (idiophonia).

Speech rate and rhythm may also be affected by an inadequate breath supply, especially one marked by quick, shallow respiration (tachypnea), rapid or panting respiration (polypnea), or difficult or labored breathing (dyspnea). Rate may be slowed or irregular and rhythm may be marked by "choppiness" if the individual utters only one, two, or three syllables per expiration.

Diagnosis

Distinguishing respiratory-based phonasthenia and speech rate and rhythm problems from other forms requires the combined efforts of an organized group of specialists. Conditions such as lung disease, enlarged heart, or various muscle diseases must be determined by appropriate medical specialists. The speech clinician may help establish the speech breathing repercussion of the underlying condition by taking the various measures referred to in Chapter 2; that is, he can determine the speech air volume, the inspiratory-expiratory speech breathing ratio, and the vegetative breathing-speech breathing transition.

Prognosis

A good deal of the prognosis in respiration-based speech symptoms depends on the amenability of the underlying condition to medical treatment. With respect to the speech symptoms, at least two factors are important regarding a favorable prognosis: (a) the amount of the speech respiratory irregularity that is due to persisting faulty patterns no longer necessary either because of successful or partially successful treatment of the underlying condition or because of degrees of spontaneous resolution of the problem (i.e., habituated respiratory irregularities), and (b) the degree of interest and drive of the client in utilizing various compensatory techniques.

Therapy

Secondary Preventive Measures. In order to minimize the effects on respiration of the underlying condition, certain respiratory hygiene practices should be recommended by the speech and hearing clinician. Among these practices are maintaining an appropriate weight level and good general muscle tonus and avoiding excessive smoking and use of alcohol.

Causal Therapy. Primary causal therapy aimed at the underlying condition is provided by the appropriate physician or surgeon. When quality-loudness and speech-time symptoms persist, the clinician begins the following program of therapy: (a) having the client progressively increase the amount of time he can sustain vowels on one expiration; (b) having the client progressively increase in frequency the number of on-off phonations on one expiration; (c) working on pitch and loudness variability exercises; and (d) working on rapid shifting from vegetative to speech breathing and on lengthening the expiratory phase of the inspiratory-expiratory speech breathing ratio. The last two therapy goals may be facilitated by having the client watch pneumographic recordings of his attempts.

Symptom Therapy. For those speech symptoms that appear to be habituated, a self-adjusting (autotherapy) approach is recommended. As previously mentioned, all forms of self-adjusting therapy are described more appropriately in Chapter 8.

Compensatory Therapy. West and Ansberry (1969, p. 232) suggested the following compensatory techniques for the asthenic voice resulting from reduced breath pressure: (a) seek a pitch level in the client that results in optimum resonance, although this level may vary from his habitual speaking fundamental frequency level; and (b) encourage the use of crisp, precise articulation.

PHONATORY EFFECTOR DISORDERS

The major purpose of the phonatory effector is to transform the airstream produced by the respiratory effector into speech tone. Pitch is varied primarily by the modification of glottic tension and mass, and loudness is varied by the alteration of subglottal pressure, airflow rate, and glottal resistance. Structures important to the phonatory function include the nine laryngeal cartilages, the intrinsic laryngeal musculature, and the extrinsic laryngeal musculature.

Background

Various general as well as relatively specific problems may affect the structure of the sound generator or larynx. (Neurogenic backgrounds for phonatory involvements are discussed in Chapter 7.)

General Conditions. Certain general conditions affect the laryngeal musculature and hence reduce its efficiency.

Fatigue or illness is usually reflected by weak voice. Family and friends make the "auditory diagnosis" of fatigue and illness quite easily when hearing the phonasthenic voice of a relative or friend. Relatedly, vocal changes such as hoarseness, lower pitch, and vocal instability have been observed in women preceding the menses (Frable, 1962).

Iatrogenic causes of voice problems have also been reported. Damste (1967) warns of the possible virilizing affects on the voices of women of androgenic compounds. Such compounds may be prescribed for tiredness, underweight, and nervousness. The main hope for reversal of the voice symptom is discontinuation of the drug upon the very first signs of virilization.

Mytonic dystrophy is ". . . a type of heredofamilial degeneration which gives rise to selective atrophy of the muscles, myotonia, and various other symptoms, such as cataract, alopecia, atrophy of the sex glands, and premature senility" (Ford, 1966, p. 1237). Onset occurs usually between the ages of 20 and 35, but the disease may occur as early as infancy. The first symptoms may be due to wasting of the muscles or to myotonia. Facial muscles are the first to be affected. In some cases the tongue, velum, pharynx, and vocal cords may be involved. The hard palate is high and narrow and the face is long and thin. "Speech is characteristically low-pitched, monotonous and often nasal" (p. 1238). Mental deficiency is common.

Weinberg *et al.* (1968) describe a 27-year-old male whose early symptom of mytonic dystrophy was a slowly progressive hypernasality. Slower-than-normal rate, articulatory deterioration when fatigued, and compensatory movements were also observed. Other symptoms manifested were: temporal muscle atrophy; bilateral ptosis; facial, masseter, and tongue weakness; dull facies; open bite; high palatal arch; and prognathism. Identification and proper referral by the speech clinician is essential when such a case is seen by the clinician first.

Myasthenia gravis "refers to a condition characterized by weakness and by abnormal fatigue of the striated muscles, which is not constantly associated with any demonstrable anatomical lesions" (Ford, 1966, p. 1259). The cause of the problem is still unknown. It usually does not develop before the age of puberty but has been identified in childhood and even infancy. Usually, the muscles innervated by the cranial nerves are affected first. Diplopia is often the first symptom and is accompanied or followed by unilateral or bilateral ptosis and by some limitation of ocular movement. Symptoms worsen as the day progresses. "As a rule, weakness of the bulbar muscles develops shortly after the ocular muscles are affected. The voice becomes weak, and, after the patient has talked for a few minutes, it becomes nasal and hoarse. Swallowing is difficult. The tongue cannot be protruded and articulation becomes indistinct" (p. 1262).

Wolski (1967) reported on a 14-year-old girl who presented hypernasality as the primary symptom of myasthenia gravis. Because speech symptoms are often the earliest symptoms of more general and serious conditions, the speech clinician must remain alert to all their possible implications.

Various other diseases such as tuberculosis, typhoid fever, tetanus, and syphilis may involve laryngeal muscles and cause muscle disease or scarring and consequently vocal repercussions. Laryngeal involvement (ulceration) and dysphonia have also been reported in cases of acute myeloid leukemia (Jones and Shalom, 1968).

Specific Conditions. Relatively specific conditions that may have vocal repercussions are discussed under the headings of neoplasms, structural anomalies, diseases and infections, and trauma.

Neoplasms of various kinds may affect the functioning of the laryngeal mechanism. Among these neoplasms are malignant tumors and various benign tumors. Among the benign types are papilloma, polyps, nodules, hematoma, and keratosis (Moore, 1971, p. 542). Contact ulcers and granuloma may also be viewed as types of benign new formations.

Structural anomalies or laryngeal malformations either present at birth or acquired at an early age may also produce vocal dysfunction. Among these structural abnormalities of the vocal organ are: hypoplasia or underdevelopment of the organ (Moore, 1971, p. 539); laryngeal diaphragm or web; vocal cord sulcus (Luchsinger and Arnold, 1965, pp. 168–175); underdevelopment of one of the vocal folds; and outward veering of the vocal processes of the arytenoids (West and Ansberry, 1968, pp. 220–221).

Diseases and infections of various kinds may also disturb the functioning of the vocal organ. Among them are: myasthenia laryngis due to vocal abuse; damage to the lateral cricoarytenoid and sternothyroid muscles of various origins (Luchsinger and Arnold, 1965, pp. 256–259); ankylosis of the cricoarytenoid joint, sometimes due to rheumatoid arthritis; laryngeal edema of various origins; and vocal cord engorgement, due to overuse of alcohol (Moore, 1971, pp. 550–551). Symptoms that may appear in cricoarytenoid arthritis are hoarseness, pain when talking, dysphagia, radiation of pain to the ears, and sensation of a foreign body in the throat (Lofgren and Montgomery, 1962).

Trauma to the laryngeal structures is also capable of producing vocal symptoms.

Luchsinger and Arnold (1965, pp. 275–281) describe three forms of injury to the laryngeal cartilages: sudden impact injuries such as may be encountered in auto accidents or during sports such as baseball and boxing or during criminal assaults; penetrating injuries from bullets or industrial accidents; and stabbing and knife cuts. Traumatic fixation of the cricothyroid and cricoarytenoid joints is also possible. Various types of trauma to the cords may also be sustained, for example, granuloma following trauma due to intubation anesthesia, excessive excision of vocal cord tissue during surgery, and spontaneous vocal cord paralysis.

Clinical Manifestations

Various types and degrees of pitch and quality anomalies may be associated with the different conditions just described.

High-Pitched Voice. Moore (1971, pp. 539–540) recognizes at least three organic reasons for a chronically high-pitched voice; in the case of a male, for example, a hypoplasia of the larynx sometimes associated with a general structural retardation, or with a familial characteristic, or with a hypogonadism. The phonodynamics behind high pitch are that small vocal cords vibrate with greater frequency and hence the resulting feminine-like voice ("gynophonia").

Abnormally high-pitched voices may also be associated with laryngeal web. The phonodynamics of the high pitch here are that the web causes a shortening of the vibrating portions of the vocal cords and hence increases the frequency of vibration of those portions. Abnormal approximation of the posterior segments of the vocal cords may also result in a high-pitched voice. This occurs when, due to a structural asymmetry, one vocal process of an arytenoid slides under or over the other, thereby damping the vibrations of the posterior segments and causing the anterior segments to increase their vibratory frequency.

Low-Pitched Voice. The phonodynamics behind abnormally low-pitched voice (baryphonia) are related to conditions that increase the mass and slow the vibration rate of the vocal cords. In the female, anything that may be responsible for hyperplasia of the larynx may be responsible for a male-like voice (androphonia). Tumors of various kinds and edema of the cords may also dampen the vibration rate and result in low-pitched phonation.

Loud and Tense Voice. Loud voice (megaphonia) may be the result of ". . . laryngeal conditions in which the voluntary act of phonation is accompanied by too tight a closure of the glottis" (West and Ansberry, 1968, p. 223). The usually loud and tense voice results from the individual being unable to send the airstream through the larynx unless he uses great pressure.

Among the conditions that may be responsible for abnormally loud and tense voices are: increase in the mass of laryngeal tissue due to edema and inflammation, excessive mucal deposits upon the vocal folds, and various benign and malignant laryngeal neoplasms.

Weak Voice. Phonasthenia has already been described under "Respiratory Speech Effector;" however, phonasthenia may also result from problems on the glottal level. For example, the vocal cords may lack the strength to allow for sufficient build-up of subglottal air pressure and hence the resultant phonasthenia. Specific laryngeal muscle weakness, as in myasthenia laryngis due to vocal strain, or muscle weakness of a more general nature, as in myasthenia gravis, may be causative factors.

West and Ansberry (1968, pp. 224–226) describe certain structural anomalies that may result in reducing the volume of the voice (microphonia). For example, narrow epiglottis, small faucial arch, and enlarged palatine tonsils.

Breathy Voice. The phonodynamics behind pneumophonia are that the vocal folds are unable to interrupt the speech airstream well enough or long enough to develop adequate subglottal air pressure; that is, either the closed phase of the vibratory cycle is short or the glottis does not close completely (Moore, 1971, p. 541).

Among the conditions that may produce pneumophonia are: fixation of the cricoarytenoid joint, myasthenia laryngis, tumors, contact ulcers, surgical removal of part of a vocal fold, swelling of the cords, tubercular or syphilitic irregularities of the vibrating edges of the vocal cords, scarring of the vocal bands due to injury or intubation anesthesia, temporary laryngitis, and underdevelopment of one of the vocal folds.

Hoarse Voice. According to Moore (1971, p. 543), the phonodynamics behind trachyphonia are as follows: "It is probable that the primary or common factor in hoarseness is noise of a relatively high frequency that is produced by transient or highly unstable vibrations." These laryngeal transients usually combine with low-pitch sounds which, in turn, result from laryngeal conditions which reduce the frequency of vocal-cord vibration. The overall effect is one of "hoarseness."

Among the conditions that may produce trachyphonia are: excessive accumulation of mucus on the vocal folds, flaccidity of the vocal cords, neoplasms, and surgical removal of vocal cord tissue.

Similar laryngeal conditions, for example, vocal nodules, may produce overlapping or different vocal symptoms at different times, depending on severity (or size), amount of phonatory effort, and the amount of compensatory ability available to the individual. The vocal symptom may range from no voice to breathy voice to hoarse voice.

Intermittent Voice. When voice is episodically interrupted during phonatory efforts it may be referred to as intermittent vocalization. The phonodynamics are similar to those presented under "Loud and Tense Voice." The reasons for the condition may also be similar.

Without Voice. A complete absence of voice (aphonia) may result from any of the previously-mentioned conditions leading to structural changes in the larynx when they are severe enough; for example, substantial injury to the laryngeal cartilages, large neoplasms, and inflammation of the larynx. The most dramatic basis for aphonia is the total removal of the larynx, usually because of a malignant neoplasm.

Diagnosis

The diagnosis of phonatory effector problems requires the close cooperation of the speech and hearing clinician, the otolaryngologist, and other medical specialists. Whenever a client presents symptoms of aphonia, intermittent vocalization, or breathy or hoarse voice to a speech and hearing clinician first, he must be referred for laryngological study. The referral is absolutely necessary to determine whether tissue pathology exists, its nature, and whether surgical or medical attention is warranted.

Hence, the speech clincian is usually not involved with determining the immediate organic cause of a phonatory deviation; that is the physician's domain. Rather, his concern is proper referral and determining the phonodynamics behind the vocal symptoms. That is, the speech clinician's diagnostic contribution begins when: (a) medical resolution of the organic pathology has taken place but the individual persists in a misuse vocal pattern; (b) the medical or surgical treatment results in some permanent laryngeal irregularity, for example, partial removal of a vocal cord; (c) an inactive but irreversible laryngeal anomaly exists; and (d) the laryngeal anomaly is due to misuse-abuse but where the effects of the abuse may be reversed by a modification in the habitual pattern of voicing.

After one of the above factors is identified, the speech clinician begins his evaluation of the phonodynamics of the vocal symptoms.

Identification of Predominant Symptom. The clinician first attempts to identify what the predominant vocal symptom is. Is it one of pitch, loudness, or quality?

Self-awareness of Vocal Symptom. Whether the client is able to identify his error voice when produced by the clinician and whether he can describe aspects of his own error voice are also determined. By this examination the clinician attempts to determine the role of audioregulation in the voice problem.

Effects of Disruption of Audioregulation of Voice. The effects on the pathologic voice of bilateral white noise sufficient to mask the individual's voice should also be studied. When such masking results in the partial or complete return of a physiologic voice, which frequently occurs, the clinician has collected important information relative to the existing potential of the vocal mechanism and also the role of audioregulatory mechanisms in the voice problem.

Voice Variability. The clinician should also evaluate the degree of pitch, loudness, and quality variability still available to the client. Upon request and following appropriate demonstration can the client assume low-, medium-, and high-pitched voices? Can he speak softly, moderately loud, and loudly? And can he alter his voice quality from breathy to hoarse to full voice? A display of such vocal variability by the client is important to the prognosis for improvement in therapy.

Prognosis

As in the case of respiration-based speech symptoms, the prognosis for improvement of larynx-based vocal symptoms depends largely on how amenable to medical and surgical attention are the underlying conditions causing the vocal symptoms.

Other important factors include: remaining voice potential following medical or surgical intervention, the client's motivation and drive for voice improvement, and the client's vocal compensatory abilities.

Therapy

Primary Preventive Measures. The public as well as various health specialists must be reminded of the vulnerability of the laryngeal mechanism to disease and trauma.

The public should be made aware of the dangers to vocal structures of: abuse of the voice; excessive smoking and alcohol usage; sudden impact injuries possibly encountered in auto accidents or while playing ball; and the possible vocal sequelae to tuberculosis, typhoid fever, tetanus, and syphilis.

Health specialists need to be reminded of the possible vocal repercussions of: intubation anesthesia, excessive excision of vocal cord tissue during surgery, and possible involvement of the inferior recurrent laryngeal nerve during thyroidectomy.

Secondary Preventive Measures. Once the laryngeal mechanism has been involved and vocal rehabilitation is underway, the client should be encouraged to maintain good eating and sleeping habits, refrain from or significantly reduce the use of cigarettes and alcohol, and avoid excessive and abusive use of the voice.

Causal Therapy. Appropriate physicians and surgeons provide the treatment aimed at the underlying cause of the vocal symptoms. However, causal voice therapy is planned when symptoms of weak voice, high- and low-pitched voice, breathy voice, and hoarse voice persist.

Increasing laryngeal muscle tonus and improving the approximation of the cords are often needed goals to strengthen weak and breathy voices and some hoarse voices and to raise some low-pitched voices.

Activities that promote *synkinetic movements* (unintentional movements accompanying volitional movements) of the laryngeal muscles are one way of improving tonus and approximation of the cords. Laryngeal synkinesis may be effected in various ways. While sitting with hands outspread on the seat at the sides of the thighs, the client simultaneously phonates and lifts himself quickly off the seat. While standing with hands clenched in front of the chest, the client simultaneously phonates and vigorously pulls each hand laterally (against the resistance of each clenched hand). Also, while standing and leaning against a wall with outstretched hands, the client simultaneouly phonates while quickly pushing off the wall with his hands. Similar techniques were introduced by Froeschels and described by Brodnitz (1959) as "pushing exercises."

Once the desired synkinetic tonus and vowel tone have been achieved, they must next be produced in a more voluntary fashion. Synkinetic vocalization may be transformed into volitional vocalization by: (a) having the client produce the synkinetic tone easily and at will and with various vowels; (b) having him practice sustaining the synkinetic phonation for about 10 seconds while "memorizing" the muscle feel; (c) having him produce the synkinetic phonation, sustain it, and memorize the feel while slowly phasing out the voluntary lift, pull, or push triggering movement; and (d) having him voluntarily produce the synkinetic tone. The new tone may then be directly applied to brief periods of conversational speech or, if necessary, more gradually applied to conversational speech units.

A program of general *physical conditioning* may also be helpful in improving laryngeal muscle tonus. For clients who are able, a suitable program of calisthenics, running, and jogging carried out two or three times a week is also recommended.

Reducing laryngeal muscle tonus and easing the approximation of the cords are often required goals to improve loud and tense voices and intermittent voice and to lower some high-pitched voices.

Work on contrasting tonus is one way of helping to develop a more appropriate laryngeal muscle tonus. This is accomplished by: (a) having the client volitionally over-tense the facial, neck, and shoulder muscles and hold and "memorize" the tense muscle feel; and (b) having him then "let go" and "memorize" the feel of reduced muscle tonus. After the client is able to volitionally increase muscle tonus in the upper region of the body and then volitionally reduce it rather easily and well, he is asked to phonate during the reduced tonus phase.

The extension of easy hum, sigh, and yawn vocalization into vowels and subsequently into speaking units is another way of learning to adopt a more appropriate laryngeal muscle tonus for speech.

Holbrook *et al.* (1974) reported on the effective use of a portable device (voice intensity controller) that provides an auditory signal contingent on excessive vocal intensity in treating patients with dysphonia related to vocal cord lesions and to laryngeal hypertension.

Symptom Therapy. Symptom voice therapy is applied in those cases where organic factors are not discernible, where structural anomalies or lesions have been surgically corrected, or where medical treatments have successfully resolved laryngeal pathologies but where there is a persisting pathologic voice. A self-adjusting approach is recommended in such cases and is more appropriately discussed in Chapter 8.

Compensatory Therapy. Compensatory voice therapy techniques are applied in those cases where congenital conditions, trauma, and so on are not amenable to medical or surgical treatment and where there is permanent reduction in voicing potential.

Creating a substitute or entirely new voice is the most dramatic utilization of compensatory voice therapy and is developed in cases of complete loss of voice due to total laryngectomy. Since an extensive literature has developed in this area (e.g., see Snidecor *et al.* (1962), Diedrich and Youngstrom (1966), and Rigrodsky *et al.* (1971)), no effort is made here to present any details on alaryngeal voice rehabilitation. The reader is also referred to another relatively brief but informative chapter by Snidecor (1971).

The problem for the laryngectomee who is usually in possession of his preoperative linguistic and articulatory skills is to develop a new sound source to articulate. He may do this by learning to vibrate the mouth of his esophagus by first "inhaling," "swallowing," or "injecting" air (or doing all three) into the esophagus and then vibrating its mouth upon releasing this air. A relatively new and as yet not widely used method of creating pseudovoice is through the Asai laryngectomy-laryngoplasty operation (Snidecor, 1971). A neoglottis is created in the operation by constructing a dermal tube that leads from the top of the tracheal stoma, turns inward directly below the base of the tongue, and ends in the hypopharynx. Either the point of turning or the mouth of the tube vibrates as the neoglottis. In order to create sound or "Asai speech," the individual occludes the tracheal stoma with a finger and forces air into the dermal tube and vibrates the neoglottis. The electrolarynx is still another way to create a new voice and may be used by individuals who are unable to develop esophageal speech. The electrolarynx has also been used to good advantage by individuals in the early stages of learning esophageal speech and as an alternative method, under certain circumstances, to esophageal speech.

Obtaining the most "speech power" from a permanently disabled voice may be attempted via various compensatory techniques. For example, in cases where speech air volume is wasted because of ineffective closure of the glottis, clients may work on increasing tidal air volume; in cases where speech intelligibility is lowered because of weak voice, the client may work on sharpening articulation, slowing rate, and using an "over-articulation" pattern while speaking.

Finding a "pitch" that provides the most voice for the least effort should also be done. Increased voice may sometimes be obtained by experimenting with and finding a particular head position or by the use of slight pressure on the right or left side of the thyroid cartilage. When such techniques are found to facilitate phonation, the client is asked to "memorize" the feel of the adjustment and attempt to reproduce it with the head in a more normal position or without the lateral displacement of the thyroid cartilage. This is sometimes possible. Even if this is not possible, such compensatory maneuvers can be used to good advantage in particular speaking situations when more voice is needed.

RESONATORY EFFECTOR DISORDERS

Amplification and modification of the laryngeal tone is the general function of the resonatory effector. Structures and areas involved in the amplification-modification process are: the hard and soft palate; the oral, buccal, and faucial cavities; and the naso-, oro-, and laryngopharynxes. The resonatory effector functions by modifying the size, shape, and tension of the pharynx and by coupling the pharynx with the mouth or nose.

Background

Problems in the resonatory effector may be related to relatively specific congenital anomalies, more general congenital anomalies, trauma, infection, and neoplasms. (Neurogenic backgrounds for resonatory involvements are discussed in Chapter 7.)

General Congenital Anomalies. By general congenital conditions is meant conditions that are usually detected at birth and that may have resulted from heritable factors, chromosomal anomalies, or unknown factors, and that include involvement of some part of the resonatory effector, for example, the palate.

Those that have already been described in Chapter 3 under "Gnosogenic Language Disorders in Children" are: "Chromosome 18" deletion (fish-like mouth, cleft lip and palate, and prominent mandible); "Oral-Facial-Digital (OFD) Syndrome" (cleft palate and lip or midline notch of upper lip); "Ring Chromosome 18" (high-arched palate, cleft palate, and micrognathia); "Cri Du Chat Syndrome" (micrognathia and occasionally cleft palate); "Otopalatodigital (OPD) Syndrome" (small, fish-like mouth with cleft palate); and "Prader-Willi Syndrome" (fish-like mouth with micrognathia).

Following are brief descriptions of observable characteristics of other congenital conditions that may include cleft palate and that have been described by Gellis and Feingold (1968).

Median cleft face syndrome, in which about 20% of the children exhibit varying degrees of retardation, presents the following characteristics: horseshoe-shaped depression of median plane of the forehead, varying degrees of hypertelorism, median clefts of the nose varying from a notch to complete division, and cleft lip and palate.

Popliteal pterygium, in which intelligence is usually normal, presents the following characteristics: bilateral popliteal pterygia, syndactyly, hypoplasia or aplasia of digits, fusion of eyelids, and various types and degrees of cleft lip and palate.

Pierre Robin syndrome, in which intelligence in usually normal, presents the following characteristics: infrequent eye anomalies (esotropia, cataracts, microphthalmia), possibly low-set ears, underdeveloped lower jaw, and varying degrees of cleft palate.

Specific Congenital Anomalies. By specific congenital anomalies is meant anomalies of the resonatory effector that are present at birth and that are relatively localized.

Relatively isolated cleft palate and lip conditions are recognized. An extensive literature has developed in this area covering classification, incidence, embryology, etiology, anatomy, physiology, evaluation, and management (e.g., surgical, orthodontic, prosthetic, otologic, dental, psychological, speech, and hearing). The speech and hearing clinician is referred to the *Cleft Palate Journal,* to chapters by Koepp-Baker (1971, Chs. 29 and 30), and to books by Morley (1966) and Spriestersbach and Sherman (1968).

Briefly and simply, clefts of the lip and palate range from a bifid uvula or a lip pit to a combination of complete cleft of the soft and hard palates and complete bilateral clefts of the lip. The incidence of congenital clefts of the palate and(or) lip is estimated at 1 in 750 to 800 live births. Genetic as well as various environmental explanations are cited in particular cases. Family histories are reported in approximately 27% of cases of isolated cleft lip, in 19% of cases of isolated cleft palate, and in 41% of cases of combined cleft lip and palate. Possible environmental causes include maternal radiation, thyroid deficiency, basal metabolism irregularity, dietary deficiency, infection, and stress. Parental age and the number and recency of color fusions in the maternal ancestry are other possible causes cited.

About 40% of the children with congenital cleft palate conditions may present hearing problems; these problems are usually attributed to infections of the upper respiratory system and to anomalies of the eustachian tubes. In any one case the child may also present degrees of language immaturity, phonatory-resonatory irregularities associated with oronasal and velopharyngeal structural anomalies, and articulatory deviations connected with chronic hearing problems and anomalies of the lip, alveolar ridge, dentition, dental occlusion, and palatal vault.

Other relatively specific congenital anomalies that may have speech resonatory repercussions include: hypoplasia of the hard and soft palates, submucous cleft, occipitalization of the atlas causing an irregular depth to the nasopharyngeal space, or widespread pterygoid plates causing an irregular width to the nasopharyngeal space. These conditions may be responsible for an increase in nasal resonance. A congenital condition that may reduce nasal resonance is a high palatal arch.

Loss of palatal tissue due to infection, trauma, or malignancy may also result in increased nasal resonance. More specifically, destruction of the soft palate by syphilitic gumma and trauma of palate and pillars during tonsilloadenoidectomy may result in hypernasality.

Obstructions or stoppages of the nares and nasal cavities may lead to hyponasality or mixed hyper-hyponasality. Frequent causes of obstructions in the anterior nasal cavities are "Swollen and irritated mucous membranes, hypertrophied turbinates, misshapen septum, elevated palatal arch . . . , broken or deformed nose, and various growths such as nasal tonsils, septal spurs, synechiae, polyps, syphilitic gummas . . ." (West and Ansberry, 1968, p. 110).

The external shape of the nose may also contribute to alteration of nasal resonance. For example, the enlarged nose in acromegaly, the immature nose in cretinism, the saddle nose in congenital syphilis, the collapsed naris in congenital cleft lip and palate, the thin, beaked nose in progeria, and "the thin nose and constricted nares of the allergic facies and the adenoid facies . . . " (Bloomer, 1971, p. 751).

Hypertrophied tonsillar tissue is another cause of disturbed nasal resonance. Obstruction of the nasopharyngeal port by enlarged pharyngeal tonsils (adenoids) may result in hyponasality, while enlarged lingual and palatine tonsils may have a "muffling" effect on oral resonance.

Transient hypernasality (about 6 weeks in duration) may result when adenoidal tissue is surgically removed; a chronic hypernasality may occur when tonsilloadenoidectomy is performed in individuals whose velopharyngeal structures are inadequate and who depend on the adenoid tissue for closure, for example, in cases of submucous cleft palate. Greene (1957) studied 377 children before and after removal of tonsils and adenoids. She found a high incidence of malarticulation in the group and considered that enlarged tonsils may be contributory. Articulation was greatly improved following surgery. She also believed that postoperative hypernasality was due to the precipitate removal of the adenoids, which, prior to the operation, prevented the velum from elevating completely, rather than to trauma or scarring of the palate.

Clinical Manifestations

Resonatory effector symptoms are characterized by: hypernasality (also positive nasality, rhinolalia aperta, rhinophonia, rhinoglossia, nasal speech); hyponasality (also negative nasality, rhinolalia clausa, stomatolalia, denasal speech); and combined hyper-hyponasality. Luchsinger and Arnold (1965, p. 658) refer to hypernasality due to palatal involvement as palatal dysglossia, hyponasality due to obstruction in posterior or anterior parts of the nose as nasal dysglossia, and mixed nasality as palatonasal dysglossia.

Hypernasality. Excessive nasality refers to the nasalization of vowels and semivowels due to inadequate velopharyngeal closure. The most important reason for organic hypernasality is congenital cleft lip and palate.

In congenital cleft conditions, complicating factors are usually found and the resulting complex may be referred to as the "cleft palate speech syndrome." The syndrome includes: (a) nasalization of vowels and semivowels, (b) reduced or absent plosive and fricative sounds due to inability to create adequate intraoral breath pressure, which, in turn, may cause nasal or pharyngeal fricative sound substitutions and glottal plosive and fricative sound substitutions; and (c) malarticulation associated with frequent concomitant anomalies of the lip, teeth, occlusion, alveolar ridge, and palatal vault. Further complications stem from frequent conductive hearing loss, nasopharyngeal snorting, facial grimacing, and nasal alar constriction.

Assimilation Nasality. When increased nasal resonance occurs only on words containing nasal sounds, the symptoms may be referred to as assimilation nasality. Two forms of this condition are recognized, anticipation and retention forms. *Anticipation nasality* describes the nasalization of a vowel preceding a nasal sound in a word, for example, the nasalization of [æ] in the word [æm]; *retention nasality* desribes the nasalization of a vowel following a nasal sound in a word, for example, the nasalization of [i] in the word [mi]. Organic assimilation nasality may be the result of minimal anomalies or dysfunction in the velopharyngeal area or of minimal residual dysfunction following medical or surgical treatment of a problem.

Hyponasality. A reduction in or absence of nasal resonance on sounds normally uttered with nasal resonance, that is, [m,n, ŋ], due to some form of obstruction is referred to as organic hyponasality. Two forms of this condition may be encountered, posterior and anterior forms. *Posterior hyponasality* describes the denasalization of [m,n, ŋ] or, in extreme form, their substitution by forms of [b,d,g], respectively, because of blockage of the nasopharyngeal port. "Clogged-nose speech" or "adenoid speech" are descriptive terms for the speech resonance heard. Conditions that may contribute to such hyponasality are hypertrophied adenoids, tumors, choanal polyps and atresias, and severe mucosal congestion from some form of chronic rhinitis. *Anterior hyponasality* describes the muffling or distortion of the nasal sounds because of blockage in the anterior nasal cavities. Conditions that may contribute to such hyponasality are deviated septum, hypertrophied turbinates, and polyps.

Combined Hyper-Hyponasality. Combined or mixed nasality is manifested whenever conditions causing hypernasality and hyponasality occur simultaneously. For example, in cases of cleft palate where closure is still a problem and where a flattened nasal ala exists, speech may be characterized by nasalized vowels and denasalized nasals.

Combined nasality may also occur when a partial obstruction in the nasal passages causes anterior hyponasality as well as eventual sluggishness of the closure mechanism, which, in turn, contributes to hypernasality.

Diagnosis

As in the case of phonatory effector problems, diagnosis of resonatory effector problems should represent the cooperative effort of the speech and hearing clinician, the ear, nose, and throat (ENT) specialist, and other medical specialists. Clinical, direct, group, and instrumental diagnostic approaches can contribute to the identification of organic rhinolalia.

Clinical Diagnosis. "Auditory diagnosis," or more accurately clinical identification of simple hypernasality and hyponasality, is usually made quickly and accurately by the experienced clinician. Assimilation nasality, posterior vs. anterior hyponasality, and combined nasality may not be so easily determined by the ear alone.

To confirm an auditory identification of hypernasality, a number of simple tests may be used. The "finger test" is done by simply placing a finger lightly on the side of the client's nose while he vocalizes a few vowels or utters a test sentence containing no nasal sounds, for example, "I like coffee." Alar vibration during these tests would indicate that nasality was present. The "mirror test" is done by holding a cold laryngeal mirror against the client's nostril while he produces non-nasal utterances; fogging of the mirror is the positive finding. The "pinch test" is done by having the client sustain vowels while the clinician pinches and releases the nostrils in an alternating fashion; positive nasality is evidenced by on-off nasal resonance during the pinching maneuver. Other signs of velopharyngeal incompetency that should attract the clinician are compensatory glottal plosive and fricative and pharyngeal fricative sound substitutions for various pressure consonants, nasal emission during production of consonant sounds, and alar constriction and facial grimacing during speech efforts.

A number of nonverbal tests of closure integrity may also prove useful. For example, the following are considered positive findings: inability to whistle, gargle, extinguish a match, inflate a balloon, and drink through a straw, and losing liquid through the nose while drinking in a head down position, as when drinking over a fountain.

Direct Diagnosis. Once the presence of some form of nasality has been confirmed, the next step is to attempt to determine its origin. Direct visual inspection of the palatal area may reveal frank cleft conditions that could certainly explain perceived hypernasality. Less obvious developmental anomalies of the oropharyngeal area and vertebral structures that may cause hypernasality may not be so easily visualized; one such anomaly that can usually be visually diagnosed is the condition known as submucous cleft. Visual inspection usually reveals a number of signs, some of which include a bifid uvula, absence of the median raphe of the velum, hypoplasia of the hard and soft palates, and a palpable notch in the horizontal palatine bones.

Numerous conditions that may explain hyponasality may also be directly observed. Mouth breathing, narrow face, narrow and high-arched palate, and dull facies may all point to long-standing, hypertrophied adenoids as the background for the perceived posterior hyponasality. The ENT specialist explores directly the possible relationships between hyponasality and polyps, tumors, deviated septum, chronic mucosal congestion, and atresias.

Instrumental Diagnosis. The speech clinician may also use various clinical instruments already discussed in Chapter 2 to confirm the presence of hypernasality. A simple nonverbal test is the oral pressure index (OPI) test. The OPI is a measure of air lost through the nose during the act of blowing. To determine the amount, a dry or wet spirometer or oral manometer may be used to establish vital capacity readings with the nostrils occluded and then with the nostrils unoccluded. The former figure is used as the denominator and the latter is used as the numerator in arriving at the index. An index of about 0.8 or less may be viewed as a positive test finding. A relatively simple verbal test is the nasal pressure index (NPI) test. The NPI is a measure of air lost through the nose during the utterance of a series of syllables. The instrument consists of nasal olives, a Y-tube, and a length of tubing leading to a U-tube filled with liquid, one arm of which is calibrated in cc. The nasal olives are fitted to the client's nostrils and he is asked to utter, for example, a series of non-nasal consonant-vowel syllables. A positive finding would be a noticeable displacement of the liquid in the U-tube during the utterances.

Adequacy of velopharyngeal closure may also be evaluated through lateral x-rays and through cineradiography. Radiography is also used to confirm the presence of developmental anomalies, residuals of trauma, and neoplasms of various kinds.

Spectrographic or acoustic studies of nasality may also be performed by the speech clinician. "The most frequent of the spectrographic corre-lates of nasality mentioned in the literature include: broadening and flattening of the peaks in the vowel spectra especially in the region of the first formant; increase in the intensity of harmonics near 250 cps and a reduction in the intensity of harmonics near 500 cps; reduction of formant one intensity, extra resonances between regular vowel for-mants; reduction of the intensity of high frequency harmonics, and reduction in the over-all intensity of the vowel" (Mysak, 1966, p. 176).

Group Diagnosis. In all cases of organic rhinolalia, a group diagnos-tic effort is required. A core team should include the ENT specialist, speech and hearing clinician, plastic surgeon, and the prosthodontist.

Prognosis

Prognosis for speech improvement of organic rhinolalias depends largely on the effectiveness of surgical and medical correction of the structural anomaly or disease process. The degree of correction follow-ing surgical and medical intervention is also qualified by the speech clinician's evaluation of how much of the rhinolalia was directly the result of the organic condition and how much was due to other factors.

The time of medical and surgical intervention is also important to the prognosis. For example, hypernasality resulting from developmental anomalies such as cleft palate is usually unchanged following successful surgical closure of the palate if the surgery was done after the child began to learn speech without benefit of an intact closure mechanism. Speech therapy is usually needed in such cases. However, in the case of an individual who suffers a palatal opening following the speech-learn-ing period, and if such a condition is corrected in a relatively short time, the surgical correction alone should eventually be sufficient. Similarly, in the case of hyponasality due to obstructions of various kinds, if the condition develops after the speech-learning period and if the condition is corrected within a reasonable length of time, speech readjustment should eventually take place without speech therapy; however, if the obstruction developed before or during the speech-learning period and is not corrected for some time, for example, after 7 or 8 years of age, hyponasality may become hypernasality following surgery because the child did not need to incorporate the closure mechanism into the speech act prior to the surgery.

Therapy

Speech therapy for organic rhinolalia is indicated when: (a) hypernasality persists following successful surgery for velopharyngeal incompetency (habituated); (b) obstructed hyponasality is surgically relieved but is followed by postoperative hypernasality, due to the lack of use of the closure mechanism while the obstruction was present; (c) surgical treatment results in some involvement of the closure mechanism, for example, as in some cases of tonsilloadenoidectomy; (d) medical or surgical intervention is contraindicated; and (e) minimal organic factors exist and speech therapy alone may possibly be effective.

Primary Preventive Measures. Parents and physicians should be alerted to the possible effects on speech resonance of unattended cases of prolonged nasal congestion, sinusitis, mouth breathing, hypertrophied adenoids, and broken or deformed nose, especially when present or incurred during the speech-sound learning period (approximately 1 to 7 years).

Since the performance of a tonsilloadenoidectomy on a child with an undetected submucous cleft may lead to a persisting organic hypernasality, ENT specialists must be reminded to examine carefully for signs of the submucous cleft and to request routinely a preoperative lateral x-ray of the velopharyngeal area at rest and during the production of an extended [s] sound. The effects of tonsilloadenoidectomies in children with undetected submucous clefts were shown in a film prepared by the author (Mysak, 1961).

Secondary Preventive Measures. Secondary preventive measures include providing optimal prespeech experiences for infants who present a high risk of manifesting a future organic rhinolalia, for example, infants with cleft palate, and attempting to reduce secondary speech symptoms arising from existing organic rhinolalia as well as social and emotional repercussions.

In cases of congenital cleft palate, the author (Mysak, 1961) advanced the idea that the hypernasality arises not only from the lack of separation of oral and nasal chambers but also from the development of abnormal air-flow patterns. Such abnormal nasopneumodynamics for speech may be a more important contributor to the resonatory problem in some cases than the actual cleft condition. Important to the discussion here is that normal oropneumodynamics for speech is apparently not completely dependent on an intact closure mechanism. Support for such an idea comes from the following: (a) development of hypernasal speech in clients despite what appears to be successful surgery, (b) occasional discovery of clients who speak almost normally despite unclosed clefts, and (c) development of adequate speech despite what appears to be an unsuccessful surgical closure. Hence, programs designed to encourage more normal oropneumodynamics in infants with palatal clefts should prove useful and increase the chances of good speech results following eventual surgical or prosthetic procedures.

More normal oropneumodynamics may be encouraged in at least three ways (techniques should be begun as soon after birth as possible). (a) The construction of an oral prosthesis with a pharyngeal bulb that could be used during suckling-swallowing activities. This allows the infant to experience negative as well as positive intraoral air pressure during feeding. (b) The occlusion of the nostrils, for example, by gently pinching them with the fingers, during the outflow phase of such signal activities as screaming, crying, and laughing. This allows the infant to experience oralized, positive-pressure air flows during signal vocalizations. (c) The occlusion of the nostrils by gently pinching them during babbling and lalling. Most importantly, this allows the child to experience the build-up of intraoral breath pressure during consonant production, and it inhibits the nasal rerouting (nasopneumodynamics) and facilitates the normal oral routing (oropneumodynamics) of the speech airstream. The nasal rerouting of the airstream takes place in the child with cleft palate during the implosive phase of pressure-sound production when the voiced or voiceless air flows are rerouted nasally from the momentarily occluded oral chamber to the always open nasal chambers. Such techniques should be carried out regularly and at least up to the time of surgical or prosthodontic closure of the palate.

Secondary speech symptoms such as alar constriction and facial grimacing during speech in certain cases of hypernasality and habitual nose-clearing noises during speech in certain cases of hyponsasality should be discouraged and eliminated.

Causal Therapy. Causal speech therapy is carried out when situations described in the opening paragraph of this therapy section prevail.

To improve velopharyngeal closure and reduce hypernasality, the following techniques may prove useful: (a) massaging and lifting of the velum with the index finger; (b) stroking along the line of the median raphe of the velum to stimulate velar elevation; (c) tapping the velum in order to elicit the palatal reflex; (d) protruding the tongue and uttering vowels such as [ɑ, u, ɛ] (thrusting of tongue stretches and stimulates palatal elevators and tensors), and regular and frequent swallowing exercises (Moore, 1971, p. 568); (e) palatal synkinesis exercises similar to those described under "Phonatory Effector System—Therapy;" (f) alternation of nasal and oral airstreams by first closing the mouth and blowing through the nose and then closing the nasopharyngeal port and blowing through the mouth (pinching of the nostrils may be done early in the exercises if there is nasal air escape); and (g) velar diadochocinetic exercises done by rapidly alternating production of [m] and [b], [n] and [d], and [ŋ] and [g]; the nose may be pinched during production of the non-nasal plosives until nasal escape is eliminated.

To increase nasal resonance in instances of reduced nasal resonance, humming nasal sounds may prove of some value.

Symptom Therapy. Symptom therapy for resonance problems is done in those cases where the organic problems have been resolved and where the mechanisms have been exercised but where the individual persists in the use of former resonance patterns. A self-adjusting approach is recommended in such cases and is described in Chapter 8.

Compensatory Therapy. When efforts at causal and symptom therapy are less than desired, compensatory therapy techniques are applied.

Techniques that are sometimes useful in reducing perceived hypernasality are exaggerated and slowed articulation patterns, locating pitch and(or) loudness levels that lessen perceived nasality, and adoption of a light-contact articulation pattern.

When these compensatory techniques prove useful, the change may be attributed to encouraging oralization of the speech airstream, modification of the vowel spectra, and minimizing the rerouting of the speech airstream, respectively.

Slowing of speech rate and "relaxed" speaking patterns are sometimes helpful techniques in reducing hyponasality.

ARTICULATORY EFFECTOR DISORDERS

Further modification of the laryngeal tone and the production of exolaryngeal speech sounds are the function of the articulatory speech effector. Lips and face and associated musculature; mandible and associated musculature; teeth, palate, and associated musculature; and the tongue and associated musculature are the major components of the articulatory effector.

Background

Mouth deformities that may have articulatory repercussions are due to numerous factors. They may be one part of more general conditions or they may reflect relatively specific conditions.

General Congenital Anomalies. Conditions that are usually identified at birth and are connected with heritable, chromosomal, endocrine, or unknown factors and include oral abnormalities are discussed here.

All general conditions that include cleft palate involvement should also be identified here since these conditions are frequently associated with anomalies of the lip, teeth, occlusion, maxillary arch, premaxilla, and palatal vault. For identification of these conditions, see "Resonatory Effector Disorders."

General conditions, including oral deformities, were also described elsewhere in the book. In "Gnosogenic Language Disorders in Children" in Chapter 3, the following were identified: "Bird-Headed Dwarf" (micrognathia, high-arched palate, absent or atrophic teeth); "de Lange's Syndrome" (fish-like mouth; narrow, high-arched palate), "Generalized Gangliosidosis" (large tongue, hypertrophied alveolar ridge and maxillary process); "Hunter's Syndrome" (large tongue); "Hurler's Syndrome" (large protruding tongue; high, narrow palate; small, peg-shaped, widely-spaced teeth); "Smith-Lemli-Opitz Syndrome" (high-arched palate, cleft uvula); "Klinefelter's Syndrome" (mandibular overgrowth, cleft palate); "Turner's Syndrome," female and male (high-arched palate, malocclusions); "Down's Syndrome" (protruding tongue, high-arched palate); "Trisomy Syndrome 16–18" (micrognathia).

Described under "Auditory Receptor Disorders" in Chapter 5 are: "Crouzon's Disease" (prognathism secondary to hypoplasia of the maxilla); "Ectodermal Dysplasia" (delayed or absent dentition); "Metaphysial Dysplasia" (prognathism, delayed dentition), "Oculoauricolovertebral Dysplasia" (unilateral hypoplasia of the mandible); and "Treacher Collins Syndrome" (fish-like mouth, high-arched palate, dental abnormalities). Described under "Visual Receptor Disorders" are: "Hallerman-Streiff Syndrome" (high-arched palate, dental irregularities, micrognathia), "Oculo-Dento-Digital Dysplasia," and "Rieger's Syndrome" (dental anomalies).

Brief descriptions of other general congenital conditions that include mouth deformities and that have been identified by Gellis and Feingold (1968) follow.

Ellis-van Creveld syndrome, in which intelligence is normal in the majority of individuals, presents the following characteristics: dwarfism with shortening of the extremities (short and stubby hands with polydactyly) and various mouth deformities (peg-shaped teeth and widely spaced, possible fistula of upper lip, and hypoplasia of maxilla).

Congenital hypothyroidism, in which intelligence varies relative to degree of thyroid insufficiency, presents the following characteristics: short extremities; broad hands with short fingers; short, thick neck; large-appearing head; broad-bridged nose; and oral anomalies (large, protruding tongue, delayed dentition).

Neonatal hypoglycemia, in which individuals are of normal intelligence or may be slightly retarded, presents the following characteristics: mild microcephaly and a large and protruding tongue.

Nevoid basal cell carcinoma syndrome, in which retardation when present is mild to moderate in severity, presents the following characteristics: skin exhibits numerous, generalized nevoid basal cell carcinomas; large head with frontal and parietal bossing; eye anomalies (hypertelorism, strabismus, epicanthal folds, cataracts, glaucoma); broad-bridged nose; and oral anomalies (jaw cysts, dental anomalies, prognathism).

Cerebral gigantism, in which retardation is usually moderate, presents the following characteristics: broad, large hands; dolichocephaly; eye anomalies (hypertelorism and antimongoloid slant); and oral anomalies (high-arched palate and prognathism).

Silver's syndrome, in which intelligence is usually normal, presents the following characteristics: short fifth finger with clinodactyly; possibly asymmetrical head with broad forehead; triangular facies; and micrognathia.

Infantile hypercalcemia, in which retardation is usually mild to moderate, presents the following characteristics: elfin-like facies; broad forehead; prominent ears; eye anomalies (hypertelorism, epicanthal folds, strabismus); and mouth anomalies (broad upper lip, small mandible and teeth).

Pycnodysostosis, in which intelligence is usually normal, presents the following characteristics: short limbs and stature; hypoplastic facial bones; brachycephaly and frontal bossing; and various oral anomalies (unerupted or malformed teeth; double row of teeth; flattened or increased obtuseness of mandibular angle).

Anomalies of Individual Teeth and Dental Malocclusions. For a good description of dental occlusion and of dental anomalies and dental malocclusions, the reader is referred to Bloomer (1971, Ch. 28). At least three kinds of dental pathologies should be of interest to the speech clinician: developmental dental malocclusion, loss of teeth due to dental evolution or involution, and arch and teeth involvements due to trauma, disease, or iatrogenic reasons.

Many types of dental malocclusions may contribute to articulatory problems. Some factors responsible for malocclusion are heredity, osseous defects, muscular dysfunctions, mouth breathing, malnutrition, and tongue thrusting. For a reminder of what constitutes normal occlusion of the dental arches, the reader is referred to "Articulatory Speech Effector—Teeth" in Chapter 1. At least six forms of dental malocclusions may be related to articulatory deviations. (The description of the different classes of malocclusion are based on Bloomer's (1971, Ch. 28) discussion of Angle's original classification of malocclusion.)

Neutrocclusion is a malocclusion in which a normal anteroposterior relationship exists between the maxilla and mandible but where anterior malocclusions of various types exist. For example, there may be anomalies of individual tooth position. Following is Lischer's system of terms to describe malpositioning of individual teeth (Bloomer, 1971, p. 729): linguoversion, toward the tongue; labioversion, toward the lip or cheek; mesioversion, mesial or anterior to the normal position; distoversion, distal or posterior to the normal position; infraversion, higher in the maxilla and lower in the mandible than the line of occlusion; supraversion, lower in the maxilla or higher in the mandible than the line of occlusion; torsiversion, rotated on its long axis; axiversion, wrong axial inclination; and transversion, wrong sequential order of position in the arch.

Distocclusion is a malocclusion in which the mandible is distal or in a posterior relationship to the maxilla (weak-jaw facies). Forms of distocclusion include extreme labioversion or protrusion of the maxillary incisors; linguoversion of maxillary central incisors and labial and mesial tipping of maxillary lateral incisors; and unilateral forms. Conditions responsible for the distocclusal effect are maxillary protraction, mandibular retraction, protrusion of maxillary incisors or retrusion of mandibular incisors, and mandibular micrognathia.

Mesiocclusion is a malocclusion in which the mandible is mesial or in an anterior relationship to the maxilla (jutting-jaw facies). The prognathic jaw is the extreme form of the condition. Conditions responsible for the mesiocclusal effect are macromandibular development, micromaxillary development, marked labioversion of the anterior mandibular teeth, and marked linguoversion of the anterior maxillary teeth.

Numerous other dental occlusal and dental anomalies that may occur in isolation or in combination with the major classes of malocclusion are: infraclusion or anterior or lateral open bite, where, for example, in anterior open bite the maxillary incisors do not normally overlap the mandibular incisors; supraclusion or anterior close bite, where the maxillary incisors excessively overlap the mandibular incisors; cross bite, where portions of the upper and lower arches cross rather than overlap normally; missing or infraverted lateral incisor; anodontia (vera or congenital absence, and senile or loss or removal in older persons); oligodontia (presence of only a few teeth); supernumerary teeth; diastema (abnormal space between the teeth); and premature loss of first or second teeth.

Maxillary Anomalies. Abnormalities of the alveolar ridge, premaxilla, and palatal vault may have direct or indirect effects on speech articulation. Maxillary anomalies may arise as a result of congenital malformations, trauma, and postsurgical residuals.

The topic of congenital palatal involvement has already been discussed under "Resonatory Effector Disorders." However, the maxilla and its components contribute also to articulatory function by separating oral and nasal chambers, by allowing for build-up of intraoral breath pressure, and by providing for various articulatory contact points (lingua-alveolar, linguapalatal, linguavelar). In addition to the more common palatal cleft conditions, whose major speech repercussions are of a resonatory nature, other conditions exist that may have articulatory consequences, for example, hypertrophied premaxilla resulting in severe distocclusion, flattened maxillary arch, and flattened or high and narrow palatal vaults.

Trauma to the palate may occur through penetration by pointed objects and bullet wounds and by crushing in car accidents.

Palatal scarring, adhesions, fistula, and growth disturbance are unfortunate residuals of some surgical procedures on the palate and related areas.

Mandibular Anomalies. Mandibular anomalies may also stem from congenital conditions, trauma, and as a result of surgery.

Developmental problems of retrognathia (mandibular retraction) and micrognathia (mandibular underdevelopment) exist. Ankylosis of the temporomandibular joint, which is often associated with micrognathia, prevents normal mandibular movement. Hypertrophy of the mandible or prognathic jaw is also found.

The mandible may also be involved with disease, necessitating total or subtotal mandibulectomies and often associated total or subtotal glossectomies.

Lingual Anomalies. Numerous deformities of the tongue may have articulatory consequences. Some of the conditions identified by Bloomer (1971, p. 748) follow: "ankyloglossia (tongue-tie); macroglossia (large tongue); microglossia (small tongue); aglossia (absence of tongue); atrophy, hypertrophy of all or a portion of the tongue; malignant or benign tumor. . . ; glossitis (inflammation of the tongue); ulceration, scarring, swelling, and painfulness to touch or movement; bifid, trifid, and lobulate tongue; . . . and partial or total glossectomy (extirpation of lingual tissue, through surgery, accident, or disease)."

Because of the common belief that tongue-tie may cause speech problems, some further thoughts on tongue-tie are in order. Tongue-tie or ankyloglossia describes a condition in which the lingual frenulum is short, thick, and fibrosed and where underlying genioglossus muscles may also be fibrosed. Open bite and mandibular prognathism may also result in cases of severe limitation of tongue-tip motion. "Although it does not cause speech defects, tongue-tie does contribute to difficulties in rate and range of articulation" (Horton et al., 1969).

Labial Anomalies. Among lip conditions that may affect speech are: neoplasms of the lips; microcheilia (abnormal smallness of lips); macrocheilia (excessive size of lips); restricted movements of the lip due to scarring; and loss of lip tissue due to trauma, disease, and surgery.

Clinical Manifestations

Numerous speech manifestations may be associated with structural anomalies of the articulatory effectors.

Labial Dyslalias. Lip muscles contribute to the production of bilabials [b, p, m], labiodentals [f, v], and to rounded vowels such as [o, u, ʊ], the semivowel [w], and to diphthongs such as [ɑ ʊ].

Following closure of congenital cleft lip, the upper lip may be short and taut and may cause some distortion of lip-round vowels, bilabials, and [r, w].

"When the lower lip is lost by injury, [b] sounds like [v], and [p] resembles a diffuse [f]; [m] is replaced by an indifferent nasal sound; [f] and [v] may be totally absent . . . . In case of a lost upper lip, the lower lip may move against or behind the upper teeth for [b], [p], and [m], as is normally the case only for [v] and [f]" (Luchsinger and Arnold, 1965, p. 644).

Dental and Dento-occlusal Dyslalias. Teeth and their occlusion have direct and indirect effects on speech production. In the formation of bilabial sounds, dental arches form a base for the compressing lips; for labiodental and linguadental sounds, the anterior teeth function as fellows with the upper lip and tongue, respectively, in constricting the oral exit so as to produce labiodental and linguadental fricative sounds; and for sibilants, the approximating arches serve as cues for the tongue and as obstructions to assist in producing lingua-alveolar or linguapalatal fricative sounds.

Sigmatism or various forms of lisping may be influenced by various dental and dento-occlusal conditions. *Interdental sigmatism* (between the teeth) may occur in cases of open bite and in cases of missing central incisors. *Lateral sigmatism* may occur in cases of flattened upper dental quadrants as in postoperative cases of palatal cleft, in cross bite, and in lateral open bite. *Addental (against the teeth) or occluded sigmatism* may appear in cases of close bite or supraclusion, linguaverted incisors, or supernumerary teeth. *Palatal sigmatism* (retropositioned tongue) may be observed in open and close bite conditions and in mesiocclusion. *Strident sigmatism* (dull or sharp whistling type) may be heard in cases of dental diastema of anterior teeth and in cases of mild infraclusion. *Labiodental sigmatism* ([f]-like lisp) may occur in cases of substantial distocclusion or substantial mesiocclusion. *Lateroflex sigmatism* (combined interdental and lateral lisping) may occur in cases of an infraverted or missing lateral incisor, as in cases of unilateral complete palatal cleft when the tongue tip and mandible may deviate toward the side of the cleft during the production of sibilants. *Edentulous sigmatism* (missing incisors or anodontia) may take the form of linguopalatal (tongue tip and anterior palate), linguoalveolar (tongue tip and upper alveolar ridge), linguolabial (tongue and upper lip), and interlabial (between the lips) fricative substitutions (Luchsinger and Arnold, 1965, p. 650). *Prosthetic sigmatism* describes sibilant distortions that may arise temporarily or more permanently as a result of ill-fitting dental caps or dentures. For good discussions of the relationships between malocclusion and speech, the reader is referred to Bloomer (1971, Ch. 28) and Luchsinger and Arnold (1965, pp. 645–650).

Betacism or difficulty in producing bilabials [b, p, m] may also be associated with dental malocclusions. An open bite that prevents the lips from readily coming into approximation may make it difficult to produce [b, p, m], and a substantial distocclusal effect may encourage labiodentally produced [b, p, m].

Thetacism or difficulty with the linguadental sounds [θ, ð] may be associated with open bite and with distocclusal relationships.

Labiodental confusion or distortion of [f, v] may also be dentogenic. Labiodental production of [f, v] with upper lip against the lower teeth may occur in substantial mesiocclusion, while labiodental distortions may occur in cases of missing upper incisors.

Rhotacism-lambdacism or [r, l] problems may be associated with severe mesiocclusion where tongue tip elevation or retroflexion may be made more difficult.

Palatal Dyslalias. As stated in Chapter 1, the role of the palate and associated musculature is to separate oral and nasal chambers and allow the build-up of intraoral breath pressure for the production of pressure sounds; to couple oral and nasal chambers for the production of nasal sounds; and to provide articulatory guide points for the production of lingua-alveolar, linguapalatal, and linguavelar sounds.

The best examples of palatally-based dysarticulation are the frequent articulatory repercussions associated with congenital cleft palate. Difficulty in producing adequate intraoral breath pressure will result in *weak pressure sounds*, especially voiceless fricatives, stops, and affricates. Inability to build-up adequate intraoral breath pressure may also lead to the unusual sound substitutions of *nasal, pharyngeal, and laryngeal plosives and fricatives*. Also, in cases of surgically-removed premaxilla, sometimes connected with habilitation of congenital cleft palate, the tongue-tip sounds [t, d, n, l] may be produced in a linguolabial fashion.

High narrow palates that do not easily accommodate the tongue may encourage interdental sigmatism.

Lingual Dyslalias. The most important articulator is the tongue and its associated musculature. The tongue contributes to speech articulation by altering the resonance characteristics of the vocal tract for production of vowels; by acting as a valve in production of linguadental and lingua-alveolar fricatives and linguapalatal fricative and affricate sounds; by redirecting the speech airstream in the production of the lateral [l] and the retroflex [r]; and by occluding the oral exit in production of lingua-alveolar and linguavelar plosives.

Ankyloglossis or shortness of the lingual frenulum rarely causes speech defects; however, *ateloglossia*, or agenesis of the tongue tip, may in extreme cases cause problems with [t, d, r, l, s, z, θ, ð] (West and Ansberry, 1968, p. 89).

Injuries to the body of the tongue may reduce tongue-tip motility and hence affect tongue-tip sounds as well as affect linguapalatal and linguavelar sounds.

Traumatic or surgical removal of the anterior portion of the tongue (*partial glossectomy*) may result in [d] sounding like [g], [t] like [k], [s] like [ʃ], and in the absence of [r] and [l].

Total glossectomy or absence of the tongue may result in the following compensatory, aglossic articulation: [d, t, n] may be produced in a labiodental fashion; [s, ʃ] may be produced by blowing through the teeth or through approximated lips; [g, k, ŋ] may be produced by contact between any residual lingual tissue and the pharyngeal wall or through the use of glottal plosives; and [r] may be produced by vibrating the uvula or vocal folds.

Macroglossia or enlarged tongue may have numerous origins, according to Bloomer (1971, pp. 749–750). Among them are congenital, acromegaly, and lingual hemangioma (tumor composed of new-formed blood vessels). Bloomer indicates that macroglossia affects the tongue-tip sounds in particular. "Consonants /t/, /d/, and /n/ are likely to be produced with the tongue tip depressed and the blade of the tongue in contact with the upper alveolar arch, or perhaps with the tongue protruded so that valving becomes lingua-incisal" (p. 749). Interdental sigmatism is also common.

Degrees of mandibuloglossectomy resulting from surgical removal of tissue due to infection or malignancy complicate lingual dyslalias because loss of portions of the mandible reduces the efficiency of an important compensatory articulator.

Diagnosis

Clinical, direct, differential, and group diagnoses are among the approaches that contribute to the determination of organic dyslalias.

Clinical Diagnosis. Important clinical information for determining organic dyslalia is the phonetic inventory. "In most instances the articulatory syndrome is to be regarded as pointing to, or suggesting, a given type of defect arising from a given cause rather than proving definitely the nature of the cause" (Kanter and West, 1960, p. 341). A "phonemodiagnosis" of a relatively specific labial dyslalia should reveal an articulatory profile where only lip sounds are involved, for example, bilabials, labiodentals, lip-round vowels, and diphthongs. The nonspeech test of labial function should indicate difficulty with bilabial movements and postures and with assuming, in an alternating fashion, lip-round and lip-neutral postures. Spontaneous compensatory sound substitutions may further support the phonemodiagnosis, for example, in the case of a short stiff upper lip, labiodental plosives may be used to substitute for the normal bilabial plosives.

A phonemodiagnosis of a particular kind of dento-occlusal dyslalia, that is, one associated with the mesiocclusal effect, serves as a second example. The articulatory syndrome should include difficulty with sibilants, labiodental sounds, and retroflex and lateral sounds. The nonspeech evaluation should reveal great difficulty or inability in voluntarily achieving more adequate approximation of the upper and lower dental arches. Compensatory sound substitutions may include inverted [f, v], labiodental (upper lip against lower teeth) sibilants, and bilabialized [r, l].

A phonemodiagnosis of the speech repercussions of the distocclusal effect serves as a final example. The articulatory syndrome should include difficulty with bilabial sounds and sibilants. The nonspeech evaluation should indicate great difficulty or inability in voluntarily achieving a more normal approximation of the dental arches. Compensatory sound substitutions include labiodental postures for bilabials [p, b, m].

Various other articulatory syndromes may be found in the discussion of palatal and lingual dyslalias.

Direct Diagnosis. Once an articulatory effector disorder is suspected, the clinician directly observes the possibly involved region. The clinician must learn to recognize the various kinds of individual dental and dento-occlusal anomalies and their common articulatory repercussions. Similarly, he must learn to recognize visually all maxillary, mandibular, lingual, and labial anomalies that may possibly give rise to articulatory deficits.

Differential Diagnosis. The diagnostician must be careful to distinguish between, for example, dental sigmatism and sibilant immaturity; dental sigmatism and audiogenic sigmatism; dental sigmatism and speech-model or imitative sigmatism; dental sigmatism and paralytic sigmatism; and dental sigmatism and psychogenic or functional sigmatism. Labial and palatal dyslalias are more readily diagnosed on a direct basis; however, many of the lingual dyslalias also need to be carefully differentiated as in the case of the dental sigmatisms.

Group Diagnosis. In cases of articulatory effector disorders, the speech and hearing clinician must be prepared to work in conjunction with at least the dentist, orthodontist, prosthodontist, ear, nose, and throat (ENT) specialist, pediatrician, and surgeon. Whenever a speech clinician is confronted with an oral anomaly that may be part of a larger syndrome, as in the case of the general congenital anomalies discussed, he must refer to the pediatrician. Joint conferences should be held with the dentist and orthodontist in cases of dental and dento-occlusal dyslalias; with the ENT specialist and plastic surgeon in cases of palatal dyslalias; and with the plastic surgeon in cases of labial and lingual dyslalias.

Prognosis

In general, the prognosis in cases of articulatory effector disorders is good. Important variables that contribute to the prognosis are the severity of the malocclusion or the maxillary, mandibular, or lingual anomalies; whether the condition is congenital or acquired and, if acquired, whether it occurred before, during, or after the speech-learning period; the efficiency of the dental or surgical intervention; and the intelligence and motivation of the client.

The time factor is critical. For example, a normal speaker who loses all of his teeth through disease, trauma, or aging should require no more than well-fitting dentures to restore his premorbid speech ability. On the other hand, a child with congenital anodontia who is allowed to use edentulous speech patterns into the speech-learning period and establishes such patterns will not automatically use standard patterns following dental habilitation. He will need follow-up speech therapy in order to unlearn the edentulous articulatory patterns and learn standard ones. Also, when error patterns are used well into adulthood before dental work and speech therapy are used, the chances are that standard articulation will be extremely difficult to achieve, if ever.

The severity factor is also operative in articulatory effector disorders. For example, rarely will labial dyslalias be important or intractable, short of the effects of complete loss of the upper or lower lip. Similarly, lingual and dento-occlusal anomalies must lean toward the severe before lasting speech repercussions occur.

The importance of the efficiency of surgical and dental intervention is clear. Most causes of articulatory effector disorder, that is, malocclusion, maxillary, mandibular, labial, and lingual problems, are more or less amenable to surgical and dental intervention, and, depending on time and severity factors, such intervention may be all that is necessary to resolve the dyslalia.

The intelligence and motivation factor is important in those cases requiring follow-up speech therapy.

Therapy

Speech therapy for articulatory effector disorders is used when (a) error patterns persist following successful dental and surgical intervention, and (b) dental or surgical intervention is unsatisfactory or cannot completely resolve the problem.

Primary Preventive Measures. Parents, pediatricians, and dentists should be reminded of the importance of dental maturation and of the integrity of labial, palatal, mandibular, and lingual structures to speech articulation. Proper diet, hygiene, and speedy attention to injuries to any of these orofacial regions should be stressed, especially before and during the speech-learning period.

Secondary Preventive Measures. The most important factor under secondary preventive measures is the time factor. When dental, dento-occlusal, maxillary, mandibular, labial, or lingual problems are discovered, they should receive attention whenever possible before 1 year of age or as soon as possible after that. This means, for example, attending to dental and occlusal anomalies of deciduous teeth. Prespeech intervention increases the chances of normal speech sound maturation, and early postspeech intervention increases the chances of spontaneous correction of articulation following sucessful dental or surgical intervention.

Causal Therapy. Primary causal therapy is represented by the dental or surgical intervention.

Speech or secondary causal therapy for a stiff or tight upper lip following surgery, for example, may include daily massage, stretching, and lip rounding and spreading exercises.

To counter the distocclusal effect, mandibular extension or stretching exercises could be used. The client is asked to approximate progressively the upper anterior teeth with his mandibular anterior teeth for 5 or 10 minutes, two or three times a day. Similarly, compensatory retrusion exercises of the mandible in cases of the mesiocclusal effect may be initiated.

For lingual anomalies, passive and active stretching, resistance, and compensatory movement techniques may be used; for example, stretching exercises for a short frenulum, pushing exercises with remaining lingual tissue in cases of glossectomy to stimulate compensatory elevation of the floor of the mouth, and practice in bringing cheek muscles against the dental arches in order to produce compensatory plosive sounds.

Symptom Therapy. When primary and secondary causal therapies have been used reasonably successfully, but articulatory error patterns persist, a self-adjusting form of symptom therapy is recommended. Principles of self-adjusting therapy are presented in Chapter 8.

Compensatory Therapy. When the results of causal therapies are limited and where standard articulation is not likely to be achieved, programs of compensatory therapy should be planned.

When bilabial contact is not possible *labiodental forms* of [p, b, m] can be stimulated. Glottal substitutions are also possible.

When lingua-alveolar contact is not possible, labioalveolar (lower lip raised behind upper teeth and making contact with alveolar surface) forms of [t, d] and of [n] can be elicited. Glottal plosive substitutions are also possible.

When normal labiodental contact (lower lip against upper teeth) is not possible, inverted labiodental (upper lip against lower teeth) fricative forms of [f, v] can be produced.

When lingua-alveolar and linguapalatal contacts are not possible, bilabial and labiodental fricative forms and sending-the-airstream-through-the-teeth forms of [s, z, ʃ] can be produced. Glottal and pharyngeal fricative substitutions are also possible.

When retroflex and lateral positions are not possible, bilabial forms of [r, l] can be produced. Uvular and glottal [r] substitutions are also possible.

When linguavelar contact is not possible, [k, g] sounds may be made by approximating and vibrating the faucial arches or in a glottal plosive fashion.

ENDOCRINOGENIC DISORDERS

Endocrines influence the speech effectors in at least two ways. (a) By permeating the muscle and associated nerve tissue of different effectors, endocrine products affect the level of activity of these effectors. (b) Endocrine products affect certain speech effectors through their role in regulating growth. Glandular organs that may influence speech are the thyroid, parathyroids, adrenals, pituitary, and the gonads (West and Ansberry, 1968, p. 19).

Background

Information on disorders of the endocrine system is drawn basically from Nelson (1964, pp. 1254–1320). Characteristics of the disorders are restricted to those more readily visualized by the speech clinician.

Pituitary Gland Disorders. *Idiopathic pituitary dwarfism* apparently results from absent or inadequate secretion of growth hormone and is characterized by the following: intelligence is usually normal; head is round; face is short and broad; nose is small, bridge is depressed and saddleshaped; eyes are bulging; mandible is underdeveloped; teeth are frequently crowded; neck is short and larynx is small; voice is high-pitched even after puberty; and extremities are well proportioned, with small hands and feet (acromicria).

Progeria, whose etiology is obscure, is a rare type of dwarfism combined with premature senility and is characterized by the following: intelligence is normal; head is large and prematurely bald; face is small; eyes appear prominent; nose is "beaked"; chin recedes; chest is narrow; and abdomen protrudes.

Pituitary gigantism and acromegaly are caused by overproduction of growth hormone. Such overproduction of growth hormone in young persons causes gigantism (in most cases abnormal growth becomes evident at puberty); in older individuals it causes acromegaly. Acromegaly is characterized by the following: increase in skull circumference; nose becomes broad; tongue enlarges and often protrudes between thickened lips; mandible grows excessively; and dorsal kyphosis may be found.

Thyroid Gland Disorders. *Congenital hypothyroidism* (sporadic cretinism), usually due to a complete absence or a rudimentary thyroid gland, is characterized by the following: mental development is usually retarded; speech is delayed accordingly and voice is hoarse; growth is stunted, extremities are short, and head appears large; eyes appear far apart, palpebral fissures are narrow, and eyelids are swollen; nose is broad and bridge is depressed; mouth is in an open posture and there is a broad protruding tongue; dentition is delayed; neck is short and thick; hands are broad and fingers short; skin is dry and scaly; and the muscles are usually hypotonic. "The specific effect of hypothyroidism in speech development is seen in its extreme form in the infantile language, meager ideation and 'thick-tongue' arrhythmic speech of the cretin" (Berry and Eisenson, 1956, p. 97).

Acquired hypothyroidism (juvenile hypothyroidism) may result from a variety of causes, for example: total or subtotal thyroidectomy due to thyrotoxicosis or cancer; removal due to anomalous thyroid (ectopic, i.e., displaced or malpositioned); deficiency of pituitary thyrotropin; or unknown causes. The extent of dysfunction and age at the onset of the disorder determine the clinical manifestations.

Goiter is an enlargement of the thyroid gland and may be congenital or acquired, endemic or sporadic. Enlarged thyroid may have no affect on thyroid function (euthyroidism) or may cause hypothyroidism (thyroid deficiency) or hyperthyroidism (thyroid overproduction). Two forms of goiter of special interest to the speech and hearing clinician are goiter and congenital deafness (Pendred syndrome) and intratracheal goiter. In the Pendred syndrome, which is heritable, there is usually normal mental and physical development, euthyroidism or mild hypothyroidism with thyroid enlargement (either barely detectable or pronounced) making its appearance during childhood, and congenital high-frequency hearing loss. The syndrome should not be confused with: (a) deaf-mutism in persons with goiter from areas of endemic goiter, and (b) mild hearing impairment in severely hypothyroid individuals. The connection between the thyroid and hearing involvement is obscure. Goiter within the trachea or intratracheal goiter may cause obstruction of the airway and, hence, respiratory repercussions.

Hyperthyroidism (thyrotoxicosis, toxic goiter, Graves' disease, exophthalmic goiter) results from excessive secretion of thyroid hormone.

Usually, affected individuals have a diffuse goiter with or without exophthalmos. Etiology is unknown. Characteristics of the condition are as follows: in children the earliest signs may be emotional disturbances, hyperactivity, irritability, excitability; tremor of fingers with arm extended; exophthalmos in majority of cases but not severe; and skin is smooth and flushed with excessive sweating.

Disorders of the Parathyroid Glands. The primary function of the parathyroid is maintenance of calcium and phosphorous balance. Hypofunction of the parathyroid glands results in tetany (sharp flexion of wrists and ankle joints, muscle twitchings, cramps, and convulsions). Congenital aplasia, surgical removal, and traumatic destruction or atrophy of the glands are causes of permanent parathyroid deficiency. *Idiopathic hypoparathyroidism* is occasionally congenital. Congenital aplasia and familial tendencies are possible backgrounds. Some of the characteristics of the condition are: muscular pain and cramps; eye abnormalities (lacrimation, photophobia, corneal ulceration); irregular and late eruption of teeth; dry and scaly skin; and thin and patchy hair. "In the pathological state of decreased blood calcium, a rapid and overly nervous speech may be observable" (Kaplan, 1960, p. 57).

Adrenal Gland Disorders. Hypersecretion of androgenic hormones causes the *adrenogenital syndrome*. Congenital defects or tumors may be causative. Characteristics of the form known as congenital virilizing adrenal hyperplasia are: in the male, precocity of sexual development including development of acne and of a deep voice; in the female there is female pseudohermaphroditism, acne, and development of a male-like voice. *Cushing's syndrome* is the result of maintenance of high blood levels of hydrocortisone by hyperfunction of the adrenal cortex. The condition may be caused by adrenal hyperplasia or by a tumor. Characteristics of the disorder include: obesity of the "buffalo type"; hypertrichosis of the face; intensely red cheeks; acne even in very young children; and a deep and coarse voice.

Disorders of the Gonads. Various forms of testicular hypofunction exist. In *primary hypogonadism*, decreased production of androgen and impaired spermatogenesis are present. Traumatic or surgical castration, congenital absence of testes (anorchia), atrophy of testes due to damage to the vascular supply, and acute orchitis resulting from mumps may cause hypogonadism; also degrees of hypogonadism are associated with Klinefelter's syndrome and Turner's syndrome in the male. Signs of primary hypogonadism that are noted only at puberty or after are: failure of development of secondary sex characteristics; accumulation of fat in region of hips, buttocks, and sometimes in breasts and on abdomen; scant or absent facial hair; and a persisting high-pitched voice. *Froehlich's syndrome* describes a form of hypogonadism that may be secondary to lesions of the hypothalamus caused by tumors, trauma, or encephalitis. Features of the condition include obesity, beardless face, and a high-pitched voice after adolescence.

Various forms of ovarian hypofunction exist. *Primary hypogonadism* in females may be due to surgical removal of both ovaries or to gonadal dysgenesis (Turner's syndrome, Bonnevie-Ullrich syndrome). The majority of patients with gonadal dysgenesis show chromosomal abnormality. Characteristics of gonadal dysgenesis are: shortness of stature, webbing of the neck, small mandible, epicanthal folds, and prominent ears.

Clinical Manifestations

Endocrine dysfunction may affect overall patterns of growth and development, including that of effector structures and cause various linguistic, auditory, articulatory, and phonatory problems, and (or) endocrine dysfunction may affect the functioning of effector muscles and cause phonatory, articulatory, and speech rhythm problems.

Endocrine Dyslogias. When overall growth and development are disturbed by endocrine involvement, as in congenital hypothyroidism and primary female hypogonadism, degrees of mental retardation and associated delay in onset or underdevelopment of language function may occur. Such endocrine dyslogias are more appropriately listed under "Gnosogenic Language Disorders in Children" in Chapter 3.

Endocrine Hypacuses. Thyroid involvement apparently is connected in some way with hearing function, as in the cases of Pendred syndrome, endemic goiter, and severe hypothyroidism. Cases of hearing loss and hyperparathyroidism have also been reported. Such endocrine hypacuses are more appropriately listed under "Auditory Receptor Disorders" in Chapter 5.

Endocrine Dyslalias. Articulatory anomalies related to endocrine-based changes in effector structures include *mesiocclusal dyslalia*, often found in acromegaly (sigmatism, lambdacism, rhotacism, inverted [f, v]); *distocclusal dyslalia*, which may be found in idiopathic pituitary dwarfism and progeria (sigmatism, labiodental bilabials); and *macroglossal dyslalias*, often found in acromegaly and congenital hypothyroidism (anterior or interdental production of tongue-tip sounds [s, z, t, d, n, l].

Articulatory anomalies possibly related to endocrine-based influences on speech muscle irritability include: *imprecise or over-elided articulation* (asaphia), due to tremors and tautness based on hyperthyroidism; and *sluggish or labored articulation* (bradylalia), due to hypotonicity based on hypothyroidism (myxedema) or hyperparathyroidism.

Endocrine Speech Dysrhythmias. Irregular speech rhythm may result from changes in speech muscle irritability due to endocrine influences. *Rapid and irregular rhythm* may be associated with hyperthyroidism or hypoparathyroidism ("There is a special type of speech retardation in which articulation is unclear because muscular responses are so hurried as to be incomplete and noncoordinated. It is thought that parathyroid deficiency may account for this type of retardation" (Berry and Eisenson, 1956, p. 98)). *Slow and labored rhythm* may be associated with hypothyroidism and hyperparathyroidism. Berry and Eisenson (1956, pp. 97–98), in speaking of the function of the adrenals, hypothesize "that the slow, poorly timed, and hypotonic muscular contractions of the speech muscles in some cases of retardation may be caused by latent adrenal insufficiency."

Endocrine Dysphonias. Various dysphonias may be related to endocrine dysfunctioning. Luchsinger and Arnold (1965, pp. 188–217) devoted a section of their book to vocal disorders of endocrine origin.

Pituitary dysphonias are marked by persisting high-pitched voice (acrophonia), as in hypofunction of the pituitary gland causing hypoplasia of the larynx in cases of idiopathic pituitary dwarfism, or abnormally low-pitched voice, as in hyperfunction of the pituitary gland causing hypertrophy of the laryngeal structures in acromegaly. In acromegaly, "marked virilization of the voice [androphonia] is often striking in women" (Luchsinger and Arnold, 1965, p. 214).

Thyroid dysphonias may appear in the form of hoarse voice (trachyphonia) and laryngeal hypoplasia in congenital hypothyroidism. Luchsinger and Arnold (1965, p. 207) report that, in cases of subclinical cretinism, there may be severe delay in language development, huskiness, high pitch, or feeble voice. Hypothyroidism in adults or myxedema may lead to vocal muscle involvement, which results in weak-hoarse voice (phonasthenia-trachyphonia). Hyperthyroidism may be associated with easy fatigue of the voice, upward displacement of speaking pitch, and tremulous voice (tromophonia). In instances where thyroid enlargement or goiter results in tracheal and (or) laryngeal compression, a downwardly displaced speaking pitch may be observed. Sonninen (1960) compared voice symptoms of individuals with toxic goiter and compression goiter. Lowering of pitch and quality changes characterized the compression goiter group, while weakness of the voice when shouting characterized the toxic goiter group.

Parathyroid dysphonias have been reported in the form of aphonia in cases of hyperparathyroidism (hypercalcemia) (Luchsinger and Arnold, 1965, p. 211). Simpson (1954) reported on three cases of middle-aged women where dysphonia and hearing involvement were associated with hyperparathyroidism. Hypercalcemia might be expected to decrease nerve excitability, and hence the voice and hearing symptoms could be attributed to decrease in nerve reactions in the ear and larynx. Symptoms were resolved in each case by removal of parathyroid adenomas.

Adrenal dysphonias may be characterized by a prematurely deep voice in males and virilization of voice (androphonia) in females, as in cases of congenital virilizing adrenal hyperplasia. Deep and coarse voices are also found in Cushing's syndrome.

Gonadal dysphonias may be marked by persisting high-pitched voice in boys, as in primary hypogonadism and in Froehlich's syndrome. Luchsinger and Arnold (1965, p. 194) discuss three forms of incomplete vocal mutation due to "slight delays in physical maturation on a constitutional basis." Chronic hoarseness and vocal weakness are the common signs of incomplete mutation in young males. Delayed mutation describes voice change that begins much later than expected; prolonged mutation describes signs of voice change that may persist over several years instead of the usual few months; and incomplete mutation describes a male voice that does not fully develop. The latter two conditions may be considered forms of puberphonia. Incomplete mutational conditions are in contrast to mutational falsetto voice in males, which describes the persistent use of the prepubescent voice although the larynx has developed normally and appears capable of producing a normal adult voice. Gonadal conditions that produce precocious puberty may lead to premature establishment of adult male or female voices in males or females or in the more irregular development of an adult male voice in the female.

Diagnosis

Diagnosis of endocrinogenic disorders of the speech effectors by the speech clinician involves differentiation of the effects of endocrinopathies on the speech effectors from other conditions of the effectors and appropriate referral. Because of the interdependence and interrelationships of the various endocrine glands, the speech clinician should avoid making guesses as to which gland may be the primary source of the disorder of a particular speech effector. "Because the glands interact in the endocrine 'ring' it is difficult to define metabolic dysfunction in terms of one gland. Because they also interact with the autonomic system, it is difficult to restrict the action even to the endocrine system" (Berry and Eisenson, 1956, p. 97).

Differential Diagnosis. The first task of the speech clinician when presented, for example, with possible endocrine dyslalias or dysphonias is to differentiate them from other possible backgrounds.

For example, acromegalic, prognathic dyslalia must be differentiated from a pseudoprognathic dyslalia resulting from an underdeveloped maxilla due to congenital hypoplasia or trauma; and hypothyroid macroglossal dyslalia must be differentiated from pseudomacroglossal dyslalia associated with a normal-sized tongue within an abnormally small oral chamber. Similarly, high-pitched gonadal dysphonias must be differentiated from forms of incomplete vocal mutation and falsetto voice, and low-pitched gonadal and adrenal dysphonias must be differentiated from various functional versions.

Group Diagnosis. When an endocrinogenic speech disorder is suspected, group diagnosis is the diagnostic approach of choice. Such a team should include the speech pathologist, ENT specialist, endocrinologist, pediatrician or internist, and the psychologist.

Prognosis

The major factor in prognosis of endocrinogenic speech disorder is the accuracy of the endocrinological diagnosis and the effectiveness of endocrinotherapy. If the primary problem is discovered during the prespeech period and if effective medical therapy is initiated early, under ordinary circumstances speech therapy should not be needed.

Obviously, the speech prognosis is always more favorable in cases where the endocrine disorder affects speech muscle irritability as opposed to cases where the endocrine disorder has affected overall growth patterns, including those of the speech effectors.

Therapy

Speech therapy for endocrinogenic speech disorders is initiated when: (a) endocrine dyslalias or dysphonias are habituated and persist even after successful endocrinotherapy; (b) endocrinotherapy is only partially successful and degrees of structural change and abnormal muscle tonus remain; and (c) endocrinotherapy is ineffective and compensatory speech therapy may offer some improvement.

Preventive Measures. Parents and health specialists must be kept sensitive to the direct and indirect effects on the speech effectors of endocrine inbalances. Early intervention should be emphasized, preferably before the speech age so that error speech patterns are not established, and in later life so that error patterns are not habituated.

Causal Therapy. Primary causal therapy is conducted by the endocrinologist. Speech causal therapy for endocrine dyslalias and dysphonias is similar to those techniques described under "Articulatory Effector Disorders—Therapy" and "Phonatory Effector Disorders—Therapy." Recommendations for symptom and compensatory therapies under those sections are also similar.

REFERENCES

Berry, M. F., and Eisenson, J., Speech Disorders: Principles and Practices of Therapy. New York: Appleton-Century-Crofts (1956)

Bloomer, H. H., Speech Defects Associated with Dental Malocclusions and Related Abnormalities. In L. E. Travis (Ed.), Handbook of Speech Pathology and Audiology. New York: Appleton-Century-Crofts (1971).

Brodnitz, F. S., Vocal Rehabilitation. Rochester, Minn.: Whiting Press (1959).

Damste, P. H., Voice change in adult women caused by virilizing agents. J. Speech Hear. Disord., 32, 126–132 (1967).

Diedrich, W., and Youngstrom, K., Alaryngeal Speech. Springfield, Ill.: Charles C Thomas (1966).

Ford, F. R., Diseases of the Nervous System in Infancy, Childhood, and Adolescence. Springfield, Ill.: Charles C Thomas (1966).

Frable, M. A., Hoarseness: A symptom of premenstrual tension. Arch. Otolaryngol., 75, 66–68 (1962).

Gellis, S. S., and Feingold, M., Atlas of Mental Retardation Syndromes. Washington, D. C.: U. S. Department of Health, Education and Welfare (1968).

Greene, M. C. L., Speech of children before and after removal of tonsils and adenoids. J. Speech Hear. Disord., 22, 361–370 (1957).

Holbrook, A., Rolnick, M. I., and Bailey, C. W., Treatment of vocal abuse disorders using a vocal intensity controller. J. Speech Hear. Disord., 39, 298–303 (1974).

Horton, C. E., Crawford, H. H., Adamson, J. E., and Ashbell, T. S., Tongue-tie. Cleft Palate J., 6, 8–23 (1969).

Jones, R. V., and Shalom, A. S., Laryngeal involvement in acute leukaemia. J. Laryngol. Otol., 82, 123–128 (1968).

Kanter, C. E., and West, R., Phonetics. New York: Harper and Row (1960).

Kaplan, H. M., Anatomy and Physiology of Speech. New York: McGraw-Hill, Book Co., (1960).

Koepp-Baker, H., Orofacial Clefts: Their Forms and Effects. The Treatment of Orofacial Clefts: Surgical, Orthopedic, and Prosthetic. In L. E. Travis (Ed.), Handbook of Speech Pathology and Audiology. Appleton-Century-Crofts (1971).

Lofgren, R. H., and Montgomery, W. W., Incidence of laryngeal involvement in rheumatoid arthritis. N. Engl. J. Med., 267, 193–195 (1962).

Luchsinger, R., and Arnold, G., Voice-Speech-Language. Belmont, Calif.: Wadsworth Publishing Co. (1965).

Moore, G. P., Voice Disorders Organically Based. In L. E. Travis (Ed.), Handbook of Speech Pathology and Audiology. New York: Appleton-Century-Crofts (1971).

Morley, M. E., Cleft Palate and Speech. Baltimore: The Williams & Wilkins Company (1966).

Mullendore, J. M., and Stoudt, R. J., Speech patterns of muscular dystrophic individuals. J. Speech Hear. Disord., 26, 252–257 (1961).

Mysak, E. D., The Unmasked Palatal Cleft. Newington, Conn: Newington Children's Hospital (1961).

Mysak, E. D., Pneumodynamics as a factor in cleft palate speech. Plast. Reconstr. Surg., 28, 588–591 (1961).

Mysak, E. D., Phonatory and Resonatory Problems. In R. W. Rieber and R. S. Brubaker (Eds.) Speech Pathology: An International Study of the Science. Amsterdam: North-Holland Publishing Company (1966).

Nelson, W. E. (Ed.), Textbook of Pediatrics. Philadelphia: W. B. Saunders Company (1964).

Rigrodsky, S., Lerman J., and Morrison, E. (Eds.), Therapy for the Laryngectomized. New York: Teachers College Press, Columbia University (1971).

Simpson, J. A., Aphonia and deafness in hyperparathyroidism. Br. Med. J., 4869, 494–499 (1954).

Snidecor, J. C., and others, Speech Rehabilitation of the Laryngectomized. Springfield, Ill.: Charles C Thomas (1962).

Snidecor, J. C., Speech Without a Larynx. In L. E. Travis (Ed.), Handbook of Speech Pathology and Audiology. New York: Appleton-Century-Crofts (1971)

Sonninen, A., Laryngeal signs and symptoms of goitre. Folia Phoniatr., 12, 41–47 (1960).

Spriestersbach, D. C., and Sherman, D., (Eds.), Cleft Palate and Communication. New York: Academic Press, Inc. (1968).

Weinberg, B., Bosma, J. F., Shanks, J. C., and De Meyer, W., Myotonic dystrophy initially manifested by speech disability. J. Speech Hear. Disord., 33, 51–59 (1968).

West, R. W., and Ansberry, M., The Rehabilitation of Speech. New York: Harper and Row (1968).

Wolski, W., Hypernasality as the presenting symptom of myasthenia gravis. J. Speech Hear. Disord., 32, 36–39 (1967).

7

Speech Transmitter System

The speech transmitter system is basically a service or passive system; that is, the system itself does not actively process or pattern speech signals, it simply conveys the code of sensory impulses generated by the speech receptors to central regions of the speech system, its cerebripetal function, or it conveys patterns of impulses generated by central regions of the speech system to the speech effectors, its cerebrifugal function. A certain amount of transmutation of these inflow and outflow patterns takes place during ascent or descent phases, but this is not a function of the transmitter system. Transmission functions are not consciously experienced by the speaker. The central division of the system is composed of upper sensory and motor tracts and their relay centers; the peripheral division is composed of lower sensory and motor nerves and associated autonomic nerves.

Problems of the transmitter system are observed in children and adults. In general, inflow problems may take the form of distorted, on-off, or no transmission thus affecting speech perception, while outflow problems may take the form of reduced, erratic, or no transmission thus affecting speech production. Discussion of problems of the speech transmitter system is divided into disorders of afferent transmission and disorders of efferent transmission.

AFFERENT TRANSMITTER DISORDERS

The primary function of the afferent speech transmitter is to convey audiovisual nerve impulses generated at the level of auditory and visual receptors to higher speech centers via lower and upper sensory neurons. The discussion here is limited to problems in auditory pathways and their relay centers. This includes: the neural auditory pathway, which is central to the organ of Corti and leads to the auditory cortices and its relay centers, including the ganglion cells within the cochlea; the ventral and dorsal cochlear nuclei, superior olive, and trapezoid body at the level of the medulla; the inferior colliculi at the level of the midbrain; and the medial geniculate body at the level of the thalamus.

Background

Disturbances of the neural auditory pathway and its relay stations may be due to generalized congenital abnormalities, heredity, neoplasms, infections, anoxia, Rh factor, trauma, vascular lesions, degenerative diseases, aging, and auditory atrophy.

Congenital Abnormalities. Certain generalized congenital conditions, for example, Down's syndrome, may include involvement of central auditory pathways (Davis, 1970, p. 127). Various cerebral palsies may also exhibit central auditory impairment.

Heredity. Involvement of the neural auditory pathway is found in cases of genetic cochlear aplasia (Goodhill *et al.*, 1971, pp. 320–321). Depending on the degree of aplasia, hypacuses as well as anacuses are presented.

Neoplasms. Brain and Walton (1969, pp. 247–248) report hearing impairment related to tumors of the midbrain or pineal body. Compression of the auditory nerve by cerebellopontine angle tumors and acoustic neurinoma, or tumors of the auditory nerve, is another neoplastic condition that affects central auditory functioning. Davis (1970, p. 127) considers brain tumors, cysts, and abscesses important backgrounds for central dysacusis.

Infections. Lesions in the central auditory pathway as well as the cochlea have been found in cases of rubella deafness (Goodhill *et al.*, 1971, p. 324). Postrubella children are also reported to present "A greater prevalence of learning disability (including aphasia) and severe emotional disturbance . . . ." The "aphasia" in many of these cases may be reflective of the involvement of the central auditory pathway. Central auditory pathways may also be involved in generalized childhood bacterial disease such as meningitis and encephalitis, as well as in "specific infections such as syphilis" (Davis, 1970, p. 127).

Anoxia. "Probably the most important cause of natal ear injury is prolonged hypoxia or anoxia of the infant" (Goodhill *et al.*, 1971, p. 326). Anoxic neural hypacusis may be manifested by various forms and degrees of sensorineural hypacusis. Background factors may include prolonged labor, disturbance in respiration, congenital cardiac and circulatory problems, and maternal sedation. Prolonged asphyxia due, for example, to nonfatal drowning accidents or carbon monoxide poisoning is also mentioned as a possible cause of central impairment (Davis, 1970, p. 127).

Rh Factor. When an Rh-negative mother gives birth to an Rh-positive infant, she may experience a build-up of Rh-positive antibodies. Such a build-up of maternal antibodies may reach a point where it will affect second-born Rh-positive children. The condition results in the destruction of red blood cells and the circulation of toxic pigment within the fetus. Kernicterus describes the neural pathologic state resulting from deposition of pigment in the pons and medulla. "Among the sequelae of kernicterus are athetoid cerebral palsy due to involvement of the extrapyramidal tracts and a specific type of central deafness due to involvement of the dorsal and ventral cochlear nuclei which has been termed 'nuclear deafness' " (Goodhill *et al.*, 1971, p. 326). Pathologic pigmentation may also occur in the cochlea, the efferent auditory pathway, and the reticular system, as well as the thalamic and cortical areas. Incompatibilities within A B O blood classifications are also considered possible backgrounds for nuclear deafness.

Trauma. Local injuries such as those incurred at birth, by skull fractures, or gunshot wounds "and the scars and adhesions resulting from these" are also possible backgrounds for central auditory impairment (Davis, 1970, p. 127).

Cerebrovascular Lesions. Cerebral hemorrhage, thrombosis, or embolism may also be etiologic in central dysacusis (Davis, 1970, p. 127).

Degenerative Diseases. Progressive diseases such as multiple sclerosis may also involve the central auditory system (Davis, 1970, p. 127).

Aging. Loss of neurons due to aging is also considered a possible factor in central impairment by Davis (1970, p. 127). "Phonemic regression" is the term sometimes used to describe the central dysacusis characterized by substantial difficulty in speech discrimination that does not correlate with results of pure tone audiometry (which often shows nearly normal thresholds up to at least 2000 Hz). Accompanying behavior patterns include short attention span and the need for greater time and special motivation before responding to certain speech stimuli. Probably the most common cause of the problem, according to Davis (1970, p. 129), is generalized cerebral arteriosclerosis.

Auditory Atrophy. Davis (1970, pp. 131–132) believes that true congenital aphasia is rare, that is, a child with a particular problem in language learning, with no significant hearing loss, and with important damage to speech areas in both hemispheres. He believes a more probable explanation of the language learning problem is an early partial hearing loss (significant loss of hearing for the middle range of frequencies important for speech perception) that goes unrecognized during the first 4 or 5 years and results in the child's disregarding sound as a means of communication.

Davis postulates that the auditory system, in order to complete its development, requires sensory input especially during the second year when speech learning usually takes place. However, because of the unrecognized special hearing loss, such stimulation does not occur and the auditory system may not fully organize even when amplification is provided later. Davis proposes the term dyslogomathia to describe a condition of special difficulty in learning speech and language that is secondary to partial sensory deprivation. Children who present such a condition usually "show some reactions to fairly loud sounds but do not spontaneously develop speech, and often have great difficulty learning speech later."

A companion concept was expressed by the present author (Mysak, 1968, p. 24) when discussing audition in certain brain-damaged children. "For example, when actual auditory problems exist and these are not detected or properly treated, the child may eventually find it unrewarding to attend auditorially, and he may begin to use less of his auditory capacity. Consequently, a type of 'auditory atrophy' may manifest itself."

Clinical Manifestations

Speech symtoms of problems in auditory transmission should be limited to those caused by disturbance in conveying impulses generated by the speech receptors to central regions of the speech system; however, since degrees of transmutation of auditory inflow apparently occur during the ascent, it is difficult to differentiate easily symptoms of auditory transmission from, for example, symptoms of problems in lower-order integration of auditory input described in Chapter 4. In Chapter 4, the function of lower-order integration is described as the automatic turning on, tuning in, and fine tuning of the speech receiving system; more specifically, the function includes arousal to, fixing and tracking of, and maintaining selective attention to the speech signal.

Auditory transmission symptoms should also be differentiated from auditory recognition symptoms, that is, where the individual apparently hears the speech signal well enough but does not recognize it as a meaningful stimulus (auditory verbal agnosia); from auditory association symptoms, that is, where the individual apparently hears the speech signal, recognizes its meaningfulness, but cannot associate it with an object, person, event, and so on (a form of auditory aphasia); and from "simple" hypacusis or anacusis.

Central organic dysacusis, central auditory imperception, and phonemic regression are the terms that have been used to describe disorders that include some of the symptoms discussed here.

Speech Learning. If prespeech children suffer from difficulty in auditory transmisssion of speech signals, they may manifest serious difficulty in speech and language learning. Such difficulty in learning speech may very well be based on the concept that faulty transmission may lead to partial sensory deprivation, which, in turn, does not allow for the full organization of the central auditory system for speech processing (auditory atrophy). Depending on severity and time of involvement, symptoms may range from severe limitation in speech comprehension to the "huh" or "what" syndrome where the child automatically requests utterances to be repeated in the absence of hypacusis.

Speech Loudness. Problems in loudness perception may also be exhibited. Hardy (1956) described children with damaged or maldeveloped auditory pathways (brain stem, interbrain, and thalamus). He said they are "aware of and are alerted by various gross sounds in the environment, that they often respond to the cessation of sound, but that there is discontinuity in their evident awareness and responsiveness." Further, some children with such problems respond better to loud than to soft sounds, or better to soft than to loud sounds.

Speech Frequencies. Perception of the frequencies of which speech sounds are composed may also be impaired. Therefore, children with minimal brain dysfunction that includes auditory involvement may confuse speech sounds that are similar. Symptoms described by Carhart (Davis, 1970, p. 129) as phonemic regression may also be discussed here. In essence, Carhart found certain elderly people who showed a disproportionate amount of difficulty perceiving speech sounds when compared to their ability to hear simple pure tones. Such individuals complain of not understanding what people say to them and have particular problems with speech when there is background noise.

The expressive result of speech signal distortion is "what-did-you-say" behavior or error responses to what the individual assumes he hears.

Speech Sequencing and Synthesis. Problems in auditory transmission may also lead to problems in putting words or parts of words together. One reflection of difficulty in speech synthesis is that individuals require speech to be spoken more slowly to ensure better comprehension. Expressive symptoms of problems in speech sequencing and synthesis are reversing syllables in certain words or producing neologisms. (This problem is more appropriately discussed in Chapter 8 as a reflection of an audiogenic sensor disorder.)

Diagnosis

Combinations of data drawn from more than one diagnostic approach are needed to help determine whether the presenting hearing-for-speech symptoms are related to disturbances of the afferent speech transmitter.

Differential Diagnosis. Auditory behavior and the secondary speech behavior resulting from afferent transmitter difficulty must be differentiated from behaviors associated with problems of the auditory speech receptor, the lower-order speech integrator (input processing function), and the higher-order speech integrator (perception-comprehension function). The task here is to differentiate auditory-speech symptoms associated with problems on at least four levels of auditory processing of speech signals. Overlapping of certain symptoms is apparent when reviewing the sections of the book that discuss these four levels of speech-signal processing. Some of the overlapping is related to the existence of lesions that affect more than one type of processing, causing mixed symptoms.

At the risk of oversimplification, the major symptoms associated with each level of auditory processing will be restated and(or) amplified. (Again, whenever secondary speech symptoms are mentioned, the reader should recognize these as reflections of audiogenic sensor disorders, which are discussed more appropriately in Chapter 8.) In general, *partial middle ear losses* cause a raising of the threshold for speech reception without important distortion of the speech signal; secondary speech problems (audiogenic dyslalia-dysphonia) may consist of low and weak voice, a tendency toward monotonous pitch patterning and hyponasality, and unvoicing of final consonants. *Partial cochlear losses* cause a raising of the threshold for speech reception accompanied by degrees of distortion of the speech signal. Secondary speech problems may consist of high and loud voice, a tendency toward monotonous pitch patterning and hypernasality, and difficulty in producing high-frequency, voiceless consonants with a tendency to omit sounds in final positions. *Problems in lower-order speech integration* (auditory centers in central auditory pathways) may be characterized by difficulty in arousing the auditory system to speech events (utterances may need to be repeated), in auditory fixing and tracking of the speech signal once arousal has occurred, or in sustaining auditory tracking once auditory arousal, fixing, and tracking have occurred. Secondary speech problems are reflected by lack of response, responses indicating incomplete comprehension, and inappropriate responses. *Problems in higher-order speech integration* (types of cortical hearing) may be reflected by: (a) a loss in auditory recognition of speech events, that is, the individual apparently hears the speech signal at a normal hearing level and hears it clearly but apparently no longer recognizes the signal as meaningful speech stimuli (auditory agnosia); and (b) a loss in auditory association, that is, the individual hears the word easily and well, recognizes its symbolic significance, but is unable to make a meaningful association with it (auditory aphasia).

These symptoms are to be differentiated from those associated with problems of the *afferent speech transmitter*. Without significant shifts in hearing levels, these individuals may have difficulty in discriminating among frequencies of which certain speech sounds are composed or may respond differentially to loud or soft sounds. Intermittent hearing or on-off hearing for speech may also be observed. A tendency toward syllable reversals and use of neologisms are some of the secondary symptoms that may be observed.

Instrumental Diagnosis. In a summary of audiometric attempts to identify central neural impairments of the auditory system, Carhart *et al.*, (1969) note the following findings: little or no reduction in sensitivity for pure tones in either ear; little or no abnormality in any monaural suprathreshold test involving pure tones; moderate to marked impairment in the ability to understand speech signals in the ear contralateral to the affected side of the brain; severe impairment in the ability to fuse coherent binaural signals; and severe impairment in the ability to separate noncoherent binaural signals.

Among the basic audiologic features of transmissive hypacuses or anacuses (lesions involving the auditory nerve and(or) the central auditory pathways) identified by Goodhill et al., (1971, p. 320) are: absent air-bone gap; variable agreement between speech reception threshold (SRT) and pure-tone air-conduction findings; variable speech discrimination (SDS) score; variable, often absent, recruitment of loudness; variable, often poor, response to amplification; low short increment sensitivity index (SISI) score; and predominantly Type III or IV Békésy audiogram. Goodhill et al. caution that mixed lesions may confuse the audiologic data and that an otologic diagnosis depends on a combination of audiologic tests as well as on a medical history, physical examination, vestibular tests, and radiographic studies.

The importance of speech testing in identification of central dysacusis is emphasized by Davis (1970, pp. 128–129): "One of the best diagnostic clues to central dysacusis is a discrepancy between the ability to understand speech and the prediction based on pure-tone audiometry." Also, "Central dysacusis is not measured in hertz or in decibels. Better dimensions are to be found in speed of perception, in synthesis, and in understanding." Newby (1964, p. 184) also emphasizes results of speech testing in identification of central auditory disorders. For example: "The ear contralateral to the lesion may perform in a markedly inferior manner to the ipsilateral ear in response to low-pass-filtered speech and to speech of faint intensity. A lesion that is not localized in either hemisphere, such as post-encephalitic or arteriosclerotic Parkinsonism, will probably result in an 'abnormal' reduction of discrimination scores in both ears when speech is subjected to low-pass filtering . . . ."

Group Diagnosis. A clear diagnosis of central organic dysacusis is dependent on neurologic corroboration of the findings of the otologist, audiologist, and speech pathologist. No single specialist may easily assume the responsibility for making the diagnosis.

Prognosis

Because of the number of possibly important factors relative to disorders of the afferent speech transmitter, no simple statement with respect to prognosis can be made. That is, if the problem is due to a degenerative disease or to pathologic aging, the prognosis is negative. On the other hand, in some young children mild bilateral amplification may make a substantial difference in their speech perception. In the cases of young children with special losses in the speech frequencies, the possible problem of auditory atrophy should be kept in mind, and hence early intervention (below 2 or 3 years if possible) should be emphasized to ensure the most favorable prognosis.

Therapy

Primary Preventive Measures. Some contributions to primary prevention of problems of the afferent speech transmitter are made: (a) by genetic counseling of individuals with backgrounds of heritable involvement of the neural auditory pathways; (b) by prevention and(or) early effective treatment of rubella, meningitis, encephalitis; (c) by making strenuous efforts to reduce anoxic repercussions associated with prolonged labor, maternal sedation, and respiratory disturbances; and (d) by desensitization to or early and effective treatment of Rh-negative incompatibility.

Secondary Preventive Measures. High-risk infants should receive early and periodic hearing checks. If auditory involvement is suspected, the benefits of speech amplification should be assessed. Sensitivity to the prevention of the possible secondary problem discussed under "Auditory Atrophy" is important here. Speech amplification may take the form of a personal hearing aid, reducing speaker-listener distance, and raising speakers' voice levels. In addition, high-risk cases should receive the kinds of stimulation outlined under "Developmental and Genetic Language Disorders—Therapy" in Chapter 3.

Causal Therapy. Causal therapy includes any medical treatment to cure or relieve the underlying condition affecting the central auditory pathways and the fitting of an appropriate hearing aid. Clinicians should keep in mind that individuals with disturbances in the auditory speech transmitter respond variably to amplification.

Symptom Therapy. As indicated under "Auditory Receptor Disorders—Symptom Therapy" in Chapter 5, symptom therapy is begun by the onset of the speech age (1 to 2 years). The guides for symptom therapy outlined in that place are also appropriate here. Expanding, improving, and correcting speech perception are appropriate symptom therapy goals.

Techniques that may prove useful in facilitating speech perception are: (a) reducing competing noise in the listening environment; (b) speaking more slowly and more precisely; (c) overarticulating; (d) varying speaking pitch and loudness and seeking the most effective combination; (e) using short, simple, and direct language; (f) allowing longer-than-usual pauses between verbal units; and (g) repeating and restructuring hard-to-understand verbal units.

Compensatory Therapy. Compensatory stimulation of auditory arousal, orienting, fixing, and tracking functions, or the turning on-tuning in process, may prove useful. That is, the speaker should attract the affected listener first, for example, by calling his name or signalling in some other fashion, thus ensuring audiovisual attention before speaking his message.

The development of compensatory speechreading, including the reading of speech-associated articulatory movements and body language is also recommended. Techniques and procedures described under "Compensatory Speechreading" in Chapter 5 are also appropriate here.

EFFERENT TRANSMITTER DISORDERS

The primary function of the efferent transmitter system is to conduct patterns of nerve impulses, organized by higher speech centers, over upper and lower motor neurons to respiratory, phonatory, resonatory, and articulatory mechanisms. Hence, the discussion is limited to those speech repercussions associated with involvement of the central or peripheral divisions of cervical nerves I to VIII and thoracic nerves I to XII (respiration); cranial nerve X (phonation); cranial nerves V, X, and XI (resonation); and cranial nerves V, VII, IX, X, XI, and XII (articulation).

Background

Involvement of thoracic, cervical, and cranial nerves may be related to congenital anomalies, infection, trauma, neoplasms, progressive diseases, nonprogressive diseases, and cerebrovascular diseases. Such conditions may affect only the upper motor neuron, only the lower motor neuron, or both.

Congenital Anomalies. Central speech tracts or peripheral speech nerves may be involved in various congenital conditions.

Central speech tracts may be affected in the group of general conditions know as *cerebral palsy*. Central thoracic, cervical, and cranial tracts and hence respiratory, phonatory, resonatory, and articulatory speech-transmitter problems may be found. Cerebral palsy speech repercussions are described by the author elsewhere (Mysak, 1971).

The various neurological conditions known as congenital cerebral palsy may be related to heritable conditions, prematurity, anoxia, brain malformations, brain trauma, and so on. The definition presented by the author (Mysak, 1971, p. 673) is the one used here, that is, ". . . disease complexes which have their inception during the period of infancy, reflect nonprogressive damage of multiple causation to cortical and subcortical areas of the brain, and which may appear in various forms and combinations of sensorimotor, perceptual, and behavioral disorders."

The cerebral variety, or that variety of cerebral palsy causing spasticity and(or) flaccidity of the speech muscles, is appropriately discussed here. The speech implications of the basal ganglia and the cerebellar varieties are more appropriately discussed under "Output Patterning Disorders" in Chapter 4.

Worster-Drought (1968), when describing speech disorders in children arising from organic disorders of the nervous system, identified a specific central condition known as *congenital suprabulbar paresis*. The developmental anomaly in this condition appears limited to the cortico-bulbar tract, that is, "the tract of nerve-fibers . . . proceeding from the motor cells of the lower part of the Rolandic cerebral cortex to the cranial nerve nuclei situated in the medulla or bulb." Varying degrees and combinations of upper motor neuron paralysis of the lips, tongue, soft palate, and pharyngeal and laryngeal muscles may result. "Speech is dysarthric, being slurred and indistinct with deficient lingual and labial sounds and is also nasalized owing to incomplete oro-nasal closure."

Worster-Drought recognized two forms of the condition, the "complete syndrome" and the "incomplete syndrome." The complete syndrome shows paralysis of lip-rounding muscle, weakness or paralysis of the tongue, paresis of the velum, possible phonatory involvement, and swallowing difficulty. Only components of the speech musculature are involved in the incomplete syndrome. Isolated weakness or paralysis of the soft palate and associated hypernasality may be found; relatively isolated lingual paralysis may also be found.

Peripheral speech nerves may be involved in the congenital anomaly known as *Moebius' syndrome* (nuclear agenesis). The syndrome presents an inexpressive facial appearance as well as frequent associated anomalies such as clubfeet and amyoplasia. "Moebius' syndrome is paralysis of the external recti (rarely only on one side) associated with paresis or paralysis of the facial musculature. . . . Other ocular muscles may be involved and many other congenital anomalies in various areas of the body may co-exist" (Paine and Oppé, 1966, p. 123). Such bilateral facial weakness or paralysis may cause difficulty with the labial group of sounds. Congenital defects of the twelfth nerve nucleus (hypoglossal) may cause paralysis and wasting of the tongue and, if bilateral, problems in articulating the lingual group of sounds (Worster-Drought, 1968).

Syringobulbia is another cause of involvement of peripheral speech nerves. Syringobulbia is generally considered to be a congenital abnormality based on defective development of the central canal of the spinal cord (Brain and Walton, 1969, p. 662; Ford, 1966, p. 985). Syringomyelia is the term used to describe the pathologic presence of long cavities surrounded by gliosis found in the central portions of the spinal cord. When the condition extends into the medulla, it is termed syringobulbia. However, the medulla may also be the primary site of the problem.

Important symptoms of syringobulbia include: facial analgesia and thermanesthesia (cranial nerve V) and paralysis of the tongue, palate, pharynx, and vocal cords (cranial nerves IX, X, XI, XII).

Infection. Various forms of infection may involve central speech tracts and peripheral speech nerves.

Central speech tracts may be disturbed in encephalitis and neurosyphilis (West and Ansberry, 1968, pp. 185–188).

Peripheral speech nerves may be disturbed by the following forms of infection.

Meningitis at the base of the brain, spreading infection from *acute inflammation of the middle ear*, and *poliomyelitis* may cause unilateral or bilateral facial-nerve paralysis (Worster-Drought, 1968). Bilateral forms of paralysis are more important to speech function since unilateral forms are frequently alleviated by spontaneous, compensatory speech behavior.

Another cause of peripheral facial paralysis is Bell's palsy or paralysis. Brain and Walton (1969) define it as "Facial paralysis of acute onset due to non-suppurative inflammation of the facial nerve within the stylomastoid foramen" (p. 168). Young adult males are most commonly affected. The onset is sudden and almost always unilateral. Some of the symptoms include: paralysis of the muscles of expression, wider palpebral fissure on affected side with inability to close the eye, overflow of tears, mouth drawn to the sound side, inability to purse lips, and difficulty with labial sounds.

Palatal paralysis may also occur as a result of infective damage to lower motor neurons. *Poliomyelitis, diphtheria,* and the *Guillain-Barré* syndrome were cited as etiologic by Paine and Oppé (1966, p. 54). *Bulbar poliomyelitis* or *diphtheria*, with consequent paralysis of the soft palate and associated hypernasality, was also described by Worster-Drought (1968).

Worster-Drought (1968) also identifies *bulbar poliomyelitis* as a possible causative agent in damage to the hypoglossal or twelfth cranial nerve. "If bilateral, the patient will have difficulty in pronouncing lingual sounds."

Trauma. Different types of trauma may disturb the functioning of central speech tracts and peripheral speech nerves.

Central speech tracts may be damaged via brain injury incurred as a result of war injuries or by automobile accidents (West and Ansberry, 1968, p. 200).

Peripheral speech nerves such as the palatal nerve may be injured during *tonsillectomy,* leaving hypernasality as a consequence. *Thyroidectomy* surgical procedures occasionally damage the recurrent nerve to the larynx, resulting in unilateral paralysis of the vocal cords with associated weak and hoarse voice. *Radical neck dissection* procedures in connection with surgical removal of laryngeal cancer may cause unilateral lingual paralysis and also lower lip weakness because of possible injury to the hypoglossal and facial nerves (Luchsinger and Arnold, 1965, p. 654). Palatal paralysis may occur following operations for closure of cleft palate.

Various combinations of paralysis of the fifth through twelfth cranial nerves were reported in sagittal bullet injuries through the face or cranial base (Luchsinger and Arnold, 1965, p. 653).

Neoplasms. By neoplasm here is meant any new and abnormal growth such as tumors, aneurysms, or abscesses. Such space-filling lesions may cause temporary disturbance of central speech tracts or peripheral speech nerves or may leave more permanent involvement following their surgical removal. These lesions cause damage either through pressure and inhibition of circulation or through direct damage of nervous tissue through cellular alteration or toxin infiltration. Neoplasms may affect central speech tracts or peripheral speech nerves.

Central speech tracts may be affected by *chronic subdural hematoma* (blood tumor under the dura mater creating pressure against cortex), *intracranial aneurysm* (sac formed within the cranium by dilatation of the walls of an artery or of a vein and filled with blood), *tumors* of nervous tissue of the brain or of its membranes, and *cerebral abscesses* (localized collection of pus in a cavity).

Peripheral speech nerves may be disturbed by a cerebellopontine angle tumor (West and Ansberry, 1968, p. 184); because of its nearness to the cerebellum and pons, such a tumor may also affect various cranial nerves. "The dysarthria begins with numbness of the face and advances until motor paralysis renders speech unmistakably paretic and ataxic." Tumors of the medulla may also produce lower-motor-neuron speech symptoms.

Gardner (1969) reported on a case of a tumor in the jugular foramen involving cranial nerves VII, IX, X, and XII. Presenting symptoms included left-sided paralysis of the vocal fold (fixed halfway between adduction and abduction), of the soft palate, and of the tongue. Speech and voice symptoms included barely audible voice, several distorted sounds, and air wastage symptoms. Following cobalt therapy and after 10 months of speech therapy, the client exhibited adequate volume and pitch.

Progressive Diseases. Various degenerative diseases may involve central speech tracts and peripheral speech nerves. Some of the degenerative diseases that could affect central speech tracts and that might be described here but that are more appropriately described under "Output-Patterning Disorders—Lower-Order Speech Integration" in Chapter 4 are: Parkinson's disease, Huntington's chorea, torsion dystonia, Wilson's disease, and various cerebellar degenerative diseases.

A progressive disease that affects lower motor neurons involved in speech is *motor neuron disease*. Information on this disease is based on material from Brain and Walton (1969, pp. 595–606). Synonyms for the disease include progressive bulbar palsy, amyotrophic lateral sclerosis, and progressive muscular atrophy. "When the lower motor neurone lesions predominate, or, as more rarely happens, occur alone, the term 'progressive muscular atrophy' is still sometimes applied to the disease, and when the muscles innervated from the medulla are predominantly involved it has been termed 'progressive bulbar palsy'" (p. 595). Darley *et al*. (1969) described the "flaccid dysarthria" in bulbar palsy (damage to lower motor neurons of cranial nerves V, VII, IX to XI, XII) as being composed of three clusters (correlated symptoms) of speech symptoms. The three clusters are: (a) phonatory incompetence (breathy voice, audible inspiration, and phrases short); (b) resonatory incompetence (hypernasality, nasal emission, imprecise consonants, and phrases short); and (c) phonatory-prosodic insufficiency (harsh voice, monopitch, and monoloudness).

Pathologic changes in nervous tissue have been found in the spinal cord, medulla, and cerebral hemispheres. Motor neuron disease usually occurs in late middle life, and the exact etiology is still unclear. Usually, the first symptoms appear in the hands (weakness, stiffness, clumsiness, wasting, or fibrillary twitching). The first symptom may be dysarthria or dysphagia when the degeneration begins in the bulbar motor nuclei. "The tongue is usually the first to waste and becomes shrunken and wrinkled and shows conspicuous fasciculation" (p. 599). Lip muscles are also involved early. Shortly afterward the tongue, palatal muscles, and the extrinsic muscles of the pharynx and larynx are involved. Intrinsic laryngeal muscles are involved later. Mandibular muscles are affected to a lesser degree than are tongue and lip muscles. Such paretic involvement of lip, tongue, and palate eventually renders speech unintelligible (bulbar anarthria).

Because the degeneration is rarely restricted to the lower motor neurons, the condition is frequently complicated by symptoms of upper motor neuron involvement. As previously stated, when lower motor neuron degeneration exists alone, the condition is termed progressive bulbar palsy; however, when upper motor neuron degeneration exists alone, the condition is termed pseudobulbar palsy. A combination of both is the most common. Pseudobulbar palsy, or lesions of both corticospinal tracts above the medulla, also leads to dysarthria and dysphagia. In contast to lower motor neuron symptoms, symptoms of pseudobulbar palsy include: spastic muscles, not wasted and hypotonic; a somewhat smaller appearing tongue, not wrinkled with fasciculation; and exaggerated jaw-jerk, palatal, and pharyngeal reflexes. Dysarthria and dysphagia are intensified when the individual shows symptoms of both upper and lower motor neuron degeneration. Speech degeneration may proceed from difficulty with lip sounds, then tongue-tip and tongue-back sounds, then be reflected by an increase in nasality, and finally by problems in voicing.

Darley *et al.* (1969) described the "mixed" spastic-flaccid dysarthria in amyotrophic lateral sclerosis (progressive degeneration of both upper and lower motor neurons) as being essentially composed of a mix of the clusters described under bulbar palsy and pseudobulbar palsy (described below) with some exceptions.

Nonprogressive Diseases. Isolated pseudobulbar palsy may be considered a nonprogressive disease of the nervous system that causes damage to central speech tracts. The condition has already been mentioned in the discussion of progressive bulbar palsy.

The condition is marked by bilateral corticospinal lesions that may be due to degeneration of both tracts, congenital anomalies (congenital suprabulbar paresis previously described), vascular lesions, tumors, and so on. Essential features of the pseudobulbar palsy syndrome are: impairment of voluntary control over emotional expression; dysphagia; exaggeration of palatal, pharyngeal, and jaw-jerk reflexes; weak and spastic articulatory muscles; and spastic dysarthria (Brain and Walton, 1969, p. 98). Brain and Walton also report finding palilalia in pseudobulbar palsy due to vascular lesions. In congenital pseudobulbar palsy, Ford (1966) adds that "Stimulation of the lips or tongue may produce reflex movements of sucking, chewing and swallowing which are termed the 'feeding reflex' " (pp. 31–32).

Darley *et al.* (1969) described the "spastic dysarthria" in pseudobulbar palsy as being composed of four clusters of speech symptoms. They are: (a) prosodic excess (excess and equal stress and slow rate of speech); (b) prosodic insufficiency (monopitch, monoloudness, reduced stress, and phrases short); (c) articulatory-resonance incompetence (imprecise consonants, vowels distorted, and hypernasality); and (d) phonatory stenosis (low pitch, harsh voice, strain-strangled voice, and pitch breaks).

Cerebrovascular Diseases. West and Ansberry (1968, p. 200) indentify various cerebrovascular accidents (CVA's) as being "notoriously productive of dysarthrias." They occur mostly in midddle life. Hemorrhages, thromboses, and embolisms are the disturbances of the arterial circulation of the brain to which West and Ansberry refer. The nature of these CVA's was discussed under "Neurogenic Language Disorders in Adults" in Chapter 3. Possible involvement of central speech tracts is expected by these CVA's. "The CVA that classically results in dysarthria is one in which the right side of the body is spastically paralyzed."

Special Syndromes of the Last Four Cranial Nerves. Because of the importance of the last four cranial nerves to speech, identification of a number of syndromes involving these nerves (due, for example, to tumors, syphilis, inflammations) should be of interest to the speech clinician.

(a) *Avellis's syndrome* is manifested by: ipsilateral paralysis of the soft palate, pharynx, and larynx with dysarthria, dysphagia, and anesthesia of the pharynx and larynx (nerve X and bulbar portion of nerve XI); and by contralateral dissociate hemianesthesia, with loss of pain and temperature sense but not of the touch and pressure senses (spinothalamic tract).

(b) *Schmidt's syndrome* is manifested by: ipsilateral paralysis of the velum, pharynx, and larynx with anesthesia of the pharynx and larynx (nerve X and bulbar portion of nerve XI); and by ipsilateral sternocleidomastoid muscle paralysis (and sometimes paralysis of part of the trapezius muscle) causing inability to rotate the head to the side opposite the lesion and inability to shrug the shoulder (spinal portion of nerve XI).

(c) *Jackson's syndrome* is manifested by: ipsilateral paralysis of the velum, pharynx, and larynx (nerve X); ipsilateral paralysis of sternocleidomastoid and trapezius muscles (nerve XI); and ipsilateral paralysis and atrophy of the tongue (nerve XII).

(d) *Tapia's syndrome* is manifested by: ipsilateral paralysis of the pharynx and larynx, and ipsilateral paralysis and atrophy of the tongue.

(e) *Babinski-Nageotte bulbar syndrome* (nerves IX and X, bulbar portion of nerve XI, part of nerve V) is manifested by: ipsilateral paralysis of the tongue, pharynx, and larynx; ipsilateral loss of taste on posterior third of the tongue; ipsilateral Horner's syndrome (miosis, ptosis, and enophthalmos); ipsilateral loss of pain and temperature sense on the face; ipsilateral asynergia and ataxia and a tendency to fall to the side of lesion; and contralateral hemiplegia (arm-leg) and contralateral dissociate hemianesthesia (loss of pain and temperature sense).

(f) *Bonnier's syndrome* is manifested by: paroxysmal vertigo (symptom of Ménière's disease); symptoms of involvement of nerves IX and X and sometimes nerves III and V; contralateral hemiplegia; occasionally somnolence; and apprehension, tachycardia, and weakness.

(g) *Hypoglossal hemiplegia alternans* is manifested by: contralateral hemiplegia, and ipsilateral paralysis of the tongue.

(h) *Vernet's syndrome* (usually result of basilar skull fracture of jugular foramen and involving nerves IX, X, XI) is manifested by: ipsilateral glossopharyngeal paralysis; ipsilateral vagus paralysis; and ipsilateral accessory paralysis.

Clinical Manifestations

In Chapter 2 the author stated that the primary role of efferent speech transmission is to convey patterns of motor impulses generated within the central speech system over upper and lower motor neurons to the speech effectors, and that transmission processes differ from lower-order integration processes since only cerebrifugal transmission of nerve impulses is implied and not transmutation of these output signals. Since in the descent of motor impulses along central speech tracts influences upon the impulses must be assumed, it may be difficult to distinguish sharply between central speech tract manifestations and speech manifestations due to problems in lower-order output patterning. (Clinical manifestations of output-patterning disorders are discussed in Chapter 4.) However, speech manifestations of problems in efferent transmission are clearly identified with involvement of peripheral speech nerves.

Disorders of the respiratory transmitter (cervical nerves I to VIII and thoracic nerves I to XII), the phonatory transmitter (cranial nerve X), the resonatory transmitter (branches of cranial nerves V, X, and XI), and the articulatory transmitter (cranial nerves V, VII, IX, X, XI, and XII) may all be termed central and(or) peripheral laloplegias or logoplegias (paralysis of organs of speech). For the sake of exposition, this section of the chapter is organized in terms of paralysis of individual speech organs; in actuality, in most cases, central and peripheral laloplegias present themselves in various combinations of paralyzed speech organs.

Pneumaplegia. *Phonasthenia* or weak voice may result from degrees of paralysis of lung function. Phrenoplegia, or paralysis of the diaphragm due to trauma to the phrenic nerve, or bulbar poliomyelitis may account for such a phonasthenia (West and Ansberry, 1968, p. 232). Tumors of the spinal cord, compression of the aorta by aneurysm, intrathoracic neoplasms, polyneuritis due to alcohol, and diphtheria are other backgrounds for damage to the phrenic nerve (Brain and Walton, 1969, p. 768).

Laryngoplegias. Paralysis of the vocal cords may be due to central tract involvement or peripheral nerve involvement of the vagus.

Central laryngoplegias are not permanent unless involvement of both upper motor neurons exist, since voicing function is served by bilateral cortical representation. *Spastic vocal paralysis* "causes the cords to be approximated too tightly during phonation . . ." (West and Ansberry 1968, p. 219). Luchsinger and Arnold (1965, pp. 252–254) report the following vocal symptoms associated with various brain diseases: *vocal monotony and spastic dysphonia* in multiple sclerosis; *monotonous groaning sound of the voice and tremor of the vocal cords* in Parkinson's disease; *low, distorted in melody, easily fatigued, and inspiratory voicing* in chorea; and *jerky and explosive voice quality and ventricular dysphonia* in cerebellar diseases.

Peripheral laryngoplegias may be exhibited by aspirate voice, intermittent voicing, or by low, weak, and rough voicing. *Aspirate voice* may be heard when the inferior recurrent laryngeal branch of the vagus is involved by aneurysm of the aorta, pathology of apex of the lungs, tumors, goiter, trauma, diphtheria, influenza, and typhoid (West and Ansberry, 1968, p. 220). According to West and Ansberry, *intermittent voicing* may result when the lesion is associated with cardiac or arterial abnormality, that is, vocal spasms may be synchronous with the pulse beat. *Low-weak-rough* voice may result from isolated paralysis of the superior laryngeal nerve, or cricothyroid paralysis (Luchsinger and Arnold, 1965, p. 220); the most common cause of the problem is post-thyroidectomy complication.

Veloplegias. Paralysis of the velopharyngeal closure mechanism may also be based on central tract or peripheral nerve involvements and may be unilateral or bilateral. In almost all cases the presenting symptom is hypernasality. *Hypernasality* may be exhibited due to, for example, lower motor neuron damage resulting from bulbar poliomyelitis or diphtheria; or *hypernasality* may be exhibited due to, for example, upper motor neuron damage associated with diseases such as Parkinson's and torsion dystonia. In some cases of central veloplegia, however, palatal spasms may occur and be reflected by episodic hyponasality.

Linguoplegias. Parlaysis of the tongue due to involvement of the hypoglossus may result from involvement of the central tract or the peripheral nerve.

Central linguoplegias are only permanent in cases of bilateral involvement of the hypoglossus, since cortical innervation of the articulators is bilaterally represented. Central linguoplegias are reflected by problems in articulating those sounds requiring action by the lingual muscles: *linguadental sounds* [θ, ð], *lingua-alveolar sounds* [t, d, n, r, s, z], *linguapalatal sounds* [ʃ, ʒ], *semivowels* [j, l, r], and *vowels* [i, i, ɛ, æ, ɑ, ɜ].

Peripheral linguoplegias, when unilateral, are sometimes considered nonsignificant with respect to speech function; however, many individuals do experience problems. Some of the sounds that may cause difficulty are [d, t, l, s, z, ʃ, gr, gl, kr, kl]; lateral sigmatism may also appear (Luchsinger and Arnold, 1965, p. 654). Severe problems with all lingual sounds identified under central linguoplegias are experienced in cases of bilateral involvement.

Labioplegias. Paralysis of the lips may be of a central or peripheral nature and may be unilateral or bilateral.

Central labioplegia of the bilateral form may be seen in certain cases of congenital neurosyphilis or cerebral palsy. Cranial nerve lesions in congenital syphilis are usually due to syphilitic meningitis. "The seventh nerve is most frequently affected but the third, fourth and sixth nerves are also commonly involved" (Ford, 1966, p. 511). Such children may show difficulty with the *bilabials* [p, b, m, w], *labiodentals* [f, v], and *lip-round vowels* such as [o, u, ʊ].

Peripheral labioplegias occur almost always in unilateral form in cases of Bell's palsy. Again, *bilabials, labiodentals,* and *lip-round vowels* may cause some difficulty; however, the individual usually learns to compensate for one-sided problems rather quickly.

Bilateral forms are much more difficult. Problems with sounds described under central labioplegia apply here as well. Luchsinger and Arnold (1965, p. 644) report that, in bilateral labial paralysis, [b] may appear as a bilabial [v], [p] may appear as a bilabial [f], [n] may be substituted for [m], and difficulty may be evidenced with lip-round and lip-spread vowels.

Combined Laloplegia. An example of a central form of spasmodic laloplegia that may involve the lungs, larynx, velum, tongue, and lips is West's phemolepsy or speech epilepsy. This neuromotor dysautomaticity or stutter-like speech arises because of episodic, uncontrolled release of electrical potential in motor speech areas of the cortex.

Diagnosis

Differential and group diagnostic approaches are used to good advantage when diagnosing possible disturbances in the efferent speech transmitter.

Differential Diagnoses. When examining for possible speech transmitter problems, the clinician attempts to make the following differentiations. (a) Are the phonatory, resonatory, and articulatory symptoms due to central tract or peripheral nerve disturbances, or are they reflections of problems of the lower-order speech integrator (output-patterning disorders) or speech effector system? (b) If the problem is one of speech transmission, is it of a central or peripheral nature? (c) If the problem is of a central or peripheral nature, is it unilateral or bilateral? (d) If the problem is of a central or peripheral nature and is unilateral or bilateral, which tract(s) or nerve(s) is involved?

Identification of which system may be responsible for the symptoms presented is made more or less easy depending on the manifested speech symptoms.

Phonasthenia resulting from pneumaplegia appears similar to, for example, phonasthenia resulting from certain basal ganglia disorders associated with the lower-order speech integrator, or from certain lung and muscle diseases associated with the respiratory speech effector. In this case, the vocal symptom alone does not contribute to making a diagnosis of which speech system is disturbed. Diagnosis depends on obtaining information regarding phrenic nerve function and on the presence or absence of basal ganglia or muscle disease in a particular individual.

Lack of voice, low-pitched voice, loud and tense voice, breathy voice, hoarse voice, or intermittent voice that may be secondary to central or peripheral laryngoplegia may be difficult to distinguish from similar vocal symptoms arising from various conditions of the phonatory effector, for example: laryngeal tumors and edema, mucal deposits upon the folds, laryngeal muscle weakness or disease, fixation of the cricoarytenoid joint, ulcers, surgical removal of a vocal fold or a part of it, irregularities of the vibrating edges of the vocal folds, and so on. A systems' distinction depends on direct laryngological evaluation of the status of the cords and on information with respect to the individual's nervous, muscle, and endocrine systems. Psychological motivations must also be taken into account.

Hypernasality secondary to central or peripheral veloplegia is indistinguishable from that which is secondary to various structural anomalies of the resonatory effector, for example, clefts of the soft and(or) hard palates, occipitalization of the atlas, or widespread pterygoid plates; or from that which is secondary to loss of palatal tissue resulting from infection, trauma, or malignancy. Diagnosis of the system responsible for the hypernasality is made after evaluation of the velopharyngeal structures and of the integrity of the associated nervous supply.

Articulatory symptoms of linguoplegias and labioplegias may be differentiated more directly by the speech clinician from articulatory symptoms associated with output-patterning disorders (disorders of lower-order integrator system) and from labial dyslalias and lingual dyslalias (articulatory effector disorders).

For example, relatively specific labioplegias and linguoplegias should be free of the following symptoms of disorders of output patterning that may include: (a) reflexogenic symptoms, where attempts at articulation may elicit concomitantly movements associated with suckling, mouth-opening, lip, rooting, biting, and chewing reflexes; (b) disorders in programing of movements, in which limitations in direction and range of movements, or significant weakness, or slowness of movements are not major contributory factors to the dysarticulation (as they are in laloplegias); (c) coordination disorders, in which, for example, difficulty may exist in coordinating articulatory and phonatory mechanisms resulting in voicing-unvoicing confusions; (d) interference with articulation due to tremor, athetotic, or choreiform movements; and (e) rhythm disorders characterized by articulatory freezing, palilalia, festination, and so on.

Labial and lingual dyslalias are distinguished from labioplegias and linguoplegias in at least two ways: (a) by evaluating the adequacy for speech purposes of lip, dental, occlusal, and lingual structures; and (b) by evaluating the range and symmetry of nonspeech movements of the lips and tongue, the at-rest posture of the lips and tongue, and the muscle tonus of the lips and tongue.

Once the speech transmitter system has been identified as being responsible for the presenting symptoms, the clinician must then establish whether the symptoms are associated with central tract or peripheral nerve involvement. Attempts at such differentiation are not easy, however, since some involvements may show combinations of central and peripheral features and some may include muscle diseases or psychological components.

Central tract involvement is manifested in the following ways. *Speech symptoms* are usually more generalized, that is, not only are phonetic lapses present but voicing and resonance symptoms may also be present. Also, depending on the nature of the central tract problem, other disorders of speech may be present, such as dysphasia. *Muscle tonus* in the involved area is usually hypertonic. *Vegetative-reflex movements*, as in swallowing and gagging, are generally unimpaired or sometimes exaggerated. *Emotional-response movements*, as in smiling or crying, are generally unimpaired but may be limited. *Voluntary nonspeech movements* of the involved muscles are impaired in the same way as they are for speech movements. *Associated sensory impairments*, when present, usually involve the special senses of audition and vision.

Peripheral nerve involvement exhibits other characteristics. *Speech symptoms* are usually more specific depending on the cranial nerves involved. For example, if only the seventh is involved, as in Bell's palsy, only the labial group of sounds is affected; if only the tenth nerve is involved, as in certain cases of surgical trauma (thyroidectomy), only voicing is affected, and so on. *Muscle tonus* in the involved area is usually hypotonic. *Fasciculation* (involuntary twitching of a group of muscle fibers due to early stages of muscle atrophy), especially of the tongue, may be observed. *Wasting atrophy* may eventually occur. *Vegetative-reflex movements* of the involved muscles are affected in the same way as these movements are affected during speech. *Emotional-response movements* of the involved muscles are affected in the same way as these movements are affected during speech. *Voluntary nonspeech movements* of the involved muscles are impaired in the same way as they are for speech movements. *Associated sensory impairment*, when present, usually involve the tactile and kinesthetic senses (complication of a transmitter problem with a sensor system problem).

Whether the disturbance is right-sided or left-sided or bilateral is also of diagnostic importance.

The diaphragm is supplied by the phrenic nerve (derived from third, fourth, and fifth cervical spinal nerves). Paralysis of this motor nerve to the diaphragm results in the loss of diaphragmatic movement on the affected side. Loss of movement is most evident in bilateral lesions.

The vocal cords may be affected in various ways unilaterally and bilaterally. When the recurrent laryngeal branch of the tenth cranial nerve is affected on one side only, all muscles of the larynx on that side are disturbed except for the cricothyroid muscle (vocal fold tensor), which is supplied by a branch of the superior laryngeal nerve. The paralyzed cord may be located in the median position, and upon phonation the vital cord tends to approximate the devital one. In such cases, a degree of phonasthenia may be manifested initially; however, depending on the compensatory activity of the vital cord, normal or near-normal voicing may eventually be reestablished. The paralyzed cord may be in more abducted positions and, in that event, the voice may show varying degrees of breathiness. "The degree of approximation achieved by the abduction of the healthy fold is inversely related to the amount of breathiness in the voice" (Moore, 1971, p. 541). When the superior laryngeal nerve is involved on one side as well as the recurrent laryngeal nerve, a state of total paralysis of one half of the larynx exists. Frequently accompanying pharyngeal and palatal paralysis on that side may complicate the speech symptoms.

When bilateral involvement of the recurrent laryngeal nerves occurs, all muscles of the larynx are paralyzed except for the main vocal cord tensors on both sides. The almost devital cords may be observed to be relatively close together, and hence voicing is possible but asthenic. Bilateral paralysis of the larynx is complete when, in addition to the recurrent laryngeal nerves, both superior laryngeal nerves are involved. Under this circumstance, the cords appear open on either side of the median position in the so-called cadaveric position. Voicing may still be possible but is weak. Again, pharyngeal and palatal paralysis frequently accompanies such complete bilateral laryngeal paralysis and may complicate the vocal symptoms.

The velum also shows unilateral or bilateral involvement. The motor fibers of the tenth cranial nerve supply all of the striated muscles of the velum except for the tensor palati (supplied by the fifth cranial). "Unilateral vagal paralysis produces drooping of the palatal arch on the affected side and the uvula and medial raphé deviate towards the normal side" (Paine and Oppé, 1966, p. 137). Phonation tends to increase the posture of the uvula toward the normal side. In some cases, unilateral palatal paralysis may result in few symptoms because of good compensatory action of the vital side of the velum. However, degrees of hypernasality are usually apparent in cases of acute unilateral lesions.

Palatal elevation is not possible in bilateral involvement. Speech symptoms are similar to those in cleft palate and include hypernasality and difficulty in creating adequate intraoral breath pressure for pressure consonants.

Involvement of the vagus may also result in pharyngeal paralysis. In unilateral pharyngeal paralysis, the pharyngeal wall droops on the affected side. A tendency for frothy mucus to collect above the opening of the esophagus is present, and this material may overflow into the larynx, eliciting efforts at throat clearing. Swallowing difficulty is also encountered. Marked dysphagia is caused by bilateral pharyngeal paralysis (Brain and Walton, 1969, p. 194).

The tongue exhibits characteristic features depending on whether unilateral or bilateral problems of the hypoglossal nerve exist. In unilateral conditions, the tongue tip may be seen to deviate toward the vital side while lying within the mouth (Luchsinger and Arnold, 1965, p. 653). Upon protrusion, the tongue always deviates towards the affected side. Also, the median raphé becomes concave towards the paralyzed side. Little atrophy and little if any deviation on protrusion may be observed in many cases of supranuclear lesions involving the tongue (Paine and Oppé, 1966, p. 141).

Protrusion is usually impossible, and the tongue lies immobilized in the floor of the mouth under conditions of bilateral paralysis of the hypoglossus.

The lips also display one-sided or bilateral disturbances of the seventh cranial or facial nerve. In unilateral conditions, the mouth is drawn towards the vital side.

The mandible reflects unilateral involvement of the fifth or trigeminal nerve by deviating towards the paralyzed side upon its extension.

Determination of which nerve or nerves are involved in any one case is done via a "phonemodiagnosis" and by direct evaluation of the cranial nerves.

Phonemodiagnosis describes analyzing phonetic inventories from an etiologic standpoint. West and Ansberry (1968, pp. 521–522) believed that studying patterns of phonetic lapses could be useful in diagnosis, especially when the problem appears related to the muscles of articulation or their lower motor neurons. Accordingly, West and Ansberry classified groups of speech sounds in terms of neuromuscular units involved in their production. "Although there is considerable overlapping between them, the critical and distinctive features of the groups are produced through the mediation of the neuromuscular units mentioned. Phonetic lapses limited to one or two of these groups are diagnostically significant." For example, West and Ansberry identified a labial group of sounds [p, b, m, w, hw, f, v, u, ʊ, o] supplied by the seventh cranial nerve, and a lingual group, for example, [t, d, n, s, z, θ, ð, ʃ, ʒ, l, r] supplied by the twelfth cranial nerve. Once the phonetic analysis is accomplished, West and Ansberry recommended that the organs in question also be tested directly. Force and vigor of voluntary movements, rate of diadochocinesis, equality of function of the two sides of the lip, face, velum, pharynx, larynx, and cutaneous esthesia of the speech muscles are the tests recommended.

Direct evaluation of cranial nerve function is done by the physician;

however, the speech clinician should be able to screen the cranial nerves more directly related to speech function, that is, the fifth, seventh, ninth, tenth, eleventh, and twelfth cranial nerves. Such screening may be done in addition to the examination procedures described under "Speech Transmitter" in Chapter 2. Certain techniques of examination and interpretation of findings are drawn from numerous sources, such as Paine and Oppé (1966, Ch. 9) and Brain and Walton (1969, Ch. 2).

The fifth nerve (trigeminal) carries both motor and sensory fibers. Its motor fibers supply the muscles involved in jaw movements and its sensory fibers serve the lips and face. The three divisions of the trigeminal nerve are the ophthalmic nerve, the maxillary nerve, and the mandibular nerve (the motor root of the nerve fuses with the mandibular nerve). The motor root supplies the temporal, the masseter, the medial and lateral pterygoids, the anterior belly of the digastric and mylohyoid muscle, the tensor tympani, and the tensor palati.

Movement, weakness, wasting, reflexes, and sensation are factors that should be evaluated by the clinician. Wasting of the temporal and masseter muscles may be observed in peripheral lesions and results in hollowing above and below the zygoma on the affected side. Weakness may be determined by palpation of the muscles when the client is asked to clench his jaw (contraction of these muscles is less forceful on the affected side). Further tests of strength of the muscles include: having the client attempt to open the jaw and to move it from side to side against resistance applied by the examiner, and having the client bite on a tongue depressor and hold on against attempts by the examiner to withdraw it. Symmetry or asymmetry of toothmarks on the stick should provide useful information on the relative strength of both pairs of the muscles. Movement of the jaw or opening of the mouth shows deviation toward the involved side. The jaw-jerk reflex is tested by having the client open his mouth somewhat, placing of the examiner's index finger on the midpoint of the client's chin, and tapping the finger with a reflex hammer. Bilateral contraction of the masseter and temporalis muscles with sudden elevation of the mandible is the normal response. Supranuclear involvement is evidenced by an exaggerated jaw jerk. Sensory function may be screened by appraising right-left touch discrimination of the cheeks, lips, teeth, alveolar ridge, tongue, and hard and soft palates. Lesions of the fifth cranial nerve may also cause pain that may be associated with cutaneous anesthesia.

The seventh cranial nerve (facial) carries only motor fibers to the lips and face; however, it is associated in part of its course with a small number of sensory fibers that reach the external auditory meatus and that excite salivary secretion and transmit taste sensation from the anterior part of the tongue.

Weakness of one side of the face may be observed by asymmetrical muscle activity. The mouth is drawn toward the vital side, the palpebral fissure is wider on the affected side, the eyebrow droops, and eyebrow raising is not possible. In peripheral nerve involvement, the upper and lower facial muscles are usually equally affected; in supranuclear corticospinal lesion, movements of the lower face are affected more severely than are movements of the upper face, and emotional and associated movements of the face are slightly, if at all, affected. In terms of sensory function, hyperacusis (painful sensitivity to sounds) is attributed to involvement of the facial nerve's motor branch to the stapedius. Certain reflexes related to function of the motor nerve may be tested. McCarthy's reflex, or reflexive closure of the eye upon sudden percussion of the supraorbital ridge, the glabella, or the margin of the orbit, is diminished or absent in lower motor neuron problems and retained or exaggerated in supranuclear varieties of facial paralysis. Reflex closing of the eyes may also be elicited in response to sudden stimulation of the palate or face, to a sudden loud noise, or to bright light shone in the eyes. On closure of the eyes, the eyeballs roll up (associated movement); this is referred to as Bell's phenomenon when an individual with a facial paralysis attempts to close the eye on the affected side. Following are some symptoms of central tract involvement of the facial nerve. Impairment of emotional facial movements (e.g., smiling, crying), but with preservation of voluntary movements of these muscles, is possibly related to disease of the extrapyramidal cortical projections, the basal ganglia or thalamus, or to the reticular part of the pons superior to the nucleus of the facial nerve. Mask-like facies is characteristic of Parkinson's disease, but in children such facies may reflect pseudobulbar palsy or a postencephalitic condition.

The ninth (glossopharyngeal) and tenth (vagus) cranial nerves contain both sensory and motor fibers. The only motor function of the ninth cranial nerve is to supply the stylopharyngeus muscle; it also provides common sensibility to the posterior third of the tongue, the tonsils, and the pharynx. "Isolated lesions of the glossopharyngeal nerve are almost unknown. It is most frequently damaged in association with the vagus and accessory nerves at the jugular foramen . . . " (Brain and Walton, 1969, p. 189). Except for the stylopharyngeus and the tensor palati, all the striated muscles of the soft palate, pharynx, and larynx are supplied by the motor fibers of the vagus.

Motor paralysis of the ninth cranial nerve may not be possible to observe. Some drooping of the palatal arch may be seen in the rest position; however, upon phonation of [ɑ], symmetrical elevation is produced.

Phonation of [ɑ] reveals unilateral vagal paralysis by failure of the paralyzed side of the velum to elevate, with deviation of the uvula toward the normal side. No elevation of the palate is possible in bilateral palatal paralysis. The palatal reflex (elevation of velum and retraction of uvula) is tested by stimulating the inferior surface of the velum or uvula with a tongue blade or cotton applicator. The palatal reflex is lost in bilateral vagal paralysis.

Pharyngeal muscle function is tested by observing the status of the pharyngeal wall, swallow activity, elevation of the larynx during swallowing, and the pharyngeal or gag reflex. The pharyngeal reflex (elevation and constriction of the pharyngeal muscles with lingual retraction) is tested by stimulating the base of the tongue, faucial arches, or pharyngeal wall. In unilateral involvement the pharyngeal wall droops on the affected side and the pharyngeal reflex is elicited on the normal side only. Bilateral pharyngeal paralysis results in marked swallowing difficulty and a bilateral loss of the pharyngeal reflex.

Vagal innervation of the larynx is estimated via voicing and breathing difficulties. Indirect laryngoscopy may be done with interpretation based on the information already provided under "Diagnosis—Vocal Cords" in this chapter.

The eleventh cranial nerve (accessory) carries only motor fibers to the sternocleidomastoid muscle and to the upper part of the trapezius. The nerve is often involved along with the ninth and tenth cranial nerves as they leave the skull through the jugular foramen.

Observation of head posture may be the only method of examination of this nerve recommended to the speech clinician. Lesions of either the upper or lower motor neurons may result in paralytic torticollis. Involuntary movements of the head may be observed in dystonia musculorum deformans, in athetosis, and in postencephalitic conditions.

The twelfth cranial nerve (hypoglossal) is the motor nerve of the tongue. Unilateral lesions of the hypoglossus results in wasting and weakness of the affected half of the tongue. Upon protrusion the tongue deviates toward the paralyzed side. A false impression of tongue deviation may be caused by unilateral facial paralysis and this must be kept in mind. Requesting the individual to protrude his tongue against the resistance of a tongue blade held by the examiner should accentuate any tendency for tongue deviation. Comparison of right-left strength is done by having the client push the extended tongue laterally against the tongue blade. Marked wasting of the tongue on both sides with inability to protrude the tongue is observed in severe cases of bilateral hypoglossal paralysis.

Group Diagnosis. Diagnosis of efferent transmission disorders needs support from other specialists. Usually the client suspected of neurogenic problems has already been examined by an internist and a clinical neurologist who determine the presence or absence of neurologic disease. Once a disease process has been established, the job of the speech specialist is to determine whether the presenting speech symptoms may also be attributed to the neurological disease and, if so, to what particular speech system or systems.

If for some reason a client presents what appears to be neurologic speech symptoms to the speech clinician first, the speech specialist should refrain from making a final speech diagnosis until information is available from medical colleagues.

Prognosis

Prognosis for speech therapy for efferent transmission disorders is variable based on a number of factors.

In certain peripheral nerve involvements, for example, Bell's palsy, recovery is expected in 6 to 8 weeks (although exceptions exist), and hence any presenting speech problems should also be resolved. However, if compensatory patterns persist, the speech clinician may intervene and the prognosis for correction is good. Peripheral nerve disturbance may also be resolved by the process of regeneration of damaged neurons.

Unilateral vs. bilateral involvement is another factor in prognosis. In some cases unilateral involvement of the lips, tongue, velum, or larynx may cause only minimal speech disturbance; however, this unfortunately is not always true. In unilateral problems the prognosis is good, however, with respect to stimulation of compensatory behavior through therapy.

In central tract involvements the factor of "spontaneous recovery" should also be remembered. That is, immediately following a CVA, edema and shock may cause a temporary dysarthria that may pass in a matter of days or weeks. Also, phonatory and articulatory mechanisms enjoy bilateral cortical representation, and hence only bilateral cortical damage should result in permanent voicing and articulatory problems of the cortical variety.

In chronic cases such as congenital cerebral palsy some improvement in respiratory, resonatory, phonatory, and articulatory function may be expected with therapy.

In progressive degeneration diseases such as motor neuron disease, the prognosis for speech improvement is, in the long run, zero. However, as pointed out under "Output Patterning Disorders—Prognosis" in Chapter 4, where rate of degeneration is variable, speech therapy may be applied and its usefulness estimated with respect to different goals. For example, speech therapy may be designed to: reduce the possibility of secondary speech problems arising from a lack of stimulation, discouragement, and so on; ensure that the client utilizes his full speech potential at each stage of the disease process; attempt to maintain the speech system at each level of degeneration for as long as possible; and finally, assist the client and his family to adjust to the changing speech potential.

In general, factors of amenability of the disease to medical intervention, and age, intelligence, and motivation of the client are important in prognosis of the usefulness of speech therapy.

Therapy

Primary Preventive Measures. The public and health specialists must be reminded of the vulnerability of central speech tracts and peripheral speech nerves to infections such as neurosyphilis, encephalitis, meningitis, poliomyelitis, acute inflammation of the middle ear, and diphtheria. Early detection and early treatment must be emphasized.

Head injuries due to car accidents may be responsible for involvement of central speech tracts and must be guarded against. Surgeons must be reminded to make every effort to spare certain peripheral speech nerves during tonsillectomy, thyroidectomy, palatal closure, and radical-neck dissection procedures.

Reminding the public of the need to minimize chances of incurring CVA's, and hence possible associated efferent speech transmission disorders, is also in order here. Proper weight, good diet, and adequate exercises should be stressed in helping to reduce the incidence of CVA.

Secondary Preventive Measures. Once efferent transmission problems are incurred, the development of further speech complications must be prevented. For example, clients with speech problems must not be allowed to suffer "communicative atrophy" because it requires an effort to speak or because it is hard for listeners to understand. Everyone concerned with the affected individual must encourage and reward efforts at speech communication.

Also, early treatment must be sought in cases of veloplegias so that various negative compensatory behaviors do not develop, for example, speech-associated facial grimacing and alar constriction, and the use of compensatory glottal plosive and fricative sounds.

Causal Therapy. Causal therapy includes special surgery to relieve symptoms of a disease process of which one symptom is a speech disturbance. Examples of such surgery would be: (a) decompression of the facial canal in Bell's palsy and hence relief of associated unilateral labioplegia; and (b) removal of tumors, aneurysms, hematomas, and abscesses that may be temporarily affecting speech tracts and nerves and causing assorted laryngoplegias, veloplegias, and linguoplegias. Plastic surgery may also be used to correct a veloplegia through a pharyngeal flap operation, for example, or laryngeal surgery may be used to fix a devital vocal cord in the midline to improve voicing, and so on. Causal therapy also includes the use of prosthetic devices such as speech appliances in certain cases of cleft palate.

Various techniques of causal therapy are also applied by the speech clinician. These techniques are designed to help initiate movement in apparently devitalized speech organs and to develop appropriate range, speed, accuracy, and coordination of movement.

In pneumaplegia, or weak voice resulting from degrees of paralysis of lung function, various techniques designed to increase lung activity may be applied. Some of these techniques have been discussed by the author elsewhere (Mysak, 1971, pp. 697–698; p. 703). A leg-roll maneuver in the supine position may succeed in making vegetative breathing deeper and more regular. With the individual in a supine position, his legs are flexed, brought toward the axillae, and then returned to the starting position. The rate of cycles of such activity might be timed with the breaths per minute (bpm) of the clinician. A "butterfly" maneuver may be used in the seated position. The individual is seated with hands clasped behind his head and knees abducted. Then the head and elbows are brought to a maximum dorsiflexion-abduction position, respectively; then a slow, steady head-thorax ventroflexion and elbow adduction movement pattern is imposed with the ventroflexed head and adducted elbows finally brought between the abducted knees, and then there is a return to the starting position.

Speech breathing patterns, or shifting from a nasal to oral inspiration mode and from a regular inspiratory-expiratory phase to a short oral inspiratory phase followed by a slow, extended oral expiratory phase, that is, shifting from a nasal-symmetrical pattern (vegetative breathing) to an oral-asymmetrical pattern (speech breathing), may be facilitated in a number of ways. One way is to resist physically with the hands the beginning of an inspiratory breathing phase for a brief period, thus causing a quicker and deeper inspiratory phase followed by a longer expiratory phase. Another way is to have the individual hold his breath for different lengths of time, thus eventually ensuring a deeper inspiratory phase followed by an extended expiratory phase. Voicing should be encouraged during the expiratory phases of these exercises.

For additional causal therapy ideas for pneumaplegia, the reader is referred to "Respiratory Effector Disorders—Therapy" in Chapter 6.

In laryngoplegias movement and muscle tonus are affected. Recommended causal therapy techniques have already been discussed in other parts of the book. Under "Phonatory Effector Disorders—Therapy" in Chapter 6, techniques designed to increase laryngeal muscle tonus and improve vocal cord approximation and techniques to reduce laryngeal muscle tonus and ease vocal cord tension are described and should be applied according to the needs of the particular case. Also recommended here are the techniques of laryngopraxis and laryngodiadochocinesia described under "Output Patterning Disorders—Therapy" in Chapter 4.

In veloplegias techniques are aimed at improving velopharyngeal closure and hence reducing hypernasality. Recommended causal therapy techniques may be found under "Resonatory Effector Disorders—Therapy" in Chapter 6.

In *linguoplegias and labioplegias* a number of techniques may be applied to improve the range, speed, and accuracy of tongue and lip movements. Some of these techniques have been described by the author elsewhere (Mysak, 1971, pp. 703–705).

Afferent stimulation of a particular efferent outflow is one way of attempting to stimulate or increase the movement of the lips and tongue. For example, bringing the client's lips together (with the clinician's fingers), holding the lips in contact, and requesting the client to break the seal by blowing through the lips is done to encourage production of bilabial sounds. Similar maneuvers can be devised to help stimulate labiodental, linguadental, lingua-alveolar, and linguavelar movements.

Resisted-movement techniques may also be applied to the tongue and lips. If the individual has difficulty in raising the tongue tip, for example, the clinician applies graded pressure in a downward direction on the tongue tip while requesting the individual to attempt to lift his tongue tip against this resistance. If the procedure succeeds in increasing tonus or triggering additional motor units, the tongue tip may show increased movement upwards after the clinician ceases his downward pressure. Three or four maneuvers by the clinician should precede each request for the client to raise the tongue tip without the presence of the downward pressure. Similar maneuvers can be applied to facilitate lip-spread or lip-round movements and mandibular flexion and extension movements.

Resisted-movement synkinesis (unintentional movements accompanying volitional movements) is another neurofacilitatory technique. For example, if tongue tip and mandibular elevation is desired, the client's head or head and thorax are ventroflexed. The client is then asked to extend the head or head and thorax while the clinician resists the movement. Hopefully, such an effort on the part of the client with the associated resistance to the effort offered by the clinician will trigger synkinetic flexor movements of the tongue and mandible.

Counteracting-response technique may also prove useful in eliciting tongue and lip movements. For example, if tongue protrusion is desired, the clinician applies a slow and steady pressure on the anterior portion of the tongue in the direction of the oropharynx. Some time during this slow inward push on the tongue a counteracting forward movement may be triggered. Similar counteracting movements may be elicited when the lips are slowly and steadily spread or when the mandible is steadily extended.

Stroking, tapping, or kneading involved muscles may also be found to improve tonus and facilitate movement.

Articulopraxis, articulodiadochocinetic, and articulatory differentiation exercises may also be used to good advantage here. These techniques are described under "Output Patterning Disorders—Therapy" in Chapter 4.

Struggle-movement exercises are also useful. For example, to facilitate lip movement, the client is asked to converse while holding his tongue between his teeth; to facilitate lip and jaw movement, he is asked to converse while holding his tongue tip against the alveolar ridge; and to facilitate lip and tongue movement, he is asked to converse with clenched teeth.

Symptom Therapy. Symptom therapy is applied for at least two reasons: (a) the individual has more voicing and articulatory potential than he exhibits, and (b) the client has not automatically incorporated into his speech patterns the increased potential for speech made possible through progress in causal therapy.

As indicated in other chapters of the book, a self-adjusting approach for symptom improvement of speech is recommended, and the principles and methods for voice and articulation symptom therapy are described in Chapter 8.

Compensatory Therapy. Compensatory techniques are planned when the results of causal and symptom work are less than desired and when a need exists to increase speech intelligibility.

Compensatory techniques for voice and resonation problems arising from pneumaplegias, laryngoplegias, and veloplegias are similar to those described under "Respiratory Effector Disorders—Therapy," "Phonatory Effector Disorders—Therapy," and "Resonatory Effector Disorders—Therapy" in Chapter 6.

The types of substitute sounds that are possible when certain sounds cannot be made by the articulators, including when they cannot be made because of linguoplegias and labioplegias, are described under "Articulatory Effector Disorders—Therapy" in Chapter 6.

Other articulatory techniques that may improve intelligibility include: (a) the use of "hard-contact" articulation, where the client is asked to attempt harder contacts between articulators during speech; and (b) the use of an "overarticulation" style of speaking.

Adams (1966) described the following forms of compensatory therapy or communication aids for patients with progressive amyotrophic lateral sclerosis: (a) in cases where phonation is not possible but where orofacial muscles are still functioning, use of the electrolarynx; (b) in cases where voice and orofacial muscles are dysfunctioning but where head movement is possible, use of a light mounted on a headband so that a patient can point the light beam on appropriate words or phrases written on sheets of paper attached to the wall at the foot of the patient's bed; and

(c) use of a specific number of eye-blinks or grunts to indicate needs.

REFERENCES

Adams, M. R., Communication aids for patients with amyotrophic lateral sclerosis. J. Speech Hear. Disord., 31, 274–275 (1966).

Brain, W. R., and Walton, J. N., Diseases of the Nervous System. London: Oxford University Press (1969).

Carhart, R., Wever, E. G., and Sooy, F. A., Research on Hearing. In Human Communication and its Disorders–An Overview. Report of the National Institute of Neurological Diseases and Stroke. Washington, D. C.: United States Department of Health, Education and Welfare (1969).

Darley, F. L., Aronson, A. E., and Brown, J. R., Clusters of deviant speech dimensions in the dysarthrias. J. Speech Hear. Res., 12, 462–496 (1969).

Davis, H., Abnormal Hearing and Deafness. In H. Davis and S. R. Silverman (Eds.), Hearing and Deafness. New York: Holt, Rinehart and Winston (1970).

Ford, F. R., Diseases of the Nervous System in Infancy, Childhood and Adolescence. Springfield, Ill.: Charles C Thomas (1966).

Gardner, W. H., Voice and articulatory defects from paralysis by glomus jugulare tumor. J. Speech Hear. Disord., 34, 172–176 (1969).

Goodhill, V., Guggenheim, P., Hoversten, G., and Mackay, D., Pathology, Diagnosis, and Therapy of Deafness. In L. E. Travis (Ed.), Handbook of Speech Pathology and Audiology. New York: Appleton-Century-Crofts (1971).

Hardy, W. G., Problems of Audition, Perception and Understanding. Washington, D. C.: The Volta Bureau (1956).

Luchsinger, R., and Arnold, B., Voice-Speech-Language. Belmont, Calif.: Wadsworth Publishing Co. (1965).

Moore, G. P., Voice Disorders Organically Based. In L. E. Travis (Ed.), Handbook of Speech Pathology and Audiology. New York: Appleton-Century-Crofts (1971).

Mysak, E. D., Disorders of Oral Communication. In M. Bortner (Ed.), Evaluation and Education of Children with Brain Damage. Springfield, Ill.: Charles C Thomas (1968).

Mysak, E. D., Cerebral Palsy Speech Syndromes. In L. E. Travis (Ed.), Handbook of Speech Pathology and Audiology. New York: Appleton-Century-Crofts (1971).

Mysak, E. D., Cerebral Palsy Speech Habilitation. In L. E. Travis (Ed.), Handbook of Speech Pathology and Audiology. New York: Appleton-Century-Crofts (1971).

Newby, H. A., Audiology. New York: Appleton-Century-Crofts (1964).

Paine, R. S., and Oppé, T. E., Neurological Examination of Children. London: William Heinemann Medical Books, Ltd. (1966).

West, R. W., and Ansberry, M., The Rehabilitation of Speech. New York: Harper and Row (1968).

Worster-Drought, C., Speech disorders in children. Dev. Med. Child Neurol., 10, 427–440 (1968).

8

Speech Sensor System

Control and monitoring of speech are the functions of the sensor system. The major function of the system is intrapersonal speech perception; a minor function of the system is interpersonal speech perception. Intrapersonal speech perception includes automatic speech control, or control that is simultaneous to and ongoing with the speech act, and automatic speech monitoring, or monitoring that follows the speech act. The interpersonal function of the system involves the capacity of the system to monitor the utterances of others.

On the intrapersonal level, auditory and tactile-kinesthetic sensors are primary sensors, and the visual sensor is a secondary sensor (supplementary); on the interpersonal level, auditory and visual sensors are primary. In the developed speaker, the intrapersonal, auditory sensor controls and monitors spoken symbols and the voicing, loudness, and rate of those symbols, while the tactile-kinesthetic sensor basically controls and monitors articulation of those symbols. Intrapersonal control and monitoring are usually on an automatic or "subconscious" level; however, under certain circumstances, for example, during speech therapy, control and monitoring functions may be made more voluntary or "conscious."

Developmental varieties of sensor-system problems are found in children, for example, premature termination of speech sound development; and dissolution varieties are found in adults, for example, jargonaphasia. Symptoms may range from subclinical aphasoid lapses, such as not correcting an error in naming or in grammar because of fatigue or illness, to complete gibberish as in jargonaphasia due to brain injury. Sensor disturbances are manifested by various types of language disorder or by problems in articulation, voicing, loudness, or speech rate and rhythm.

Because the sensor system is not a separate but a multisystem, components of which have dual functions, the portion on background of pertinent diseases and disorders that was found in previous chapters is not presented here. Such a discussion would overlap with background information presented in connection with the perception-comprehension function of the higher-order speech integrator, the input-processing function of the lower-order speech integrator, the afferent function of the speech transmitter, and the auditory-receptor function of the speech receptor.

CLINICAL MANIFESTATIONS

Clinical manifestations of auditory and tactile-kinesthetic sensor disorders are discussed here.

Auditory Sensor Disorders

On the intrapersonal level, the auditory sensor system is responsible for simultaneous auditory control of running speech as well for postutterance monitoring. In the developing speech system, the auditory sensor is responsible for control and monitoring of verboacoustic events as well as for the articulation, voicing, rate, and rhythm of those events. Theoretically, as the total system develops, a division of labor of sensor responsibility slowly occurs and the tactile-kinesthetic sensor eventually assumes an important amount of responsibility over control and monitoring of articulation.

Problems of the auditory sensor system may be of a developmental or dissolution nature.

Auditory Sensor Disorders of Developmental Origin. The development of auditory control and monitoring of speech begins at about the second half of the first year of life and extends through about the tenth year. After about the tenth year, control and monitoring of oral symbols and their production is rather well established. The developmental sequence may be temporarily interfered with because of simple immaturity or more lastingly involved by dysmaturity of the various components of which the sensor system is composed.

Auditory sensor immaturity describes symptoms related to specific developmental factors in the absence of known pathology. Such symptoms should disappear with time.

Paleovocal behavior such as lalling, echolalia, and jargon may be protracted in some children. Extension of such protocommunication behavior may be due to problems in formulation of oral symbols (as described in Chapter 3) but may also reflect a retardation in the maturation of the sensor system.

For example, lalling may be viewed as the vocal expression of the establishment of audiovocal feedback. Audiovocal feedback allows the individual to auditorially examine self-produced sounds or sound combinations. During the echolalia phase of prespeech behavior, the audiovocal loop allows the individual to evaluate the accuracy of his reproduction of sounds as made by others. Prespeech sensor development is prerequisite to speech sensor development. Also ". . . it is assumed that during the closing and closed audiovocal loop periods, associations are being formed between the auditory events and the accompanying articulatory touch and movement sensations which produce them" (Mysak, 1966, p. 37). These associations eventually allow tactile and kinesthetic backflow to serve as supplementary, complementary, or substitute sensor stimuli.

Paleoverbal behavior such as repetitive speech behavior (physiologic verbal perseveration) and intraverbalizing (self-talk) may also be extended in some children because of slowness in the maturation of the sensor system.

Physiologic verbal perseveration may be viewed as the child's way of trying out and learning a new word or phrase by repeating it many times, watching the reactions of listeners to the new word or words, or doing it just because he enjoys the sound and feel of the new verbal events. Such physiologic verbal perseveration also reflects the development of audioverbal feedback. Audioverbal feedback allows the individual to examine auditorially the accuracy and appropriateness of the spoken symbols being uttered.

Intraverbalizing or accompanying one's activities with self-talk represents a level of perceptual-linguistic development (approximately 18 months to 3 years). During this self-talk period, the child uses speech to vocalize his perceptual processes. Such self-talk may also be viewed as inner speech or verbal thinking in-the-making. Intraverbalizing also reflects the further development of audioverbal-loop monitoring of outer and inner speech.

Speech-sound learning processes may also be inefficient during the developmental period. The author (Mysak, 1966, pp. 71–72) described the speech-sound learning process by the following sequence: (a) auditory *orienting* (complemented by vision) toward the source of human sounds, that is, toward the face and mouth of speakers; (b) auditory *scanning,* or the careful scrutiny of distinguishing features among sounds; (c) auditory *tracking,* or the attempt to reproduce particular speech sounds or auditory events; (d) auditory *comparing,* or the comparison by the speaker of his version of the sound with the model sound; (e) auditory *approximating,* or the gradual reduction of discrepancies between the model sound and its reproduction. Approximating ceases when the speaker judges his reproduction as being equal to the model sound.

Incomplete development of certain speech sounds may occur because of an inefficient comparing process. Efficient comparing depends on a developed, recurring speech loop. If the child fails to detect error factors or discrepancies between the model sound and his version, premature cessation of speech-sound learning may occur and the child may, for example, retain a developmental form of [s]; that is, he may retain an interdental version. This situation represents arrestment of [s] development based on an inefficient feedback or comparing process.

Voice-pattern development depends on the establishment of audioregulation of laryngeal function. Finding, controlling, and monitoring an individual voice pattern were described by the author (Mysak, 1966, pp. 65–66) in this way: (a) A parental model tone is progressively incorporated and is manifested, first, by the child ceasing whimpering in response to a human voice early in life; second, by his smiling in response to the maternal voice; and third, by his showing meaningful motor responses to the calling of his name. (b) Personal vocalization is progressively established concurrently with the incorporation of the model tone and is manifested, first, by unmonitored crying and screaming; second, by the use of more organized vocalization and the beginning of awareness of this vocalization by, for example, certain facial expressions; third, by the continual production of organized vocalization and the establishment of infantile audioregulation of voice as evidenced by the ability to repeat self-produced sounds; and fourth, by the ability not only to repeat self-produced sounds but also to reproduce sounds made by others.

Feedback-based voice anomalies may be caused by problems in the development of the internal audiovocal loop (reproduction of self-produced vocalization) or of the external audiovocal loop (reproduction of model vocalization).

Regulation of speech rhythm also depends on the early development of audiovocal and audioverbal loops.

"Automaticity of utterances of articulatory cycles proceeds from syllablic, to word, to phrasal to full cycle levels" (Mysak, 1966, p. 86). Slowness in the maturation of speech-automaticity mechanisms may be reflected by protracted repetition behavior at the sound and syllable or part-word levels.

Auditory sensor dysmaturity describes symptoms related to particular pathologic factors that interfere with the development of sensor control and monitoring.

Verbal anomalies of various kinds may be attributed to pathologic involvement of central neural mechanisms devoted to language function. Some symptoms of genetic language dysmaturity discussed in Chapter 3 which may be based on a sensor system disorder are syllable reversals, grammatical confusions, and difficulty in forming sentences. A symptom of neuropathic language dysfunction discussed in Chapter 3 which may be based on a sensor system disorder is pseudoeuphasia, a symptom in children with minimal brain dysfunction due to arrested hydrocephalus, where a great deal of speaking takes place but where the child is unaware of the significance of much of what is said. This may be viewed as a problem in the internal audioverbal loop. Other possible sensor-based symptoms include: asyntacticism (difficulty in combining and recombining known words), dysgrammatisms, verbal perseveration, and pathologic echolalia and jargon. Overlap exists among symptoms of immaturity, dysmaturity, and neurogenicity. At least two reasons for this overlap are (a) common mechanisms may be involved, and (b) there is difficulty in differentiating among the possible backgrounds in childhood language deficits.

Some of the language symptoms in childhood psychosis may also be viewed as sensor-based. For example, symptoms in "Psychogenic Language Disorders in Children" in Chapter 3 included: intrapersonal logophobia, or the fear of hearing oneself verbalize; autoecholalia, or a form of verbal autostimulation; and verbal perseveration.

Vocal-articulatory anomalies of various kinds are also found in cases of ear involvement. Chapter 5 describes the many primary and secondary speech problems associated with various types of hearing impairment. The following secondary symptoms may be interpreted as sensor-based:

Children with high-frequency losses who show problems in perceiving voiceless, high-frequency consonants such as [s, θ, f, k, p, ʃ, tʃ, h] also show difficulty in controlling and monitoring such sounds. Also, serious hearing loss which affects self-hearing may be reflected by omitting sounds in final positions and presenting voiced for voiceless sound substitutions.

One of the clinical manifestations of problems in auditory transmission of speech (discussed in Chapter 7) is in speech sequencing and synthesis, or putting words or parts of words together. The expressive reflection of this problem is the occurrence of syllable reversals and neologisms.

Disturbed audioregulation in significant conductive losses may be reflected by low and weak voice, monotonous speech melody, and a tendency toward hyponasality; and in sensorineural losses by high and loud voice, monotonous speech melody, and hypernasality. Problems in audioregulation may also result in the manifestation of paraphonic sounds such as noisy breathing, grunting, and clicking.

Persistence of hypernasality in certain cases of congenital velopharyngeal incompetency has sensor-system implications. For example, if a child develops a substantial amount of speech before his incompetency is surgically or prosthetically corrected, his auditory sensor system may equate hypernasal-resonance speech with normal-resonance speech. This takes place because during the speech-learning period it may have been impossible for the child to produce normal-resonance speech. This error functioning of the auditory sensor for resonance control and monitoring usually persists even after successful surgical or prosthetic treatment of the problem. Such children require speech therapy for the purpose of readjusting their auditory sensor system for appropriate control and monitoring of speech resonance.

Persistence of malarticulation in certain cases of childhood involvement of the articulatory structures also has sensor system implications. For example, if a child learns to produce sibilant sounds poorly during the speech-sound learning period because of the presence of a distocclusion, those poorly-formed sibilants usually persist following orthodontic correction of the distocclusion for the reasons given above.

Speech rhythm disturbances are also found in cases of certain types of auditory involvement (audiogenic dysautomaticity). Physiologic delay in the recurrent speech loop, due to the effects of anxiety for example, may elicit excessive speech repetitions and prolongations. Stuttering phenomena may also be observed in individuals who overmonitor fluency aspects of their speech ("Johnsonian effect"), who have overloaded auditory sensors, or who lack a dominant ear in the auditory sensor.

Auditory Sensor Disorders Based on Dissolution. Various pathologic processes may cause a deterioration of speech control and monitoring. Disturbances in the control and monitoring function may be manifested in verbal, phonatory, articulatory, and speech-rhythm forms.

Verbal problems are observed in different types of adult neuropathology. In aphasia, problems in auditory comprehension may eventually disturb the intrapersonal-audioverbal loop and cause secondary verbomotor problems in the form of paraphasia, which may lead eventually to jargonaphasia. Schuell (1969, p. 121) described the contribution of disturbed auditory feedback in aphasia. She stated that "when feedback mechanisms are disrupted the patient has difficulty recognizing his errors, even when he has produced jargon." Verbomotor repercussions in such cases may not be considered true aphasias since they are secondary to the primary comprehension aphasia. Uncorrected mistaken utterances are also considered a sensor form of "secondary aphasia." Rochford (1974) believes that jargon dysphasia is secondary to a more primary state of pathological arousal and lack of control of behavior probably due to involvement of the nondominant hemisphere.

Verbal symptoms possibly associated with sensor involvement have also been observed in various types of progressive neuropathology. Included among those symptoms are: paraphasia, jargonaphasia, apotheosis (incompletion of sentences begun), palilalia, and verbal perseveration.

Symptoms discussed under the section, "Psychogenic Language Disorders in Adults" in Chapter 3, which may be based on auditory sensor involvement include: singsong speech, senseless rhyming, acataphasia (problems in syntax), catalogia (automatic repetition of expressions in meaningless sequence after using them correctly), echophrasia, dysphrastic alliteration (use of series of words containing the same consonant sounds), intraverbalizing (thoughts-out-loud symptom), verbomania (manic verbosity), onomataphobia (morbid dread of hearing a certain name or word), endophasia (silent reproduction of a word or words), and embolophrasia (insertion of meaningless words into speech). Many of the symptoms appear to be related either to a need for excessive stimulation of the auditory sensor or to disengagement of the auditory sensor.

Voicing problems may appear in adults who suffer hearing loss as described in "Auditory Sensor Disorders of Developmental Origin." Low and weak voice, monotonous speech melody, and a tendency toward hyponasality may follow significant conductive losses; while high and loud voice, monotonous speech melody, and a tendency toward hypernasality may follow significant sensorineural losses.

Changes in vocal quality may also follow special hearing loss, for example, complete unilateral loss in the dominant ear and certain high-frequency hearing losses.

Articulatory problems may also appear in long-standing hearing losses. When adults experience serious loss of hearing the tactile-kinesthetic sensor may be sufficient to maintain good articulation; however, with the passage of time some individuals may begin to show signs of articulatory deterioration.

Tactile-Kinesthetic Sensor Disorders

The tactile-kinesthetic sensor has a major responsiblity for control of ongoing articulation in the mature speaker. Under the section on the "Speech Sensor System" in Chapter 1, it is stated that the tactile-kinesthetic sensor contributes to the control and monitoring of speech articulation by processing touch, movement, and position sensations. The sensory backflow into the sensor system may take at least two routes: (a) the cortical, or conscious and voluntary route, and (b) the cerebellar, or subconscious and automatic route. In terms of speech, the cortical sensor system is engaged when learning a new sound or sounds, that is, the child first listens to his reproduction of a new sound or sounds and consciously feels the associated tactile-kinesthetic sensations. Control and monitoring of the new articulatory pattern progresses from (a) primarily the auditory sensor, to (b) primarily the conscious, cortical sensor system, and finally to (c) primarily the subconscious and automatic cerebellar sensor system.

Problems with the tactile-kinesthetic sensor may also be of a developmental or dissolution nature.

Tactile-Kinesthetic Sensor Disorders of Developmental Origin. Factors that interfere with the sequential development of auditory control and monitoring of speech articulation, to cortical-tactile-kinesthetic, and, finally, to cerebellar-tactile-kinesthetic control may cause problems with the accuracy, consistency, and automaticity of speech articulation.

Articulatory accuracy suffers when the child is unable to associate the auditory feedback of a sound with concomitant and consistent touch, movement, and position feedback. Absent, reduced, or distorted tactile-kinesthetic feedback weakens control and monitoring of articulation. The child's best chances of maintaining a good level of articulatory accuracy rests on his ability to disregard confusing tactile-kinesthetic feedback or to focus on the auditory feedback. Concentration on auditory sensor control of articulation means that the expected division of labor between auditory sensor and tactile-kinesthetic sensor functioning may not take place and may cause overload of the auditory sensor system.

Speech learning or relearning is greatly affected when there is "a lack of sense of position and movement of the articulators and/or a lack of esthesia of the surfaces of the tongue, fauces, palate, velum and pharynx. . ." (West and Ansberry 1968, p. 183).

Articulatory consistency also suffers when tactile-kinesthetic feedback is disturbed. Under circumstances of disturbed tactile-kinesthetic feedback, an individual may produce a given sound adequately at any given time but may not at other times. Inconsistency of articulation is one of the features of disturbed tactile-kinesthetic sensor control.

Articulatory automaticity or the relatively rapid and smooth production of articulatory cycles also suffers when the tactile-kinesthetic sensor is involved. When the sensory backflow associated with the completion of articulatory contacts is lacking, reduced, or distorted, the automaticity of speech articulation is disturbed. More specifically, when the sequential maturation of articulatory control and monitoring does not reach the subconscious cerebellar level but remains at the auditory or the conscious cortical level, some form of articulatory dysautomaticity (somesthetic dysautomaticity) may be presented.

Tactile-Kinesthetic Sensor Disorders Based on Dissolution. Adults may incur trauma or disease to cortical and(or) cerebellar sensor systems and consequently show signs of disturbance in control and monitoring of articulation and speech automaticity.

Articulatory lapses were identified by Schuell (1969, p. 121) who described sensorimotor impairment as part of aphasia. Occasionally "impairment is so severe that no imitation of linguistic patterns is possible initially." Also, "The most persisting errors are confusions between phonemes with similar articulatory patterns such as p-b-m, t-d-n-l, f-v, k-g, et cetera." Along these lines, Luria (1974) states: "Destruction of the lower parts of the postcentral zone of the major hemisphere results in a kinesthetic apraxia and 'afferent' (kinesthetic) break-down of articulemes with a series of secondary disturbances of speech."

Some of the symptoms described in "Output Patterning Disorders" in Chapter 4 may be related to involvement of the tactile-kinesthetic sensor system. For example, under "Cerebellar Disorders" the general symptoms of dysmetria and disintegration may also be applied to speech articulation.

Articulatory dysmetria or poorly measured movements of the articulators manifested by articulatory inaccuracy (slurring) may be attributed to deficient guidance brought about by disturbed tactile-kinesthetic feedback. Articulatory disintegration, or the loss of articulatory movements that were once acquired, may also be attributed to absent, reduced, or distorted tactile-kinesthetic feedback. This is based on the fact that articulatory movements are not learned or maintained but only their associated sensations. Hence, if sensory patterns associated with certain articulatory movements weaken or become distorted, those articulatory movements will also disintegrate.

Articulatory dysautomaticity was described by West and Ansberry (1968, p. 182) who stated that "Most lesions of cranial nerves involved in articulation impair not only motion but also kinesthesia and often cutaneous esthesia as well." Because of deficient reporting to the Central Nervous System (CNS) of the completion of certain articulatory contacts speech automaticity is disturbed. Similarly, "parietal stuttering" has been attributed to damage to the somesthetic area of the brain.

Some of the symptoms reported in cerebellar speech dysrhythmias may be based on deficient tactile-kinesthetic feedback. Scanning speech and episodic tonic blocks are representative of such symptoms.

DIAGNOSIS

Attributing verbal, articulatory, phonatory (quality, loudness, pitch) resonatory, and speech-time (rate, rhythm) symptoms to involvement of the auditory sensory may require various diagnostic approaches. General clinical, by treatment, instrumental, and provocative approaches are among those that may be used.

Verbal Symptoms

Verbal symptoms may occur as a result of delay, retardation, or arrestment of verbal development; a need for abnormal self-stimulation of the auditory sensor; or a disengagement of the auditory sensor.

For example, extended use of repetitive speech behavior (physiologic verbal perseveration) and self-talk (inner speech in-the-making), both prerequisites for more advanced interverbalizing, may be symptomatic of an overall retardation in the development of audioverbal feedback.

Whereas, the use of autoecholalia, verbal perseveration, and excessive self-talk in a child developing normally, except in the socioemotional sphere, may reflect a symptom of regression from intercommunication to intracommunication and(or) gratification from abnormal stimulation of the auditory sensor. The avoidance of a certain word or the use of a replacement neologism by such a child may reveal the fear of stimulating the auditory sensor with that word, which is another type of sensor system problem.

In contrast to symptoms caused by an immature sensor, or a need to overstimulate the sensor, or a fear of stimulating the sensor, symptoms of paraphasia and jargonaphasia in adults may be related to a disengagement of the auditory sensor. Auditory sensor-based paraphasia and jargonaphasia may be identified by the client's apparent unawareness of his error speech as compared to the aphasic who misnames or misspeaks, shows recognition of the error by facial expressions or utterances, and attempts to correct his speech.

General clinical observation of verbal behavior is the diagnostic approach described above.

Articulatory Symptoms

In relatively simple misarticulation, that is, in cases where everything appears equal in the child except for his interdental lisp for example, the role of the auditory sensor may be evaluated rather easily. The clinician may tell the child that while they are talking he, the clinician, will make mistakes on certain sounds and that the child should signal whenever he hears the error. The clinician proceeds to talk and occasionally inserts the child's error version of the [s] sound. Once the child is able to detect the error sound rather easily the clinician then tells the child that during the next period of talking he, the clinician, wants the child to listen to his own sounds very carefully as they talk and to stop talking every time the child becomes aware of a mistake or error sound. Depending on the age and motivation of the child such a clinical procedure may shed some light on the sensitivity of the child's auditory sensor to error-sound production.

In children who show certain articulation profiles, for example, malarticulation of voiceless, high-frequency consonants, the phonemodiagnosis of audiogenicity is supported through an instrumental diagnosis, that is, through audiometric confirmation of a high-frequency hearing loss. Omission of sounds in final positions and substituting voiced for voiceless sounds may also implicate auditory sensor functioning, and again the condition is confirmed by audiometric evaluation.

In cases of clients about 10 years and older, where the clinician suspects sensor immaturity, that is, incomplete transfer of articulatory sensor function to the tactile-kinesthetic division, the clinician may assess the effects of bilateral, white-noise masking on the child's articulation. Does elimination of auditory sensor function worsen articulation or improve it?

The use of some simple clinical tests may be useful in determining whether the articulatory lapses under investigation are related to involvement of the tactile-kinesthetic sensor. Simple right-left, touch-discrimination ability of the client may be tested by applying a light touch stimulus to right and left portions of the lips, to the alveolar ridge behind right and left upper central incisors, to right and left portions of the hard palate where it joins with the soft palate, and to either side of the median raphe of the tongue at its tip, blade, and dorsum. The client identifies the side touched by raising his right or left hand.

An estimate of lingual kinesthetic function may be obtained by asking the client to hold his mouth in a relatively wide open position and applying a touch stimulus to the center of the upper and lower lips, to right and left corners of the mouth, and to various teeth in the upper and lower arches and asking the client to quickly and accurately locate with his tongue tip the points touched.

Tests for articulator-position sense may also be useful in assessing the integrity of the tactile-kinesthetic sensor. The clinician first demonstrates lip-spread and lip-round postures; mandible-open, mandible half-closed, and mandible almost-closed postures; and tongue-up, tongue-down, and tongue-right and tongue-left postures. The clinician then requests the client to assume quickly and maintain any of these postures upon command.

Articulatory deterioration in the client during requests for increased rate of speech may indicate degrees of dysfunction of the subconscious sensor (cerebellar system). Examining for positive speech changes under speaking conditions that alter speech sensor function may also yield useful diagnostic data. For example, the client may be asked to concentrate on the touch, movement, and position sensations associated with his talking; or he may be asked to exaggerate his articulatory movements while he speaks or to overarticulate; or he may be asked to speak in a slow-motion pattern; or he may be asked to speak by making hard contacts between his articulators. Improvement in articulatory accuracy or speech intelligibility under such conditions may be interpreted in at least three ways: (a) gearing-down of speech rate in a speech system unable to maintain premorbid speech rates, (b) amplification of tactile-kinesthetic feedback in an involved tactile-kinesthetic sensor, (c) shifting from an involved, subconscious sensor (cerebellar system) to a noninvolved, conscious sensor (cortical system).

Phonatory Symptoms

Pitch, loudness, and quality attributes of voice may be deficient because of involvement of the auditory sensor. Useful diagnostic information may be gathered by altering or modifying voice feedback. Modifying the speech feedback of an individual may be viewed as a diagnosis by treatment approach or a provocative diagnostic approach.

Certain cases of dysphonia appear to be resolved when the client is subjected to a bilateral, masking level of white noise. When substantial improvement or normal voicing is achieved under this masking condition, at least three interpretations are available (two of which were given in Chapter 2, "Speech Sensor"). (a) Masking-induced stress alters respiratory-laryngeal myodynamics in a positive direction and hence, improved voicing; (b) eliminating, through masking, an auditory sensor that has been maintaining a pathologic voice for some reason allows the reemergence of the physiologic voice; or (c) the masking of a deficient auditory sensor elicits a compensatory and more effective proprioceptive regulation of voicing. The two latter explanations are pertinent to the topic under discussion here.

The influence on the dysphonia of a dominant ear in auditory sensor function may also be tested. A dominant-ear sensor problem is suggested if voice improvement occurs when only one ear is masked or when the client's voice is fed back through earphones into only one ear. Left-ear masking and voice feedback to the right ear should yield the best results when a question of a dominant-ear sensor exists.

The improvement of voice through enriched auditory feedback also has implications for sensor-based voice disorders. Enrichment may be accomplished by feeding back the client's voice after it has been modified through electronic filtering. Another enrichment technique has been described by the author (Mysak, 1966, p. 68) elsewhere. The technique involves the use of a special amplifier with two microphones and two earphones. The instrument is adjusted so that the client's voice (phonating deficient [ɑ] sound) is fed back into the left earphone and the clinician's voice (appropriately voiced [ɑ] sound) is fed into the client's right earphone. Then, while the client is receiving both error voice (his) and correct voice (clinician's), the clinician uses a fader control that gradually attenuates the error voice in the left ear and amplifies the correct voice in the right ear. Under this condition, the client's voice may be observed to modify in the direction of the correct voice. If such modification occurs, support is provided for the contribution of the auditory sensor in the dysphonia under investigation.

Microphonia (possibly secondary to middle-ear hearing loss) and megaphonia (possibly secondary to inner-ear hearing loss) may be confirmed through audiometric evaluation.

Speech-Time Symptoms

Rate and rhythm symptoms may occur because of problems in the auditory sensor or in the tactile-kinesthetic sensor.

Hypersensitivity of the auditory sensor may be supported when increased disfluency is elicited in a client who is following verbal instructions by the clinician to the client to listen more carefully to his own speech in order to control disfluency. On the other hand, if, in children about 10 years old or older, instructions to them to pay more attention to the feel of the articulators during speech elicit greater fluency, then one may hypothesize that some delay in transference from auditory to tactile-kinesthetic sensor control of speech rhythm may be present.

When bilateral, white-noise masking induces fluency in certain stutterers at least two interpretations are possible. The induced fluency is the result of (a) simple distraction or (b) the elimination of a hypersensitive, overloaded, or deficient auditory sensor for the regulation of speech rhythm, and the transference, therefore, from a deficient auditory sensor regulation of speech rhythm to a more efficient tactile-kinesthetic regulation. The latter explanation is relevant to the present discussion.

Facilitation of fluency under unilateral, white-noise masking suggests a problem in dominant-ear sensor function.

The facilitation of fluency in the stutterer under conditions of delayed auditory feedback (DAF) also has pertinent interpretations. DAF-induced fluency may be the result of (a) simple distraction, (b) the improved functioning of a deficient auditory sensor for rhythm control when speech rate is reduced through DAF, and (c) forced transference of speech rhythm control to a more mature or less loaded tactile-kinesthetic sensor.

SELF-ADJUSTING THERAPY

This section describes sensor-based therapy regimens. Procedures described here are symptom-therapy procedures and may be referred to as self-adjusting forms of therapy. Since self-adjusting approaches to various symptom therapies are the ones advocated by the author, the reader was referred to this chapter when symptom-therapy programs were recommended in Chapters 5 to 7.

In discussing principles of a psychiatric theory of communication, Ruesch (1959, p. 898), referring to cybernetic concepts of Wiener, states, "Feedback, therefore, refers to the process of correction through incorporation of information about effects achieved. This function is basic to all learning, correction, and self-correction."

To facilitate the discussion of self-adjusting therapies for language, voice, resonance, articulation, and fluency disorders, general concepts in self-adjusting therapy are presented first.

General Concepts

Following are terms and definitions that are important to the development and description of self-adjustment therapy programs for various types of error-speech output. Those interested in pursuing further the application of feedback theory to speech pathology are referred to "Speech Pathology and Feedback Theory" (Mysak, 1966).

Positive and negative speech feedback refers to error-free speech or error speech, respectively. The author is aware that the terms positive and negative feedback may be used in just the opposite way by some writers. Here positive feedback means correct-operation feedback, while negative feedback means incorrect-operation feedback.

Delayed speech feedback describes a state of electronically-induced retardation in the air-conducted return of a speaker's voice to his own ears. Instruments are now readily available that produce such delays at various delay times. Some stutterers who have been asked to adjust their speech rate to coincide with the speech delay have become more fluent as a consequence.

Delayed speech feedback may also mean simply recording a client's speech and playing it back. The playback speech constitutes the delayed version.

Amplified speech feedback describes conditions where speech is fed back to the speaker in amplified form. For example, a speaker may speak through an individual amplifier and receive his voice through earphones. Speech feedback may also be amplified by having individuals speak through loudspeakers or bullhorns, insert their fingertips into their ears, or speak into "speaking tubes" directed back to their ears.

Tactile-kinesthetic feedback may be amplified through the use of slow-motion, hard-contact, or exaggerated articulation.

Attenuated, deleted, or masked speech feedback may be accomplished on the auditory level by having the client use soft voice, whisper, or no voice; by feeding back electronically-attenuated voice to the speaker through earphones; or by introducing masking levels of noise into the speaker's ears while he speaks.

Attenuating tactile-kinesthetic feedback may be accomplished by having the client use light-contact or slide-type speech. Anesthetizing the articulators is a way of eliminating tactile feedback. The application of vibrators to the articulators may mask proprioceptive feedback.

Filtered or distorted speech feedback usually means modifying the speech signal of an individual by sending it through low- or high-pass filters and then back to the individual through earphones. Such filtered-speech feedback has facilitated fluency in certain stutterers.

Enriched speech feedback describes modification of the voice feedback of an individual in a positive way. For example, an individual's voice quality may be enhanced by having the speaker vocalize in an area with certain reverberation characteristics. Electronic treatment of a voice signal may also succeed in producing a richer quality to an individual's voice feedback. The hope is that such enriched feedback will modify laryngeal function in a positive way, or, in other words, trigger the "ear-larynx matching reflex."

Shunted speech feedback is accomplished by making either auditory feedback or tactile-kinesthetic feedback the "figure" feedback and the other the "ground" feedback. Shunting to a different dominant feedback channel can be done by applying the techniques described under the headings of "Amplified" and "Attenuated Speech Feedback."

Reversed speech feedback is accomplished in at least two ways: (a) evoking neuronal activity associated with the production of certain words by imposing upon the client, via the motokinesthetic approach, the touch and movement sensations associated with those words; and (b) requesting random articulatory movements of the client, which may result in spontaneous production of true words.

Accelerated speech feedback may involve the electronic acceleration of the air-conducted return of a speaker's voice to his ears. Under such a condition, speaking rate may be increased. Speech acceleration may also be achieved by having the client attempt to track a speeded rate of speech used by the clinician.

Anticipatory speech feedback means developing a set within the speaker to anticipate the return of certain speech. For example, the clinician may tell a lisper to get ready to hear his own lisp as they converse and to signal immediately before the occurrence of the lisped [s].

Contradictory feedback is accomplished by electronically attenuating the individual's voice feedback and substituting a different or new voice feedback. For example, the client and clinician may be connected to the same amplifier via separate microphones and headsets while vocalizing the same sound: [ɑ]. Then the clinician adjusts the amplifier so that the client's personal voice feedback is attenuated or eliminated while the clinician's vocalization is sent to the client's earphones instead. Such a maneuver may cause the client's voice to shift in the direction of what is being heard, as described under enriched speech feedback.

Another technique involves introducing random speech into a speaker's ears while he attempts to converse with the clinician. Attempting to speak while hearing two feedbacks (one matching and one not) requires additional effort and concentration by the speaker. Paradoxically, when such "noise" is added to an already noisy system like, for example, the aphasic's, speech function may improve. Increasing a problem for some individuals, then, may trigger suprathreshold verbal capacity not usually manifested.

Complementary or supplementary speech feedback may be provided in different ways. For example, a client may be asked to focus visually on his articulators as he converses with the clinician through a mirror (supplementary) or he may be asked to concentrate on the sound as well as the feel of his speech (complementary).

Struggle speech feedback describes a technique where an individual is asked to talk while restraining one of the articulators. For example, the speaker may be asked to speak while holding the tongue tip against the alveolar ridge, thus triggering compensatory labial and mandibular activity. Or he may be asked to hold his mandible in a closed position while he attempts to speak, thus triggering compensatory lingual and labial activity. Or he may be asked to hold his lips in a closed position while he attempts to speak, thus triggering compensatory lingual and mandibular activity. After such struggle work, the articulators of some dysarthrics may be observed to function better.

Unilateral speech feedback indicates sending different feedback to each ear. For example, a lisper may be directing lisped words into his left ear through a speech tube while the clinician simultaneously directs the same words but produced correctly into the client's right ear.

Regenerative speech feedback is experienced by a speaker when what he is saying is obviously interesting or being enjoyed by the listener. Such signals from the listener usually cause the speaker to continue speaking and possibly to increase his intended speech output.

Double speech feedback is experienced when a client is told to expect to hear certain words spoken by the clinician, to watch the articulators of the clinician very carefully, and to attempt to speak the words simultaneously with the clinician, or to slave or shadow speak. Under those circumstances the client receives auditory and visual feedback from the clinician's speech system and auditory and tactile-kinesthetic feedback from his own speech system. Echo speech is a delayed form of double speech feedback and may be experienced by the client by having him echo his own words (autoecholalia) or by having his words echoed by the clinician. Many stutterers experience fluency when slave or shadow speaking.

Imaginal or inner speech feedback describes inner speech experiences. For example, a clinician may request a stutterer to engage in inner fluent speech and hear it with his mind's ear and feel it with his mind's articulators; or a voice case to practice using a good voice with his mind's voicebox and hear it with his mind's ear. Such imaginal speech feedback may positively condition the individual's speech system.

Language Habilitation

Self-adjusting techniques may be designed to prime the language pump, so to speak, of those children whose spoken language has not begun, is developing too slowly, or appears to have stopped developing.

Only techniques aimed at the sensor system are described here; for other therapy procedures for language-disturbed children, the reader is referred to Chapter 3 "Developmental and Genetic Language Disorders— Therapy," "Neurogenic Language Disorders—Therapy," "Gnosogenic Language Disorders—Therapy," "Psychogenic Language Disorders— Therapy."

Prespeech Feedbacks. Prior to true speech feedback, a child experiences certain prespeech feedbacks composed of auditory and tactile-kinesthetic sensations associated with certain types of vocalization, as well as kinesthetic sensations from body, hands, and face movements associated with those vocalizations. For example, during the first one or two months of life the child signals unpleasant interoceptive sensations (e.g., hunger) and exteroceptive sensations (e.g., wetness) by reflexive vocalization or crying and screaming and generalized body movements. Primary feedbacks during this *body-language stage 1* are auditory from the reflexive vocalization and kinesthetic from the associated body movements.

From one month up to about six months, the child may be heard to respond to speech or good feelings by cooing, gurgling, snorting, grunting, chuckling, laughing, and with more organized body movements. Primary feedbacks during this *body-language stage 2* are auditory as well as tactile-kinesthetic from the more differentiated vocalization, and kinesthetic from the more differentiated body movements.

During the time up to about nine months, the child may be noted to repeat self-produced sounds or sound combinations and to associate his vocalizations with bilateral hand gesturing and early facial expressions. True auditory feedback of vocalization is experienced during this *hands-language stage* as well as the early association of this auditory feedback with the concomitant tactile-kinesthetic feedback from the articulators and the kinesthetic feedback from the hand gestures.

From about 9 to 12 months, the child may be heard to imitate sounds made by others and to exhibit unilateral hand gestures and more refined facial expressions. During the *face-language stage* the child experiences true auditory feedback of utterances initiated by others, tactile-kinesthetic feedback associated with the auditory feedback, and kinesthetic feedback from the face associated with the auditory and tactile-kinesthetic feedback associated with the utterances.

The *face stage* is critical to the development of *mouth language,* or true speech, which is reached some time during the second year of life. At this time utterances are "figure language"; and supportive facial expressions, hand gestures, and body postures are "ground language".

Depending on the language status of the child, the clinician should attempt to stimulate the kinds of feedbacks associated with prespeech body, hands, and face languages.

For example, encouraging the child to move about, to use communicative body postures, hand gestures, facial expressions, and to accompany all this activity with whatever utterances are available to the child, that is, babbling, lalling, echolalia, jargon vocalization, would provide important prespeech feedbacks to the child's sensor system. Such activity may be elicited through modeling by the clinician and significant others. Application of the techniques of reverse speech feedback, or encouraging as much random articulatory activity as possible; regenerative speech feedback, or showing interest and enjoyment and rewarding the child's communicative attempts; and double speech feedback, or echoing the utterances and body language manifested by the child, should encourage the continuance of prespeech activities and hopefully move the child closer to spontaneous production of true speech.

Speech Feedbacks. Various techniques aimed at the sensor system may also be applied to stimulate those children who are just beginning to speak or who are moving along too slowly.

Imaginal feedback may be facilitated by the clinician or significant others. A good example of this technique is found in Chapter 3, "Neurogenic Language Disorders in Children—Therapy." More specifically, the technique is found under the heading "Verbal Thinking Processes."

Enriching feedback in young children who are exhibiting little or no intraverbalizing may be done in at least two ways: (a) the clincian and others when near the child may accompany their activities with appropriate out-loud speech (self-reporting); and (b) the clinician and others may report out loud the activities of the child. Hopefully, such self-reporting and reporting of movements and activities by others will stimulate self-reporting behavior in the child.

Another form of enriching speech feedback is through verbal expansion and expatiation techniques referred to in Chapter 3. Expansion means echoing children's immature or telegraphic utterances in more developed form, while expatiation means to echo an enlarged version of the child's utterances.

Providing supplementary speech feedback by having the child watch his attempts at communication before full-length mirrors; and providing amplified speech feedback by giving the child the opportunity to speak through speech tubes, loudspeaker arrangements, or in echo rooms may also be useful in stimulating increased speech output.

Language Rehabilitation

Some of the feedback techniques described here for use with adults who have lost their language ability have already been mentioned in Chapter 3, "Neurogenic Language Disorders in Adults—Therapy."

Conditioning feedback work is designed to keep active recurrent speech loops or audioverbal feedback in individuals whose aphasia has significantly reduced or eliminated spontaneous verbalization. The sensor system of these individuals during this period is either not stimulated or is being stimulated by the client's disorganized speech attempts. In order to keep the sensor system in "condition" and, hopefully, to trigger spontaneous propositional speech, the client should be required to stimulate his sensor with whatever organized speech of which he is capable.

For example, he may be able to produce minor speech ((emotional utterances, social-gesture speech (e.g., hi, so-long, good morning, I'm fine, etc.), and memorized speech (e.g., counting, days-of-the-week, alphabet, poems, songs, etc.)), or he may be able to echo the clinician. Such minor speech should be articulated as often as possible during each day.

Delayed feedback in certain forms may be used to good advantage with aphasics. The delay techniques described here are used to offset pathologic involvement of the automaticity of speech.

In order to compensate for reduced automaticity of comprehension and formulation in the client, he may be asked to: (a) repeat questions and instructions aloud and silently before he makes a final decision with respect to what is being asked; and (b) refrain from attempting a verbal response until he formulates the response in his mind and scans it for accuracy. The latter technique is a form of *imaginal or inner speech feedback*.

Reverse feedback work refers to reversing the language-paralanguage, figure-ground relationship. That is, aphasics who are having difficulty producing spoken language may be asked to lead attempts at spoken language with appropriate body language (postures, gestures, facial expressions). In normal speech, body language accompanies or supports spoken language.

For example, a client who is struggling to ask to make a phone call should precede or accompany his attempt with the appropriate body language of reaching out for an imaginary phone, lifting the receiver, and pretending to dial. Such activity often facilitates retrieval of the desired words.

Inner feedback may be stimulated or maintained through the techniques of interreporting and intrareporting, similar to the techniques described under "Language Habilitation—Enriching Feedback."

In the case of adults, the techniques of interreporting and intrareporting are more appropriately viewed as serving to stimulate inner speech or verbal thinking.

Interreporting involves the periodic out-loud reporting in simple phrases by the clinician or others of the activities of the client. For example, "Jim is reaching for the comb . . . He is combing his hair . . .

He puts the comb down." The client is also encouraged to lead all his activities with attempts at self-reporting.

Contradictory feedback is designed to provide additional stress on the sensor in the hopes of evoking more physiologic verbalization. For example, as the aphasic speaks, he receives simultaneous and nonsimilar speech in his ears through headsets. The client is asked to attempt to "speak over" the *contradictory feedback*. Attempts to over-ride the contradictory feedback may actually facilitate the speech system. The clinician must be careful not to cause too much stress in the individual and must remain sensitive to the client's tolerance level for such work.

Unilateral feedback may be utilized by aid of a portable speech amplifier with headsets. The equipment is adjusted so that as the aphasic converses into his microphone he receives his speech feedback in only his left or right ear. One-ear sensing may be found to facilitate oral language.

Comparative feedback may be accomplished by having the client's speech signal return to only one of his own ears, while the clinician simultaneously provides a more organized signal into the client's opposite ear. During this comparative work the client's signal may be attenuated.

Amplified feedback is achieved by simply having the client speak through a portable amplifier adjusted so that his feedback is returned to him bilaterally and amplified.

Complementary or supplementary feedback and *imaginal speech feedback* techniques may also be applied to good advantage with aphasics.

Articulation Therapy

When using a self-adjusting approach to articulation therapy, the clinician must remember that it is a symptom therapy, and he must determine that the client is capable of producing the standard version of the sound under correction. Otherwise, such techniques could prove frustrating and counterproductive to the client.

The major goal of the self-adjusting approach is to introduce and develop a therapeutic error signal (TES) within the individual's speech system until the TES automatically triggers speech-corrective activity. The approach differs from more standard ones in a number of ways: (a) whenever possible, the conversational mode is used during therapy, (b) the standard sound is not "taught," and, therefore, (c) assimilation of the new sound into running speech should not require drillwork.

Error-Sound Sensing

Introduction of the TES into the client's speech system or activating the intrapersonal sensor to the error sound is begun by first activating the client's interpersonal sensor for error-sound appreciation. This is accomplished by at least four ways: (a) *Professional confirmation of the existence of an error sound, for example, lateral* [s]. The clinician through discussion with the client identifies and confirms the presence of the error sound. (b) *Professional service for the error-sound correction.* The clinician should indicate why the error sound is one that requires professional attention if it is to be modified. (c) *Professional demonstration of the error sound.* As the discussion of the error sound proceeds, the clinician should periodically demonstrate the client's version of [s], that is, the error version, and compare it to the correct or standard version. Such a demonstration not only adds to the client's developing error sensitivity but should also demonstrate to the client that, just as the clinician may adopt the client's error [s], so too, he, the client, can adopt the clinician's standard version. (d) *Full activation by the clinician of the client's motivation to correct the error sound.* Time should be spent on eliciting within the individual all the motivation possible for correcting the error sound. The advantages of correct speech in social relationships, job interviews, personal image, and so on, should be discussed. If at all possible such discussions should bring the client to the point of "champing-at-the-bit" to get on with therapy.

Error-Sound Measuring

After the error sound has been introduced to the client, at least on an interpersonal level, and after the client has been "fired up" to correct the error, the clinician activates the intrapersonal-sensor function through measuring techniques. The specific goal here is to intensify the TES to the point where the individual no longer produces his error sound quickly and easily.

Measuring the error factors of any particular error sound may be done for at least three dimensions, auditory, visual, and tactile-kinesthetic.

Auditory-Error Measuring. On the interpersonal level, the client is asked to listen carefully during conversational exchanges with the clinician for the occurrence of the error sound in the speech of the clinician. So that only the auditory dimension is presented, the clinician, while speaking to the client, either turns out of the client's visual field or covers his mouth.

The task of the client during his conversation with the clinician is to interrupt him every time the clinician produces a word containing the error sound. The client may signal the occurrence by saying, "Stop, error sound in word soup, you said, 'soup.'" At the time the client says, "You said, 'soup,'" he may be asked to exaggerate the production of the error sound, for example, the lateral [s]. During this period, the clinician may insert the error sound in words in which it appears in different positions and he may speak such error words in conversations held at different rates of speed.

This phase of the work is complete when the client consistently identifies the error words during conversational exchanges with the clinician.

On the intrapersonal level, the task of the client is to identify the occurrence of the error sound in his own speech. After-error sound, during-error sound, and before-error sound techniques may be used here.

After-error work is done by recording portions of conversation between client and clinician and then during playback having the client identify the error sound every time it occurs. He may be asked to stop the recorder each time he hears himself produce the error sound, identify the error word, and reproduce it in exaggerated form as he did previously. Asking the client to repeat or echo words containing the error sound during running speech is another after-error technique.

During-error work is done by having the client converse through a personal amplifier so that his speech is fed back to him over earphones at an amplified level. He is asked to signal each time he produces a word containing the error sound by identifying the error word and reproducing it in exaggerated form. Having the client speak at a louder than usual level, or through a speaking tube, or while holding one finger in one ear, or with a finger in each of his ears are other ways of amplifying feedback of the error sound.

Before-error work is done by asking the client to scan ahead during his conversation with the clinician and attempt to predict when a word containing an error sound is about to occur. Signaling of this about to happen error sound is done in the same way as before. How well this part of the work is done depends on the age, intelligence, and motivation of the client.

Visual-Error Measuring. Visual-error measuring is done when the error sound has a rather easily detectable visible component, for example, if during production of the lateral [s] concomitant jaw lateralization and lip depression are observed.

On the interpersonal level, the client is asked to watch very carefully, during conversational exchanges, the mouth of the clinician for the occurrence of the error sound. So that the visual dimension receives additional attention, the clinician, while speaking to the client, uses whispered voice and exaggerates the visual-error dimension whenever he utters the error sound. Signaling of the occurrence of the error sound by the client is done in the manner described under "Auditory-Error Measuring."

On the intrapersonal level, after-error, during-error, and before-error techniques may be used.

After-error work is done by videotaping portions of conversation, playing them back without voice, and having the client identify error sounds as produced by himself. Signaling by the client is done as already described.

During-error work is done via mirror talking. The client and clinician converse in whisper voice or no voice, if possible. The client is asked to signal every time he sees himself produce the error sound.

Before-error work is also done through mirror talking and as described under "Auditory-Error Measuring."

Tactile-Kinesthetic-Error Measuring. Measuring tactile-kinesthetic error factors may also be done on interpersonal and intrapersonal levels.

On the interpersonal level, the client is asked to concentrate not on what he hears or sees the clinician doing while the talks, but on the "feel" of his touching and moving articulators. In order to highlight the touch and movement dimensions, the clinician uses whisper voice and slightly exaggerates all articulatory movements. In addition, the client is asked to slave speak or follow simultaneously whenever possible the movements of the clinician's articulators. The clinician assumes a slower rate during this time, and if the client still has difficulty "mouthing" the clinician's speech the clinician may occasionally say a phrase containing the error sound, pause, and have the client reproduce only the movements associated with the error utterance. The client signals the presence of error speech in the manner already described.

On the intrapersonal level, after-error, during-error, and before-error techniques may also be used.

After-error work is done by having the client converse in echo fashion, with whisper voice, and with eyes closed. That is, the client is asked to respond to the clinician in repeated phrases or "double talk." For example, if the clinician asks the client's age, the client responds by saying, "I am 15 years old, I am 15 years old." The client should not only repeat all phrases he utters, but he should also utter them slowly and in an exaggerated manner concentrating on their feel. The client is asked to study each echoed utterance for the presence of error touch and movement factors and signal as before if they are present.

During-error work is done in various ways. The client may be asked to continue conversing with whisper voice but without the echo pattern. He should use a slower rate and an exaggerated articulatory manner, keep his eyes closed, and concentrate on the feel of his articulators. He could also be asked to use a slow-motion form of articulation or a hard-contact form in order to accentuate the touch-movement dimension of his articulation. Whenever he senses the error feel he signals in the prescribed manner.

Error-sound sensing and measuring work is designed to develop the

TES to the point where the client's sensor system triggers the rejecting process. If all is proceeding well then, some time during the sensing and measuring phases of self-adjusting work the client's sensor should become activated and should reject the error sound and trigger its replacement by the standard sound. However, the error sound may be so rutted that this self-adjustment phase is not triggered, even after successful sensing and measuring. In such cases, the clinician may have to prime the rejecting process.

Error-Sound Rejecting

The rejecting process may be primed in at least two ways. The techniques are applied with clinician and client in a normal face-to-face conversational relationship. An active rejecting process is manifested in the client by his negative facial expressions, head gestures, or utterances during or immediately following the production of the error sound.

Auditory-Error Rejecting. To prime auditory rejecting, have the client speak under amplified speech feedback and each time the error sound occurs require him to interrupt his speech flow, identify the error word, and repeat the error word in a louder fashion.

Tactile-Kinesthetic Rejecting. To prime tactile-kinesthetic rejecting, (a) have the client speak under amplified speech feedback conditions, that is, have the client use a slow-motion pattern and(or) a hard-contact pattern; (b) each time the error sound occurs require the client to interrupt his speech flow, identify the error word, close his eyes, and reproduce the error word exaggerating articulatory movements to an even greater degree.

Hopefully, priming of the rejecting phase will trigger rejection and replacement of the error sound. If this is still not the case, the additional technique of correct-sound seeking is used.

Correct-Sound Seeking

One purpose of seeking work is to require the client's speech system to produce the error sound in different ways, which tends to "unrut" the error sound and facilitates the eventual replacement of it by the standard sound.

Variable Speech Feedback. One way to increase the client's repertoire of, for example, [s] production, is to ask the client directly to produce [s] sounds in as many different ways as he can during conversation. He may be shown that [s] sounds can be made with the tongue tip rolled back in the mouth, against the lower teeth, or between the anterior teeth. During conversation he is required to assume one of these positions or any that he can think of. Such work should also reinforce error sensitivity, measuring, and rejecting processes.

Struggle Speech Feedback. If the client is having difficulty with the variable speech feedback technique, struggle speech feedback may be tried. He is asked, for example, to converse with clenched teeth or with his tongue tip held against the alveolar ridge. Under such conditions, the client is forced to produce his error sound in a different fashion. At this stage it does not matter whether the various forms of [s] produced are standard or closer to standard ones.

Such seeking work should facilitate rejecting and replacing of the error sound. If self-adjustment still does not occur, correct-sound approximating work is begun next.

Correct-Sound Approximating

Approximating techniques are the last to be used in the self-adjusting approach.

Reinforced Speech Feedback. The approximating process is facilitated whenever the client during his seeking efforts is reinforced by the clinician when some of the client's different productions of [s] come closer to or approximate the standard.

Contradictory Speech Feedback. Contradictory speech feedback may be accomplished through the use of the special amplifier previously described. The client is placed under phones and speaks to the clinician through a microphone. Once the error sound is uttered by the client he is asked to stop his speech flow and slowly repeat his error. While the error sound is slowly produced the amplifier is adjusted so that the client's speech is directed to his left earphone, while the clinician's simultaneous utterance of the error word produced in standard form is directed to the client's right ear. The clinician further adjusts the amplifier so that the client's version of [s] is attenuated and his version is amplified. This contradictory feedback may trigger self-adjustment attempts by the client.

Imaginal Speech Feedback. The approximating process may also be served by a special conversational technique. The client is asked to precede each utterance during a conversation with inner-speech rehearsal of it. Whenever the utterance contains the error sound, he is asked to rehearse it and make the correct sound with his mind's articulators before he actually speaks the phrase.

Voice Therapy

A self-adjusting approach to voice therapy is recommended in those cases where organic factors are not present or where organic factors have been medically resolved but the pathologic voice persists.

As with articulation therapy, the major goal of the self-adjustment approach to voice therapy is to introduce and develop the TES until the TES automatically activates vocal self-adjustment. Only the auditory sensor is involved in this type of voice therapy.

Error-Voice Sensing

Just as in articulation work, the initial phase in activating error-voice sensing is through clinician confirmation of the existence of an error voice, assurance that the condition requires professional attention, demonstration of the client's error voice, and efforts at eliciting the client's motivation for correcting the error voice.

Error-Voice Measuring

Next, the clinician attempts to activate correct auditory-sensor function through measuring techniques. The goal is to develop the TES until the individual finds it uncomfortable to produce his error voice. Error factors to be measured are pitch, quality, and intensity dimensions of voicing.

Interpersonal Measuring. The first task of the client is to interrupt the clinician during conversational exchanges whenever the client believes that the clinician has adopted his error voice. The client is asked simply to say, "Stop, you used error voice on the phrase, 'go to work.'" He is then required to describe how the speaking pitch, loudness, or quality varies from more normal voicing. Once the client is able to identify the error voice consistently as produced by the clinician and to describe its error factors, intrapersonal-measuring work is begun.

Intrapersonal Measuring. Intrapersonal measuring of error voice is done via various techniques.

Reverse speech feedback refers to altering the usual tonal-symbol, figure-ground relationship during speech. This is necessary because most individuals consciously monitor the language they are speaking and only subconsciously monitor the voice that carries that language. To facilitate intrapersonal measuring of error factors in the voice, the client is required to produce nonpropositional or nonsense speech. Reading backwards, reading units of nonsense speech prepared by the clinician, or babble-talk between client and clinician are suggested ways of getting the client to "speak" without language. After-error and during-error techniques may be planned using such "desymbolized" voice.

After-error work is done by recording portions of such "talk" and during playback having the client identify and describe the error pitch, quality, or loudness dimensions.

During-error work is done by having the client's "talk" fed back to the client through a portable amplifier, or through a speaking tube, or by having the client vocalize while holding a finger in each ear. Periodically, the client is required to stop phonating and describe the error dimensions.

Sensing and measuring work is designed to develop the TES to the point where the auditory sensor begins to reject the error voice. Concomitant with the activation of error-voice rejecting is the beginning of vocal self-adjustment. If the rejecting and self-adjustment processes are not activated the clinician moves to the next phase of work.

Correct-Voice Seeking

Goals of correct-voice seeking include getting the client to increase his vocal repertoire and to "forget" his error voice. Emergence of the client's physiologic voice is facilitated through the achievement of such goals.

Variable-Voice Feedback. To increase vocal variability and hence prepare the client to adopt a new and more appropriate vocal pattern, the client is asked to vocalize in as many different ways as possible. He may first speak at a lower pitch, at a middle pitch, and then at a high pitch; then at a soft level, a moderate level, and a loud level; and then with a breathy voice, a hoarse voice, and a full-quality voice. Such variability work is done until the client is able to modify his voice easily and until his habitual pattern is less stable, that is, until the client begins to indicate that he is "forgetting" his habitual voice.

Delayed-Speech Feedback. Vocal variability may also be increased with delayed voice feedback. Under DAF conditions, vocal changes such as increased loudness and a rise in pitch level may be noted.

Correct-Voice Approximating

If vocal self-adjustment has not occurred after sensing, measuring, and seeking work, the clinician uses techniques designed to facilitate directly the emergence of correct-voice.

Reinforced Speech Feedback. During vocal-seeking work the clinician should reinforce those voice patterns that appear to be suitable replacements for the pathologic voice. Appropriate replacements are those voices that provide the most voice for the least effort.

Masked Speech Feedback. Masking the speech of individuals with voice problems with high-level white noise often causes vocal modification in the direction of a more physiologic voice. A possible interpretation of such an event is that for some reason audioregulatory mechanisms have been maintaining the pathologic voice and that auditory masking, which disturbs audioregulation, allows the voice to return to a more physiologic status.

If physiologic voice is elicited through auditory masking, the client should be asked to "memorize" the "feel" of the vocal adjustment that is producing the voice. Such "memorizing" may eventually develop a compensatory, proprioceptive control over the voice.

Enriched Speech Feedback. Positive vocal adjustment may also be influenced by having the speaker's voice fed back to him after being "electronically treated" through a system of filters. Similar vocal adjustment may be observed when the individual speaks in a room or box with positive reverberating characteristics. The phenomenon is a form of reversed feedback. Simply put, the technique attempts to stimulate laryngeal adjustment to match the enriched tone returning to the speaker's ear. If this occurs, the speaker should be asked to memorize the "sound" and "feel" of the "enriched" voice.

Contradictory Speech Feedback. Modified voice may sometimes be induced through a technique of unilateral, contradictory feedback. The technique is done using the autospeech therapy instrument already described.

With this apparatus, the clinician can feed the client's sustained [ɑ] into the client's left ear, while he feeds his, the clinician's, more appropriately voiced [ɑ] into the client's right ear. Then the clinician gradually fades the client's error voice while simultaneously amplifying the clinician's model voice, thus causing a mismatch between laryngeal function and the vocal pattern being heard, or a disturbance of the client's vocal homeostasis. One way for the client to reestablish vocal homeostasis is to adjust his voice to match the voice he hears, and this type of automatic self-adjustment may be observed clinically. When the vocal adjustment occurs, the client is asked to memorize the sound and "feel" of the modified voice.

Imaginal Speech Feedback. Once physiologic voice is elicited by the various techniques described, and the client is asked to memorize its sound and "feel," he is also asked to practice this voice with his mind's voice as often during each day as possible. He should "hear" this new voice with his mind's ear and "feel" it with his mind's voicebox especially before entering a speaking situation as well as occasionally during actual speaking situations.

Correct-voice approximating work should facilitate error-voice sensing, measuring, and rejecting, and hence the automatic adoption of a physiologic voice.

Therapy for Resonance Problems

A self-adjusting approach may also be designed in certain cases of resonance imbalance, for example, in cases where hypernasality persists in a child who has received appropriate surgical or prosthetic attention and where it is determined that the child is capable of effecting adequate velopharyngeal or prosthetic closure. One interpretation of such persisting hypernasality is that closure potential was actualized after audioregulation of the hypernasal voice was established. Under such circumstances, the "ear" has adjusted so that it accepts hypernasal voice as "correct" voice. The major goal of self-adjusting therapy is to get the ear to reject hypernasal voice and to allow the new potential for non-nasal voice to manifest itself.

Procedures outlined here are similar to those described under "Voice Therapy."

Error-Resonance Sensing

Initial work in sensing error resonance is identical to that listed under "Articulation Therapy" and "Voice Therapy." Also, since hypernasality is basically "undimensional," measuring and sensing techniques have been combined under sensing work.

Interpersonal Sensing. The child's first job is to become an expert at sensing when the clinician during conversational speech produces error-resonance phrases. The child may signal such "nose talk" as compared to "mouth talk" by pointing to his nose or by saying, "nose talk." To facilitate the discrimination of nose talk in the early phase of work the child may be allowed to place his finger lightly on the side of the clinician's nose.

Intrapersonal Sensing. After the child consistently identifies "nose talk" as produced by the clinician, it may be assumed that a TES is developing regarding his own nose talk. TES for hypernasality is further developed through intrapersonal sensing work.

After-error work may be done in various ways, for example, the child is asked to answer simple questions and to echo his responses. During the echo, for example, "I am six, I am six," the child is asked to listen hard and "feel" his nose talk (he may place his own finger lightly on the side of his nose during the echo utterance) or portions of the client-clinician conversation may be recorded and played back. Each time the child's speech is heard the child is asked to raise the volume and "listen hard" to his own nose talk.

During-error work is done by having the child speak through a personal amplifier which feeds back his amplified nose talk, speak through a speaking tube which directs his speech back to his right or left ears, or speak with a finger in his ear or in both ears.

Such intrapersonal feedback may also be accentuated by connecting plastic tubing to nasal olives, inserting the olive(s) into the child's nostril(s), and leading the tubing back to one of the external auditory meatuses of the child; or by simply having the child speak while holding a finger lightly on the side of his nose.

Error-Resonance Comparing

Since the child may rather easily produce near normal resonance by simply holding his nares closed with his fingers while speaking, comparing techniques may be used to further develop the TES.

After-Error Comparing. During a recorded conversation with the clinician, the child is asked to watch the clinician for a signal before responding to the clinician. For example, the clinician may ask a question and before the child responds he may point to his nose. The signal means that the child should talk with his customary nose talk; however, if the clinician points to his mouth the child should hold his nostrils closed before talking and hence produce mouth talk. After a few minutes of such recorded conversation, the conversation is played back. During the playback the child is asked to listen carefully to his utterances and to signal whether he hears nose or mouth talk either by pointing to his nose or mouth or by saying "nose" or "mouth."

During-Error Comparing. During-error work is done using the same signaling techniques described under "After-Error Comparing" and the same amplification techniques described under "During-Error Sensing."

Such sensing and comparing work should have developed a TES that causes the individual to reject his habitual hypernasality and to replace it with balanced nasal resonance. When this does not occur in any consistent fashion approximating work is done.

Correct-Resonance Approximating

Approximating work includes daily periods of talking while holding the nostrils closed, as well as the use, with appropriate modifications, of contradictory and imaginal speech feedback work as described under "Correct-Voice Approximating."

Stuttering Therapy

The major goals in a self-adjusting approach to stuttering therapy are: (a) the saturation of the individual's speech system with fluent speech; and (b) the use of more efficient feedback channels for control of speech rhythm.

Correct Fluency Feedback

The first goal in therapy is to provide the client with speaking experiences that are associated with fluency as many times each day as possible. Hence, the stutterer should produce at least twice as much fluent as disfluent speech on each talking day. In short, he should begin to anticipate fluency instead of disfluency each time he is about to speak.

Solo Speech Feedback. For those stutterers who do not stutter when alone a number of speaking assignments may be made: (a) self-reporting one's activities, that is, when alone preceding one's activities with a verbal description of them; (b) free, verbal-association work, that is, when alone speaking aloud anything that comes to mind; and (c) controlled, verbal association, that is, when alone describing aloud the events of the day. Speaking to animals and infants are other forms of "solo" speech feedback that may be used.

Novel-Pattern Speech Feedback. Fluency may be facilitated when a stutterer is asked to assume a foreign or regional dialect, speak in sing-song fashion, change his vocal pitch or quality, or speak through a puppet.

Imaginal Speech Feedback. To further increase the sense of correct speech feedback, when stutterers are in places where out loud or solo speech is not possible, they should be encouraged to hold imaginary, fluent conversations with difficult listeners with their mind's articulators. They should be asked to "memorize" the feel of this flowing inner speech.

Altering Sensor Control of Fluency

Sensor-based stuttering may be due to an inefficient, overloaded, or overcorrecting auditory sensor; to a delay in the development of tactile-kinesthetic sensor control; or to other kinds of problems in the sensor. Hence, techniques designed to alter sensor control are frequently useful self-adjusting techniques.

Delayed Speech Feedback. When speaking under conditions of delayed auditory feedback, stutterers may become more fluent.

At least two interpretations for such fluency are possible. (a) The delay in feedback usually results in a reduction of speaking rate and a prolongation of syllables. Under such conditions, a deficient auditory sensor may be able to perform its rhythm control function more efficiently. (b) The disturbing delay may cause the individual to reject the sound of his speech and to concentrate on the feel of it. Primary control over fluency by the tactile-kinesthetic sensor may produce fluency when an offending auditory sensor is present.

Attenuated Speech Feedback. Speaking under white-noise masking may induce fluency in many stutterers. One sensor explanation of the phenomenon is the elimination of an immature auditory control of fluency and the activation of a more mature and efficient tactile-kinesthetic control.

Auditory feedback may also be attenuated or eliminated with whisper voice or no-voice speech.

Double Speech Feedback. Slave or shadow talk and echo talk are two forms of double talk.

In order to slave talk the stutterer must concentrate on the movements of the lead speaker's articulators and on the tactile-kinesthetic feedback of his own articulators. Thus slave talk may facilitate the fluency of those with auditory sensor problems.

Interpersonal echoing (echoing the clinician) or intrapersonal echoing (echoing oneself) are the other forms of double talk. When these forms of talk facilitate fluency, fluency may be interpreted as the result of the ability of an inefficient auditory sensor to operate under these special conditions.

Amplified Speech Feedback. Tactile-kinesthetic feedbacks are "amplified" or highlighted by having the client intentionally focus on the touch and movement sensations of his articulators, exaggerate articulatory movements, or use a "struggle" technique while speaking (for example, holding the tongue tip against the alveolar ridge while talking).

When such techniques facilitate fluency, one sensor explanation is that the individual is using a more efficient tactile-kinesthetic sensor for fluency control.

Concluding Comments

The idea that endings are only new beginnings echoes loudly as this book comes to a close. Just as the "systems" approach to speech and hearing provides additional understanding of speech and hearing processes, disorders, and management, it also exposes large areas of unexplored territory. Much more knowledge is needed of the systems themselves, especially of the higher- and lower-order integrators and sensor system. It is also clear that clinicians need to know much more about the diseases and anomalies that may affect these systems and about the speech and hearing manifestations of these abnormalities. In the same vein, it is essential that greater collaboration occur in clinical work and research between the speech and hearing clinician and his health colleagues. Finally, further development and study is required of the range of procedures and techniques described to evaluate and treat the speech systems. In fact then, this work is not ending but is ongoing.

REFERENCES

Luria, A. R., Language and brain. Brain Lang., 1, 1–14 (1974).
Mysak, E. D., Servo theory and stuttering. J. Speech Hear. Disord., 25, 188–195 (1960).
Mysak, E. D., Speech Pathology and Feedback Theory. Springfield, Ill.: Charles C Thomas (1966).
Rochford, G., Are jargon dysphasics dysphasic? Br. J. Disord. Commun., 9, 35–44 (1974).
Ruesch, J., General theory of communication in psychiatry. In S. Arieti (Ed.), American Handbook of Psychiatry, Vol. 1. New York: Basic Books (1959).
Schuell, H., Aphasia in adults. In Human Communication and Its Disorders—an Overview. Report of the National Institute of Neurological Diseases and Stroke. Washington, D. C.: U. S. Dept. of Health, Education and Welfare (1969).
West, R. W., and Ansberry, M., The Rehabilitation of Speech. New York: Harper & Row (1968).

Appendix A
Summary Table of Composition of the Speech Systems

System	Components	Nervous supply	
		Nerves and tracts	Centers
Receptor system			
Auditory	Auricle, auditory meati, eustachian tube, tympanic membrane, ossicular chain, tensor tympani and stapedius muscles (and associated peripheral branches of the trigeminal and facial nerves), cochlea		Organ of Corti
Visual	Eyelids; eyeballs; and rectus and oblique muscles	Peripheral cranial nerves: III, IV, VI	Retina
Transmitter system			
Afferent			
Auditory		Peripheral and central cranial nerve: VIII; and lateral lemniscus	Cochlear ganglion; dorsal and ventral cochlear nuclei (medulla); pons; inferior colliculi (midbrain); and medial geniculate body (thalamus)
Visual		Peripheral and central cranial nerve: II	Lateral geniculate body (thalamus); and superior colliculi (midbrain)
Efferent			
Respiratory		Peripheral and central cervical nerves: I–VIII; and thoracic nerves: I–XII; and lateral corticospinal tract	Cortex, pons, and medulla

Phonatory	Peripheral and central cranial nerve: X		Cortex, pons, and medulla
Resonatory	Cranial nerves: V, X, XI		Cortex, pons, and medulla
Articulatory	Cranial nerves: V, VII, IX, X, XI, XII		Cortex, pons, and medulla
Lower-order integrator system			
Afferent	Reticular activating system projection fibers		Reticular cells of medulla, pons, midbrain, and thalamic and hypothalamic nuclei
Efferent	Extrapyramidal projection fibers		Basal ganglia, medulla, cerebellum, midbrain, and minor hemisphere.
Higher-order integrator system	Cerebral associative, commissural, and corticothalamic projection tracts	Left middle cerebral artery; vein of Labbé	Major hemisphere (speech comprehension and formulation): posterior cortical speech area (Wernicke's area), anterior cortical speech area (Broca's area), superior cortical speech area (Penfield's area); minor hemisphere (speech comprehension); temporal lobe, hippocampal structures (speech memory); and thalamus
Effector system Respiratory		*Nasal and oral cavities; pharynx, larynx, trachea, bronchi, lungs; spinal column, rib cage, pectoral and pelvic girdles; inspiratory muscles:* diaphragm, and pectoralis, subclavius, serratus anterior, intercostals, costal elevators, serratus posterior of thorax, and sternocleidomastoid, scalenes of neck, and latissmus dorsi	

System	Components	Nervous supply	
		Nerves and tracts	Centers
	and sacrospinalis of back; *expiratory muscles:* obliques, transversus, rectus of abdomen, and transversus, subcostals, internal intercostals of thorax, and iliocostalis dorsi, quadratus lumborum of back		
Phonatory	*Laryngeal cartilages:* thyroid, cricoid, epiglottis, arytenoid, corniculate, cuneiform; *extrinsic laryngeal muscles:* digastric, stylohyoid, mylohyoid, geniohyoid, sternohyoid, omohyoid, thyrohyoid, sternothyroid; *intrinsic laryngeal muscles:* lateral cricoarytenoid and interarytenoid (adductors); posterior cricoarytenoid (abductor); and thyroarytenoid and cricothyroid (relaxer-tensors)		
Resonatory	*Oral, buccal, nasal cavities; fauces; velopharyngeal closure mechanism:* velum, nasopharynx, oropharynx, laryngogopharynx, and related musculature, levator and tensor palatine, palatoglossus, palatopharyngeus of velum, and superior, middle, and inferior constrictors of pharynx		
Articulatory	*Lips and related musculature:* orbicularis oris, transverse, angular, and vertical muscles; *face muscles:* buc-		

cinator, risorius, quadratus labii superior, zygomatic, quadratus labii inferior, mentalis, triangularis, canine, incisivis labii superior, incisivis labii inferior; *mandible and related musculature*: digastricus, mylohyoid, geniohyoid, external pterygoid (depressors); masseter, temporalis, internal pterygoid (elevators); *teeth and dental arches; palate and related musculature*: levator and tensor palatine, salpingopharyngeal, superior pharyngeal constrictor (effect velopharyngeal closure); *tongue and related musculature*: genioglossus, styloglossus, palatoglossus, hyoglossus (extrinsic muscles); superior and inferior longitudinal, transverse, vertical (intrinsic muscles).

Sensory system			
Auditory	Same as auditory speech receptor	Same as auditory speech receptor and auditory speech transmitter	Same as auditory speech transmitter plus reticular system, hypothalamus, and posterior cortical speech area
Tactile-kinesthetic	Lips, face, mandible, tongue, palate and related musculature; and teeth	Peripheral and central sensory neurons: trigeminal, glossopharyngeal, and palatine nerves; medial lemniscus; thalamocortical fibers (cortical system); spinocerebellar tract and cerebellar tracts to brain stem and cerebral cortex (cerebellar system)	Ventroposterior medial nucleus of thalamus; postcentral gyrus of parietal lobe (cortical system); cerebellum; red nucleus; reticular system; pre-motor and motor cortex of cerebrum (cerebellar system)

Appendix B
Form for General Examination of the Speech Systems

System	Notations (e.g., within normal limits, negative, degrees of difficulty, scores, etc.)

Higher-order speech integrator
  Major speech brain
    Earedness
    Eyedness
    Tonguedness
    Carotid-amytal test
  Speech perception-comprehension
    Automaticity and complexity factors during informal conversation
    Automaticity and complexity factors during contextual testing
  Speech formulation-production
    Automaticity and complexity factors during informal conversation
    Automaticity and complexity factors during contextual testing
  Verbal thinking
    Retention
    Recall
    Sequencing
    Association
    Elaboration
    Interpretation
  Verbotype
    Autoplastic
    Alloplastic
    Regenerative
    Degenerative
    Hostile
    Authoritarian
    Disjunctive
    Pseudocommunication
    Noncommunication
    Resistant
Lower-order speech integrator
  Input processing
    Audiovisual arousal, localizing and fixing, tracking
      Quickness and accuracy factors
    Selective attention to audiovisual events
      With background music
      With background speech
  Output patterning
    Development or status of:

System	Notations (e.g., within normal limits, negative, degrees of difficulty, scores, etc.)

Breathing
Feeding reflexes
Articulatory differentiation
Laryngopraxis
Articulopraxis
Articulolaryngeal diadochocinesia
Tonal and body paralanguage
Speech system compensation during concomitant motor activity
Automatic speech behavior
  Social gesture speech
  Memorized speech
  Emotional utterances
Speech receptor
 Auditory
  Auricles, meati, drums
  Pure tone air conduction thresholds
  Pure tone bone conduction thresholds
  Speech reception threshold
  Speech discrimination score
  Impedance test
  ABLB test
  SISI test
  Tone decay test
  Bekesy test
 Visual
  Binocular balance, eye movements
  General acuity and fields
  Acuity and fields for articulatory postures
  Tracking of articulatory movements
Speech effector
 Respiratory
  Adequacy of skeletal framework
  Patency of respiratory passage
  Respiratory movements
  Vegetative breaths per minute (v-bpm)
  Speech breathing inspiratory-expiratory ratio (sb-i/e ratio)
  Speech air volume (sav)
  Vegetative breathing-speech breathing (vb-sb) transition
 Phonatory
  Vocal folds at rest
  Vocal folds during voicing
  Pitch variability
  Loudness variability
  Vowel duration variability
 Resonatory
  Nasal chambers
  Nasopharynx
  Oral chamber
  Faucial area
  Velum
  Uvula
  Oropharynx

System	Notations (e.g., within normal limits, negative, degrees of difficulty, scores, etc.)

Ah-test
Oral pressure index (opi)
Consonantal nasal pressure (cnp)
Articulatory
  Lips and face
  Mandible
  Teeth
  Palate
  Dental arches
  Tongue
  Bilabial posture and movement
  Labiodental posture and movement
  Mandibular posture and movement
  Linguadental posture and movement
  Lingua-alveolar posture and movement
  Linguapalatal posture and movement
  Linguavelar posture and movement
  Phonetic inventory
    Spontaneous articulation
    Nonspontaneous articulation
Speech transmitter
  Afferent
    Site-of-lesion audiometry
      Bekesy test
      Tone decay test
      SISI test
      Distorted speech test
  Efferent
    Respiratory muscle tonus
    Respiratory reflexes
    Voluntary respiratory movements
    Vegetative breathing-speech breathing shift (vb-sb shift)
    Phonatory muscle tonus
    Glottic closing reflex
    On-off voicing
    Velopharyngeal muscle tonus
    Palatal and pharyngeal reflexes
    Non-nasal, nasal sound shift
    Specific articulatory movements
    Swallow and pharyngeal reflexes
    Emotional responses
    Specificity of involvement
    Articulatory muscle tonus
Speech sensor
  Auditory
    Internal verbal monitoring
    External verbal control and monitoring (intrapersonal)
    External verbal monitoring (interpersonal)
    Interpersonal voice monitoring
    Intrapersonal voice monitoring
    Altering function of auditory sensor
      White noise
      Delayed auditory feedback

System	Notations (e.g., within normal limits, negative, degrees of difficulty, scores, etc.)
Tactile-kinesthetic	
Touch discrimination	
Lips	
Alveolar ridge	
Palate	
Tongue	
Lingual kinesthetic function	
Cortical vs. cerebellar sensor function	

Author Index

Ruesch, J., 252
Rusalem, H., 163

S

Schinsky, L., 139
Schuell, H., 52, 110, 111, 245, 247
Schwartz, E. R., 84
Settlage, C. F., 102
Shalom, A. S., 174
Shanks, J. C., 173
Sherman, D., 182
Shervanian, C. C., 99, 101
Silverman, A. J., 17
Silverman, S. R., 151, 156
Simpson, J. A., 205
Skelly, M., 139
Smith, R. W., 139
Smithells, R. W., 95
Snidecor, J. C., 180
Sonninen, A., 205
Sooy, F. A., 214
Sperry, R. W., 26, 28
Spiegel, R., 51, 120, 121, 122, 123, 125
Spriestersbach, D. C., 51, 182
Starbuck, H. B., 162
Steer, M. D., 39
Stoudt, R. J., 55, 171
Strauss, A. A., 86
Strauss, H., 110

T

Taylor, L., 26, 28
Teuber, H., 39

Thompson, G. N., 112
Tiffany, W. J., 114
Travis, L. E., 122

W

Wada, J., 17
Walton, J. N., 13, 82, 83, 107, 108, 109, 111,
133, 134, 135, 136, 210, 218, 219, 221, 222,
224, 230, 231, 232
Weaver, A. T., 36
Weinberg, B., 173
Weinskin, E. A., 112, 113, 124
Weller, H. C., 84
Wepman, J. M., 52, 130
Wertz, R. T., 139
West, R. W., 13, 14, 48, 59, 65, 69, 83, 101,
107, 114, 120, 152, 153, 172, 174, 176, 183,
197, 201, 219, 220, 222, 224, 225, 230, 247,
248
Wever, E. G., 214
Winitz, H., 97
Wolski, W., 174
Wood, N. E., 85, 86, 91, 101, 102
Worster-Drought, C., 85, 86, 136, 218, 219
Wyburn, G. M., 1, 3, 5, 7, 8, 38
Wyke, B., 140

Y

Young, E. H., 5
Youngstrom, K., 180

Z

Zemlin, W. R., 10, 29, 33, 36, 60

Subject Index